Women Confined

By the same author

Sex, Gender and Society (Temple Smith, 1972)
The Sociology of Housework (Martin Robertson, 1974)
Housewife (Allen Lane, 1974)
Becoming A Mother (Martin Robertson, 1979)

co-editor with Juliet Mitchell
The Rights and Wrongs of Women (Penguin, 1976)

Women Confined

TOWARDS A SOCIOLOGY OF CHILDBIRTH

Ann Oakley

Schocken Books • New York

First published by Schocken Books 1980
10 9 8 7 6 5 4 3 2 1   80 81 82 83

Library of Congress Cataloging in Publication Data
Oakley, Ann.
Women confined.
Includes bibliographical references.
1. Pregnancy—Psychological aspects. 2. Childbirth—Psychological aspects. 3. Childbirth—Social aspects. 4. Mothers. 5. Obstetrics—Social aspects. I. Title.
RG560.025   618.4'01'9   79-26267

Manufactured in the United States of America

for EMILY AND LAURA

Contents

Note on Tables and Tests of Significance

A chi square test of significance was used in the analysis of data presented in the following pages. Either the precise value of X^2 was calculated and the probability level for that value taken from R. A. Fisher and F. Yates *Statistical Tables for Biological, Agricultural and Medical Research* (London: Oliver and Boyd, 1963), or, in the case of many 2×2 tables, it was derived from D. J. Finney, R. Latscha, B. M. Bennett and P. Hsu *Tables for Testing Significance in a 2×2 Contingency Table* (Cambridge: University Press, 1963). Percentages are given in the tables without decimal points and are rounded up.

... there is a Persian myth of the creation of the world which precedes the biblical one. In that myth a woman creates the world, and she creates it by an act of natural creativity which is hers and which cannot be duplicated by men. She gives birth to a great number of sons. The sons, greatly puzzled by this act which they cannot duplicate, become frightened. They think, 'Who can tell us, that if she can give *life, she cannot also* take *life.' And so, because of their fear of this mysterious ability of woman, and of its reversible possibility, they kill her.*

[Fromm-Reichmann and Gunst, 1974, p. 88]

Introduction

This book is about one particular aspect of women's lives: their reactions to childbirth. In it I have tried to show how the first experience of childbirth is an example of general change in people's lives, and how women's responses to the advent of motherhood can be seen in these terms. My other major concern has been with the contribution of medical maternity care to women's feelings about becoming mothers. I have asked the question whether there is any connection between the two, and provided a partial answer.

Women Confined is thus not a book about women 'in general' – though I hope that what it has to say will contribute to an understanding of how women's situation is differentiated from that of men in modern industrialized society today. By focusing on one area of gender differentiation, that of female emotional responses to childbirth, I have not undertaken a general commentary, but rather a narrow exercise in the dissection of relationships between various social, psychological and medical factors in the management and context of first childbirth. This exercise makes up Part II of the book, which is devoted to describing and discussing my own research on the transition to motherhood carried out in London in 1974–6. Part I is a little broader in scope than this. It discusses literature, research and practice in the reproductive field with particular reference to the models of femininity that have dominated it to date (a version of this was published as 'A Case of Maternity: Paradigms of Women as Maternity Cases', Oakley, 1979a). In a concluding chapter (chapter 11 'Mistakes and Mystiques') I turn to the wider cultural context of motherhood, and speculate about the ways in which women's treatment as mothers is associated with their oppression as women. 'Proposing the Future' suggests some changes in the institution of motherhood and its medical control that would make becoming and being a mother a more comfortable experience.

The need to summarize and present so much data in such a

small space has forced a somewhat dense and uncompromising style upon me. I hope I will be forgiven for this. The subtitle of the book, 'Towards a Sociology of Childbirth', is intended to convey the fact that there has been very little in the way of a sociology of childbirth so far, and that what the study of reproduction has overwhelmingly lacked is an appreciation of its *social* character. Everything that is done to, and by, women having babies has a cultural base – from the preference of American doctors for forceps and of their Swedish counterparts for vacuum extraction as alternative ways of getting a baby out, to the amount of time a mother (or a father) spends with a new baby and the way she (or he) feels about it. This is one of the senses in which I mean to propose that a 'sociology' of childbirth is the only valid way to arrive at an understanding of what happens, why and with what consequences to women having babies in any culture, including that of twentieth-century industrial capitalism. For this reason I hope that the book will reach at least a few of the 'experts' whose responsibility it is to manage birth and its aftermath.

The second way in which I view this book as being 'towards a sociology of childbirth' is that it is a move towards correcting a tendency within sociological approaches to reproduction to import old paradigms rather than develop new ones. The trouble with childbirth (sociologically speaking) is that it only happens to women. But this does not mean that women's reactions to it can be explained in terms of their womanhood, their adherence to certain standards of feminine personality and behaviour. The trouble with women is that they are also people, and it is this status that is so easily forgotten in both sexist and anti-sexist types of analysis. It has long been clear that the task of a feminist consciousness in social science is not only the exposition of sexism but its correction, and in the pursuit of this end it is essential to develop fresh modes of thinking about women, a new conceptual apparatus. The trouble with sociology (as with many other academic subjects) is that it is not merely sexist on the surface but deeply and pervasively so. Bias against women as people equal in stature to men cannot therefore be expunged piecemeal: a fundamental process of revision must be engaged in. In *Women Confined* I offer one suggestion as to how this revision, in the case of women and reproduction, might be begun. My starting point is women's *human* character and the restoration of this to the centre of our thinking about women that must occur for progress, both social and sociological, to be made – hand-in-hand, naturally, with an enlarged understanding of the particularity of women's social situation; for it is by seeing how women are both different from and the same as other human beings that the prospect of a less gender-divided sociology will be realized.

This book could not have been written without the generous cooperation of the women who were interviewed for the Transition to Motherhood project, or without the valuable help of the medical, midwifery and nursing staff at the hospital involved. I am grateful also to the Social Science Research Council, who funded the research. A number of people have read the manuscript and offered many helpful comments on it: I would like to thank in particular George Brown, Iain Chalmers, David Martin, Robin Oakley and Margaret Stacey for performing this role – although of course the book in its final version is my responsibility alone.

PART I

Paradigms of Women as Reproducers

Having a baby is a biological and cultural act. In bearing a child, a woman reproduces the species and performs an 'animal function'. Yet human childbirth is accomplished in and shaped by culture, both in a general sense and in the particular sense of the varying definitions of reproduction offered by different cultures. How a society defines reproduction is closely linked with its articulation of women's position: the connections between female citizenship and the procreative role are social, not biological. Cultural attitudes both to women and to reproduction are marked by certain paradigmatic representations (OED 'pattern', 'example'; 'paradigmatize' – 'to set forth as a model'). These abound in commonsense understandings of women and motherhood, but medical, psychological and social science are their main repository. It is from the 'scientific' representation of women as maternity cases that the character of mothers is deduced. 'Science' has hidden curricula of moral evaluations that masquerade as fact: it is these 'facts' that must be probed to expose the typical paradigms of women as reproducers that characterize the culture of the contemporary industrial world.

CHAPTER 1

Medical Maternity Cases

'Where's my baby?' asked Martha anxiously.
'She's having a nice rest,' said the nurse, already on her way out.
'But I haven't seen her yet,' said Martha, weak tears behind her lids.
'You don't want to disturb her, do you?' said the nurse disapprovingly.
The door shut. The woman, whose long full breast sloped already into the baby's mouth, looked up and said, 'You'd better do as they want, dear. It saves trouble. They've got their own ideas.' [Lessing, 1966, p. 167]

Childbirth stands uncomfortably at the junction of the two worlds of nature and culture. Like death and disease it is a biological event, but the defining feature of biological events in human life is their social character. The way people are born and die, their assignations with illness and health, cannot be explained and predicted purely on the basis of knowledge about the biological functioning of the human organism. Bodies function in a social world, and the parameters of this world supply an influence of their own.

But the components of nature and culture are more potently and ambiguously mixed in the case of reproduction than in other physiological states. Having babies must be deeply natural, since the architecture of the female body fits women for this role, the production of children follows naturally from that other human occupation, heterosexual congress, and the replacement of the population is necessary for human survival. Yet at the same time, and because of these features, reproduction is a cultural activity: it has far-reaching consequences for the life of a society. Particular childbirths create or break families, establish the ownership of property and entitlement to poverty or privilege; they may alter the statuses, rights and responsibilities of persons, communities and nations.

The other paradox is that only women are the true dramatis personae of childbirth. They thus personify the union of nature (biological reproducer) and culture (social person) directly. The association between a biological emptying of the uterus and the social character of its product, a child, poses a cultural dilemma, but so also does the very existence of women. Levi-Strauss (1969) has argued that the demarcation of boundary lines between nature and culture is the crux of the human social order: in such a manner is the territory in which human beings may fully experience their humanity marked out. But the division is fragile, and the core difficulty is that women are culturally anomalous, tied as they are by their reproductivity to a continuing and necessary natural function (see Ortner, 1974).

It can be argued that the cultural subjection of women derives from the fact that because they have wombs they are caught in the trap of a collective need to control the natural forces of reproduction. Where the social order is ruled by men, women become the embodiment of an alternative government, which must be avoided at all costs. Two modes of avoidance are historically evident: separation and incorporation (these are discussed in Oakley, 1976). According to the logic of the first, the business of reproduction is given over exclusively to women. Its practice and control are divided off from the rest of social life, so that no pollution of one by the other is possible. But according to the logic of incorporation, women must give up their reproductive autonomy, their own right of control over reproduction, which is then 'mastered' by members of the dominant social group: the social, professional and gender elite of male dominated medicine. In this way reproduction comes to be the legitimate subject matter of medicine. Medicine diagnoses, prescribes and prognosticates about women as maternity 'cases' and the reproductive experiences of women are shaped by medical messages. Yet in becoming a repository of 'knowledge' about reproduction, medical science is not some kind of ultimate truth. It hides an ideological face. The products of science in general can be regarded as specific cultural representations, as theoretical strategies arising in distinct cultural milieux (see Kuhn, 1962). Such an approach to medicine is necessary if the aetiology and influence of medical paradigms about reproduction and women as its agents are to be exposed.

MEDICAL MASTERY

As Martha Knowell in Doris Lessing's *A Proper Marriage* becomes aware, the medical managers of childbirth have 'their own ideas'. The organization and routinization of hospital maternity work reflect these ideas, but the ideas themselves, whether about the separation of mother and baby or about the motives of women in having children, are rarely explicit. One important aspect of medical attitudes to childbirth is thus their *concealment* behind a screen of what purport to be exclusively clinical concerns.

In a joint analysis of data from our two different but overlapping research projects on childbirth, Hilary Graham and I suggest that:

> In talking about the different ways in which doctors and mothers view pregnancy, we are talking about a fundamental difference in their perspective on the meaning of childbearing. It is not simply a difference of opinion about approach and procedures – about whether pregnancy is normal or pathological, or whether or not labour should be routinely induced. Rather, we are suggesting that doctors and mothers have a qualitatively different way of looking at the nature, context and management of reproduction. We use the concept of a frame of reference to indicate this difference. 'Frame of reference' embraces both the notion of an *ideological perspective* – a system of values and attitudes through which mothers and doctors view pregnancy – and of a *reference group* – a network of individuals who are significant influences upon these sets of attitudes and values. [Graham and Oakley, forthcoming]

We identify five major features of the medical frame of reference:

(a) the definition of reproduction as a *specialist* subject in which only doctors are experts in the entire symptomatology of childbearing;
(b) the associated definition of reproduction as a *medical* subject, as exactly analogous to other pathological processes as topics of medical knowledge and intervention;
(c) the selection of *limited criteria of reproductive success*, i.e. perinatal and maternal mortality rates;
(d) the *divorce* of reproduction from its *social* context, pregnant patienthood being seen as a woman's only relevant status;
(e) the restriction of women to maternity – their derived *typification* as 'by nature' maternal, domesticated, family-oriented people.

I shall consider each of these dimensions in turn, drawing out their manifestations and consequences in terms of the stereotyping of women as maternity cases both within obstetric medicine and in its interrelationships with general cultural ideologies of womanhood. A third actor in the drama of medical maternity care is the midwife, who receives little attention in what follows, not because her role is insignificant but because the argument at this point is concerned with male medicine as a sender of messages about women's behaviour as reproducers. Midwives' attitudes and responsibilities have historically been tremendously important and continue to be so. An expansion of their function in the future is likely to be one direction of change in the cultural manipulation of reproduction.[1] But that is the subject of another book.

(a) Doctor Knows Best

> You decide when to see your doctor and let him confirm the fact of your pregnancy. From then onwards you are going to have to answer a lot of questions and be the subject of a lot of examinations. Never worry your head about any of these. They are necessary, they are in the interests of your baby and yourself, and none of them will ever hurt you. [*Family Doctor Publications, 1977, p. 8*]

These admonitions, from a British Medical Association publication on pregnancy, are intended to console. Their tone is patronizing and their message clear: doctors know more about having babies than women do. (An alternative, and less charitable, construction would be that women are fundamentally stupid and doctors are inherently more intelligent.[2])

Obstetrics, like midwifery, in its original meaning describes a female province. The management of reproduction has been, throughout most of history and in most cultures, a female concern; what is characteristic about childbirth in the industrial world is, conversely, its control by men. The conversion of female-controlled community management to male-controlled medical management alone would suggest that the propagation of particular paradigms of women as maternity cases has been central to the whole development of medically dominated maternity care.[3] The ideological element, as would be expected, is not part of the agenda in conventional medical histories chronicling the rise of male obstetrics – for example H. R. Spencer's *The History of British Midwifery from 1650 to 1800* (1927). Spencer terminates his discussion in a tone characteristic of the genus when he says:

> In conclusion it may be said that during the hundred and fifty years since Harvey published his 'De Generatione Animalium', a great advance had been made in the science and art of midwifery. This was due chiefly to the introduction of male practitioners, many of whom were men of learning and devoted to anatomy, the groundwork of obstetrics. [p. 175]

The achievements of male obstetrics over those of female midwifery are rarely argued empirically, but always a priori, from the double premise of male and medical superiority. More recent investigations of this argument are now revealing a different picture, in which the introduction of men into the business of reproductive management brought special dangers to mothers and babies. The easier transmission of puerperal fever in male-run lying-in hospitals is one example; the generally careless and ignorant use of technology another (see Oakley, 1976; Versluysen, n.d.). In Britain in the eighteenth and early nineteenth centuries many of the male midwives' innovations were often fatal for both mother and child. The forceps, in particular, which are frequently claimed to be the chief advantage of male medicine, were not used in more than a minority of cases attended by male midwives, and had little effect on infant mortality except perhaps to raise it further (Versluysen, n.d.). In the 1920s in America, where female midwifery was to be most completely phased out, doctors had to contend with the fact that midwifery was obviously associated with less mortality and morbidity than the interventionist character of the new obstetrical approach (Barker-Benfield, 1976).

Improvements in knowledge and technique do not in retrospect justify male participation in midwifery during the eighteenth and nineteenth centuries, and if they did so at the time it was the ideological power of the claim to greater expertise that had this effect. The success of the claim seems to have had a great deal to do with the propagation of certain notions of womanhood. The nineteenth century was a crucial period both for the evolution of modern woman's position and for the consolidation of the male obstetrical takeover. Medical writing about women's diseases and reproductive capacity during this period was characterized by a curiously strong 'emotionally charged conviction' in relation to women's character (Wood, 1974, p. 1). Women were also seen as the 'carriers' of contagion, an intrinsic threat to the health of society. Class intersects with sexism here, for it was working-class women who were seen as 'sickening' in this sense (Duffin, 1978).

'It is almost a pity that a woman has a womb', exclaimed an American professor of gynaecology in the 1860s (Wood, 1974). This statement neatly summarizes the low regard in which the medical profession held its female patients; through its ideological construction of the uterus as the controlling organ of womanhood, it effectively demoted reproduction as woman's unique achievement to the status of a pitiable handicap. Such a construction presented women essentially as reproductive machines, subject to a direct biological input. It enabled physicians to assert a role in the mechanical management of female disorder, thus justifying the particular techniques of drastic gynaecological surgery and obstetrical intervention, and therefore establishing the 'need' for a male medical ascendancy over the whole domain of reproductive care.

All sorts of claims were made about the womb, and its associates, the ovaries, as the site and cause of female inferiority, from physiological pathology to mental disorder, from personality characteristics to occupational qualification (or, rather, disqualification). It was not simply the process of reproduction that was perceived as disabling, but the possession of the apparatus, which evidenced its presence in a monthly flow of reminders about the incapacity of women to be anything other than slaves to their biology (Barker-Benfield, 1976; Delamont and Duffin, 1978; Bullough and Bullough, 1977; Haller and Haller, 1974; Delaney, Lupton and Toth, 1977).

Doctors contended that a woman's reproductive organs explained her femininity in a double-bind sense: women were ill because they were women, but also if they tried to avoid being women by choosing to follow masculine occupations. Medicine thus outlined the contours of woman's place – in nature, not culture, safely outside the limits of masculine society.

How and why male medicine came to assume control over the care of women in childbirth in Britain and America over the last hundred years is, of course, a complex question. But its general location is within this framework of medical concerns about the essential character of women. There are important parallels between medical and social ideologies of womanhood, yet medicine plays a particular role as social ideology. The reason for this is that the theoretical foundations of patriarchy lie in the manipulation of women's biology to constitute their social inferiority. Medicine, as the definer of biology, holds the key to its 'scientific' interpretation, and thus its cultural consequences. The power of medical ideology stems from the incorporation of social assumptions into the very language of physiological theories. The sent and received message hence has a holistic appearance (Jordanova, 1978). To deduce the ideological component is a difficult exercise.

Ehrenreich and English (1973) demonstrate how the exclusion of women from obstetrics followed a long process of staged decline in the female community health care function. They argue that male medical hostility to women is based on a fear of female procreative power – hence the corroding impact of male obstetrics on female midwifery, whether to its virtual extermination, as in North America, or to its definition as a secondary status health profession, as in Britain. Barker-Benfield's thesis is that the assault on midwives, the rise of eugenic interest in women as breeders, and the coterminous development of destructive gynaecological surgery, can only be understood as aspects of 'a persistent, defensive attempt to control and shape women's procreative power' (1976, p. 66). Among the many pungent anecdotes included in Barker-Benfield's book is his account of how J. Marion Sims 'discovered' the speculum. Sims said 'Introducing the bent handle of a spoon into a woman's vagina I saw everything as no man had ever seen before . . . I felt like an explorer ... who first views a new and important territory.' And a contemporary commentator caught up the colonial metaphor: 'Sims' speculum has been to diseases of the womb ... what the compass is to the mariner' (quoted in Barker-Benfield, 1976, p. 95). Sims saw himself as a Columbus; his New World, and that of his male gynaecological successors, was the vagina.

The tools used by traditional female midwives lack documentation, but it seems likely that they also used an instrument such as the bent handle of a spoon to examine the vagina and cervix. But the routinization of the speculum-assisted vaginal examination by doctors facilitated an opposition between male medical knowledge of women's bodies and women's own knowledge.[4] Throughout obstetricians' long fight to establish themselves as experts, in possession of *all* the resources necessary to the care and control of women in childbirth, this clash has remained the most vulnerable link in the chain of medical command.

The conflict between reproducer as expert and doctor as expert may have five outcomes: the reproducer may accept the doctor's definition of the situation; the doctor may accept the reproducer's; the reproducer may challenge the doctor's view; the doctor may challenge the reproducer's; or the conflict between them may be manifested in a certain pattern of communication between doctor and patient that indicates the presence of unresolved questions to do with what has been termed 'intrauterine neocolonialism' (Swinscow, 1974, p. 800). In a large series of doctor–patient encounters observed for the Transition to Motherhood study (see chapter 4, p. 106), this latter outcome was much more common than direct confrontation. The woman's status as an expert may be accorded joking recognition:

DOCTOR: *First baby?*
PATIENT: *Second.*
DOCTOR [laughing]: *So you're an expert?*

Or:

DOCTOR: *You're looking rather serious.*
PATIENT: *Well, I am rather worried about it all. It feels like a small baby – I feel much smaller with this one than I did with my first, and she weighed under six pounds. Ultrasound last week said the baby was very small, as well.*
DOCTOR: *Weighed it, did they?*
SECOND DOCTOR [entering cubicle]: *They go round to flower shows and weigh cakes, you know.*
FIRST DOCTOR: *Yes, it's a piece of cake, really.*

But frequently, patients concur in the doctor's presentation of himself (most obstetricians are male) as the possessor of privileged information:

MALE DOCTOR: *Will you keep a note in your diary of when you first feel the baby move?*
PATIENT: *Do you know – well, of course you would know – what it feels like?*
DOCTOR: *It feels like wind pains – something moving in your tummy.*

At the same time, a common feature of communication between doctor and patient is a discrepancy between their labelling of significant symptoms. The medical dilemma is that of discerning the 'presenting' symptoms of clinically significant disorders; the patient's concern is with the normalization of her subjective experience of discomfort. Of 677 statements made by patients, 12 per cent concerned symptoms of pain or discomfort, which were medically treated either by being ignored, or with a non-serious response, or through a brief and selective account of relevant physiological/anatomical data.

DOCTOR: *Feeling well?*
PATIENT: *Yes, but very tired – I can't sleep at all at night.*
DOCTOR: *Why is that?*
PATIENT: *Well, I'm very uncomfortable – I turn from one side to the other, and the baby keeps kicking. I get cramp on one side, high up in*

my leg. If I sleep on my back I choke myself, so I'm tossing and turning about all night long, which isn't very good.
DOCTOR: *We need to put you in a hammock, don't we?* [Reads case notes] *Tell me, the urine specimen which you brought in today – when did you do it?*

PATIENT: *I've got a pain in my shoulder.*
DOCTOR: *Well, that's your shopping bag hand, isn't it?*

PATIENT: *I get pains in my groin, down here, why is that?*
DOCTOR: *Well, it's some time since your last pregnancy, and also your centre of gravity is changing.*
PATIENT: *I see.*
DOCTOR: *That's okay.* [Pats on back]

Such abbreviated 'commonsense' explanations are one mode in which doctors talk to patients. The contrasting mode is to 'technicalize' – to use technical language as a means of keeping the patient in her place. In maternity consultations this interactive pattern particularly characterizes those encounters in which a patient contends equality with the doctor:

DOCTOR: *I think what we have to do is assess you – see how near you are to having it.* [Does internal examination] *Right – you'll go like a bomb, and I've given you a good stirring up.*[5] *So what I think you should do, is I think you should come in.*
PATIENT: *Is it possible to wait another week, and see what happens?*
DOCTOR: *You've been reading the* Sunday Times.[6]
PATIENT: *No, I haven't. I'm married to a doctor.*
DOCTOR: *Well, you've ripened up since last week and I've given the membranes a good sweep over.*
PATIENT: *What does that mean?*
DOCTOR: *I've swept them – not with a brush, with my finger.* [Writes in notes 'give date for induction']
PATIENT: *I'd still rather wait a bit.*
DOCTOR: *Well, we know the baby's mature now, and there's no sense in waiting. The perinatal morbidity and mortality increase rapidly after forty-two weeks. They didn't say that in the* Sunday Times, *did they?*

A second classic area of dispute between reproducers and doctors is the dating of pregnancy. Six per cent of the questions asked and 5 per cent of statements made by mothers in the antenatal clinic concerned dates, mothers usually trying to negotiate the 'correct' date of expected delivery with the doctor, who did not see this as a subject for negotiation – as a legitimate area of maternal expertise. The underlying imputation is one of feminine unreliability:

DOCTOR: *Are you absolutely sure of your dates?*
PATIENT: *Yes, and I can even tell you the date of conception.*
[Doctor laughs]
PATIENT: *No, I'm serious. This is an artificial insemination baby.*

DOCTOR: *How many weeks are you now?*
PATIENT: *Twenty-six-and-a-half.*
DOCTOR [looking at notes]: *Twenty weeks now.*
PATIENT: *No, twenty-six-and-a-half.*
DOCTOR: *You can't be.*
PATIENT: *Yes I am, look at the ultrasound report.*
DOCTOR: *When was it done?*
PATIENT: *Today.*
DOCTOR: *It was done today?*
PATIENT: *Yes.*
DOCTOR [reads report]: *Oh yes, twenty-six-and-a-half weeks, that's right.*
[Patient smiles triumphantly at researcher]

Perhaps it is significant that increasingly the routine use of serial ultrasound cephalometry is providing an alternative medical technique for the assessment of gestation length. A medical rationale for the inflation of medical over maternal expertise is thus provided. It is important to note that although the efficacy, safety and technical superiority of ultrasound is widely assumed within the medical frame of reference, this does not rest on a 'scientific' basis. No randomized controlled trials have, for example, been conducted that evaluate the usefulness of routine ultrasound versus more traditional methods of clinical examination and maternal report in assessing gestation length and foetal well-being.[7] Laboratory investigations of the physiological effects of ultrasound on developing embryonic and foetal cells are limited and contradictory. Longitudinal follow-up of children subjected to ultrasound while in the womb is sparse and restricted to a six-year period, the kind of time span known to be inadequate in showing up the long-term effects of other procedures inflicted on foetuses, such as X-rays and the administration of hormones. In animal experiments, intrauterine ultrasound has been shown to have a long-term effect on immune responses in the young (J. Rosser, 1978).[8]

Similar kinds of scientific caveats can be levelled at other medical techniques generally used in the treatment of women as maternity cases today (see, for example, Chalmers and Richards, 1977; Richards, 1975; Stewart and Stewart, 1976). Unbridled medical enthusiasm for new techniques is a general feature of modern medicine and it may be not so much that obstetrics is a special case but that medical attitudes see female reproductive patienthood as a particularly passive and appropriate site for their introduction.

(b) Medicalization

> Normally patients come to the hospital because they're ill. Pregnant women aren't ill and illness is a reason for *not* coming to the hospital.

The consultant who made this statement did so to make his colleagues laugh – but it is not really a laughing matter. This paradoxical situation in which a large number of healthy people are treated with a barrage of medical and pharmacological techniques in surgeries, hospitals and clinics for a 'natural' and 'normal' condition has to do with the general social function of medicine, as well as with its specific management of reproduction. The obstetrical claim to expertise is an aspect of the medicalization of life: the ascendancy of doctors as arbiters of human concerns. As Eliot Freidson puts it, it is characteristic of our culture that 'The medical profession has first claim to jurisdiction over the label of illness and anything to which it may be attached, *irrespective of its capacity to deal with it effectively*' (1970, p. 251; my italics). The medicalization of reproduction as a potentially abnormal activity is the theme of much medical writing and practice. It is only by an ideological transformation of the 'natural' to the 'cultural' that doctors can legitimate reproduction as a medical speciality. For example:

PATIENT: *I'm a hairdresser, I only do three days a week – is it alright to go on working?*
DOCTOR: *Up to twenty-eight weeks is alright on the whole, especially if you have a trouble-free pregnancy as you obviously have. After that it's better to give up.*
PATIENT: *I only work three days a week. I feel fine.*
DOCTOR: *Yes, everything* is *fine, but now you've got to this stage it's better to give up, just in case.*

DOCTOR: *It'd be difficult to get you off now – I think you ought to come in for rest and to do some more water tests, and then we can start you off. The baby isn't growing as fast as it was.*
PATIENT: *What do you mean, come in?*
DOCTOR: *Really it's a matter of when you come in. Sunday, I should think, and then stay in.*
PATIENT: *Stay in until it's born, you mean?*
DOCTOR: *Yes.*
PATIENT: *I don't fancy that very much.*
DOCTOR: *If you'd been ready, I would have started you off today. You see, on the ultrasound it's not growing as well as it was, and on the water tests the oestriols are falling. It's not bad, but you should come in and have some water tests, get some rest, and then we can start you off sometime next week probably, when you're ready.*
PATIENT: *If my husband wanted to come and talk to you about inducing me, can I make an appointment for him?*
DOCTOR: *I don't think anything your husband said would affect our decision one way or the other.*
PATIENT: *No, but he would like to talk to you.*
DOCTOR: *Yes, well, he can talk to whoever's on duty, but there's nothing he can say that will affect us: it's a medical question.*

DOCTOR: *This is Mrs Taylor.*[9] *She's due in four weeks. Very scientific, aren't we – she used to be a botanist. Did we do a alphafetoprotein for the previous spina bifida?*
PATIENT: *Yes.*
DOCTOR: *The risk is about one in twenty of the same thing happening again, but in fact we know it's alright, and she's not going to have one, don't we.*
PATIENT: *Yes, they said it was normal.*
DOCTOR: *Four weeks to go. You last had ultrasound – today? When are you going to have it again?*

PATIENT: *They said it was up to you.*
DOCTOR: *I think you'd better have another. We'll make you an appointment.*
PATIENT: *Does it seem alright?*
DOCTOR: *Yes, it's fine.*
PATIENT: *It's just routine?*
DOCTOR: *It isn't that we suspect anything abnormal, we're just being cautious.*
PATIENT: *I see.*
DOCTOR: *Come here next week and then in two weeks you can go to ultrasound before the clinic – that'll save you another visit.*
PATIENT: *Thank you, doctor.*

Other signs of medicalization are that in the sample of 'normal' primigravidae interviewed in the Transition to Motherhood study, 100 per cent took drugs of one kind or another in pregnancy, 100 per cent had blood and urine tests, 68 per cent were given ultrasound, 19 per cent X-rays and 30 per cent other tests; the average number of antenatal visits was thirteen. Of a series of 878 questions asked the researcher by the women in this study 24 per cent concerned medical procedures – about which women felt deprived of information or in need of reassurance. In nearly half the doctor–patient encounters observed in the research hospital, there was at least one reference to technology – to one testing procedure or another. Of the questions asked by patients 29 per cent concerned technology (ultrasound, induction, blood tests and so forth), as did 17 per cent of the statements they made to doctors.

These are some aspects of the medicalization of women as maternity cases; they are reinforced by the later treatment of women in the delivery room, where a birth without medical intervention is now virtually unknown in many industrialized countries (see International Federation of Gynaecology and Obstetrics and International Confederation of Midwives, 1976). Home births may escape this, but the medical ideology of maternity care is such as to pre-empt the advisability of all non-institutional confinements.[10]

But obstetricians must also come to terms with the self-evident fact that childbearing *is* natural – 97 per cent[11] of the female population are able to deliver babies safely and without problems. The process of reconciliation exposes the contradiction:

> Difficulties may arise if it is forgotten that, however natural the processes of pregnancy, delivery and the puerperium should be in an ideal world, the fact remains that in no aspect of life is the dividing line between the normal and the abnormal narrower than in obstetrics. Seconds of time, an ill-judged decision or lack of facilities, experience or skill, can separate joy from disaster. The safety and efficiency of a maternity service depends largely on recognition of these facts. [Stallworthy, 1972, p. 353]

Much of the antenatal literature in current British use illustrates this ambivalence. Pregnant women are told that pregnancy is a 'natural function' or a 'perfectly normal event' during which mothers enjoy 'the best of health'. They are nevertheless instructed to visit the clinic or doctor regularly, pay careful attention to medical advice and follow the doctor's orders, with the implicit message that the 'natural' function of childbirth can only be accomplished within a circumscribed medical context (Graham, 1977a).

The importance of the medical context is established by the *routinization* of technological, pharmacological and clinical procedures during as many stages of the reproductive process as possible and in as many patients as possible. To reserve these for a small proportion of maternity cases would emphasize the probability of normality: to use them for the majority of patients stresses the probability of abnormality, and the need for women to be dependent on medical care. Mary Cousins is a comptometer operator married to a greengrocer; she had had a termination of pregnancy in the past and had been (unknowingly) included in a research project designed to see whether regular vaginal examinations are of any use in preventing abortion due to cervical incompetence following a termination:

DOCTOR [entering examination cubicle]: *Okay, dear, pop up on the couch.* [Patient does so]
DOCTOR [consulting case notes]: *Mrs Cousins?*
PATIENT: *Yes.*
DOCTOR [palpating abdomen]: *I want to do an internal examination now. Open your legs and relax.*

PATIENT [begins to obey instructions, then suddenly realizes what the doctor intends to do and closes her legs]: *Oh no, please doctor, no doctor.*
DOCTOR: *Why not?*
PATIENT: *The doctor last time, he hurt me and I had a lot of bleeding afterwards – he promised he wouldn't do it again.*
DOCTOR [visibly angry]: *I don't care a damn what the doctor promised last time. If you lose the baby it's up to you. Do you know why we do these examinations?*
PATIENT: *I thought it was to tell the size of the baby.*
DOCTOR: *No, it's nothing to do with that. You've had a termination, and this can damage the neck of the womb and cause prematurity, and we look to see if the womb is opening up. If it is, we put a stitch in.*
PATIENT: *I'd rather not, doctor.*
DOCTOR [still evidently cross]: *Okay. Well, everything else appears to be alright. We'll see you in two weeks.*

The purpose of the regular internal examinations had obviously not been explained to Mary before, and it was only through a direct challenge that the covert character of the examination was revealed.

One important norm within the culture of the medical profession is that judging a sick person well is more to be avoided than judging a well person sick (Scheff, 1963). This 'medical decision rule' is applied to obstetrics as it is to other branches of medicine; the doctor views reproduction as a potentially problematic condition, reserving the label 'normal' as a purely retrospective term. Every pregnancy and labour is treated as though it is, or could be, abnormal, and the weight of the obstetrician's medical education acts against his/her achievement of work satisfaction in the treatment of unproblematic reproduction. Thus doctors in the research hospital openly declared their preference for working in the 'special clinic' where high risk cases are seen, as it 'makes life a bit more interesting'. The consequence of this attitude is of course that 'normal' reproduction becomes an anachronistic category:

CONSULTANT: *Interesting, very interesting, most unusual.*
REGISTRAR: *You mean it was a normal delivery?*
CONSULTANT: *Yes – pushed the baby out herself!*

The equation of 'normal' with 'unusual' illustrates the medical rationale, for if this equation did not hold obstetricians would presumably have no valid role in managing reproduction. A further device that labels women as medical maternity cases is the *fragmentation* of reproductive care through the separation of obstetrics from paediatrics and its alignment with gynaecology, the *diseases* that women, by virtue of their special biology, exhibit.

(c) INDICES OF SUCCESS

'Successful' reproduction in the medical frame of reference is measured in terms of concrete statistical indices: perinatal and maternal mortality rates. Certain limited indices of morbidity are also used, for example the physical condition of the baby in the immediate postpartum period. But the prevention of death remains the chief yardstick by which the obstetrician judges the value of his/her work, being particularly concerned with the concept of 'avoidable' death, the most prominent meaning of which is death for which the practitioners of reproductive medicine could hold themselves, or be held, responsible.

This statistical preoccupation has a historical aetiology. In the later decades of the nineteenth century, a moral and eugenic concern with the wastage of human life represented by high infant mortality (around 160 per 1000[12]) generated a movement for infant welfare. This hoped to improve the mortality figures by focusing on the improvement of feeding methods and physical aspects of baby care. When it failed to achieve this end, maternal welfare became an official concern, providing a final justification for the consolidation of medical reproductive management (McCleary, 1933). Both this ideology and its statistical base were relatively new (1874 was the first date at which births were compulsorily notified in Britain, though some national figures had been obtainable since the late 1830s), and both have influenced the practice of obstetrics ever since.

It might seem obvious that only mortality statistics can offer any objective base for judging the success of reproductive management. But in fact the form this argument has taken has generated two basic errors. In the first place, the reproductive 'performance' of women deduced from the mortality statistics has often been directly attributed to the impact of obstetric medicine. In the second place, the limited notion of success entailed by statistical criteria has not always reflected success from the reproducer's point of view. Here is a further arena of conflict between, on the one hand, the medical frame of reference, which has imposed certain paradigmatic representations of womanhood on people having babies, and on the other, the outlook of those who have the babies and experience the meaning of reproduction at first hand.

Taking the point about the relationship between obstetric medicine and mortality statistics first, it is evident that this is an example of a general tendency within medical history – to pre-empt the primacy of non-medical influences by asserting the exclusive right of doctors to improve health.[13] As Cassell has recently phrased it:

> The rise of modern technological medicine has so closely paralleled the disappearance of the infectious diseases of the past and the fall in infant and childhood mortality that it is generally assumed that doctors and their technology are responsible for the health our society enjoys today. Unfortunately, there is little evidence to support the assumption that the health of a population is primarily a result of its medical services – and much to contradict it. [1976, p. 17][14]

McKeown (1971) has shown that the decline in mortality during the latter half of the nineteenth century in Britain was due to a rising standard of living, especially improvements in nutrition, and to the amelioration of national hygiene via improved water supplies and more sanitary methods of sewage disposal. Mortality began to decline long before the causal organisms of many infectious diseases became known and medically treatable; the decline in tuberculosis deaths between 1840 and 1870 is a particularly clear illustration of this. A similar exercise can be carried out in the obstetric field. The problem with using crude mortality rates to assess the value of obstetric innovation is that these rates conceal secular changes in maternal age, parity and thus obstetric risk (Chalmers and Richards, 1977). On the whole, the fertility of high risk mothers has declined most in the last twenty years, so that perinatal and maternal mortality have improved regardless of the consequences (beneficial or not) of medical innovation.

Where the advantages of a particular innovation in reducing mortality are claimed as the basis for extending its use, evidence for this claim is often difficult to find. Chalmers has shown that an increased use of induction of labour together with antepartum monitoring using urinary oestrogen assay and serial ultrasound cephalometry in Cardiff over the period 1965–73 had no beneficial effect on the statistics of perinatal death (Chalmers *et al.*, 1976). Analysis of data on hospital confinement rates in relation to perinatal mortality produces the same kind of conclusion – although widely seen within the medical frame of reference as beneficial, the move towards the goal of 100 per cent hospital confinement has not consistently reduced the mortality of British babies since the mid 1960s (Ashford, 1978).

Such figures point to the importance of non-medical determinants of reproductive 'performance' as well as to the iatrogenic potential of modern obstetric practice. Support for the first argument can be drawn from many sources, but one striking example is the widening gap between the perinatal mortality rates of different social classes. In Britain, women of low socio-economic status are about four times more likely to lose their babies than their counterparts at the opposite end of the socio-economic spectrum (Chamberlain *et al.*, 1975). Differential exposure to medical care does not explain this increased risk, since no research has been conducted that could establish a causal relationship between poor, or non-existent, antenatal care and perinatal mortality. Nevertheless, many doctors and medical decision-makers argue that the primary responsibility for perinatal death lies with the mothers themselves, who stubbornly refuse to accept medical advice by smoking too much, attending antenatal clinics too little, and insisting on their right to give birth in unsuitable places (DHSS, 1977).

So far as the iatrogenic possibilities of modern obstetric styles are concerned, these are well-documented. Induction of labour, for example, is associated with an increased incidence of foetal distress, uterine rupture, preterm infants and therefore more neonatal problems such as respiratory distress syndrome (Chalmers and Richards, 1977). But the 'real' incidence of these in large populations is not known because no methodologically appropriate study has been carried out comparing their incidence in similar groups of induced and non-induced labours. The problem of causal inference in obstetrics (from the statistics to the practice) is, as I have said, not restricted to this branch of medicine, but the issue *is* considerably more complex in this field, because of the fact that most of the 'patients' are not ill and do not require medical treatment in the first place. Small babies are one highly significant 'cause' of perinatal mortality – about 7 per cent of British babies weigh less than 2500g at birth and they make up 70 per cent of perinatal deaths (Chalmers and Richards, 1977). A reduction in risk in this group associated with technological innovation could very substantially alter the perinatal mortality picture, but, at the same time, if applied unselectively to the reproductive population could result in higher mortality in normal, mature babies. It is this balancing of benefits and hazards to two different populations of mothers and babies, those who need medical care and those who do not, that represents the unique dilemma of medical maternity care.

Contemporary obstetric medicine has its roots in the 'scientific' and technological domination of male midwives over the empiricist and 'natural' methods of traditional female midwifery. What has consequentially followed is a style of medicine that decisively emphasizes the physical rather than the social or psychological. This type of medical ideology and practice fits very well the notion that success can be judged quantitatively via mortality statistics, rather than (or as well as) through the medium of the *quality* of life that mothers and babies experience during and after the medical manipulation of reproduction. The restricted meaning of successful reproductive outcome in the medical model implies (i) that a woman's own satisfaction with her childbirth experience should be complete if she emerges from childbirth alive and with a live, healthy infant, and (ii) that other more broadly based indices of health (the woman's emotional reactions to the experience of childbirth and its management, the way in which motherhood is integrated with a woman's life-style, her satisfaction/dissatisfaction with the baby and with the mother–baby relationship) are not relevant measures of reproductive success.

Again, this concern should be placed in the general context of medical care, where keeping people alive has become the primary medical goal and the quality of the lives thus extended has seemed a secondary consideration. Live babies who are brain-damaged or have had their health impaired in other ways through the circumstances of their birth present particular problems to their mothers, and may alter their capacity to 'adjust' to motherhood. In some cases a mother may feel it would have been better for all concerned had the child not survived. One such case history stands out in the series observed for the Transition to Motherhood study. A single woman had an IUCD fitted before having intercourse with her boyfriend and immediately became pregnant with twins. She was told by the doctor to give up work in order to allow the babies to grow more satisfactorily, but because she had no income aside from her employment, did not intend to get married and was planning to have the babies adopted, she saw the advice to devote herself exclusively to the task of gestation as quite counter to her own interests.

This is an extreme instance of clash between the index of statistical survival and mothers' own assessment of reproductive success; in most cases, the goal of a live baby is, of course, one that mother and medical staff share. But achievement of this goal is not necessarily equated by mothers with reproductive success. Other negative experiences may intrude: a 'bad' birth, a difficult baby, severe postnatal depression. Doctors and mothers may have different views of whose achievement the birth is. For mothers, successful childbirth is often contingent on certain ideas being realized about how birth should be accomplished. If obstetricians block the realization of these ideas, they may prevent maternal feelings of success and make more likely a pervasive sense of personal failure in the act that is culturally held out to be the primary achievement and proof of womanhood. Women evaluate the success of their childbirths in a more holistic way than the medical frame of reference allows.

(d) PREGNANT PATIENTS

This leads in to the next point: that the medical control of reproduction assigns a specially limited status to the pregnant woman. The opening of a chapter on 'The Induction of Labour' illustrates the dominant medical mode of 'conceiving' women:

> The fascination of the uterus to pharmacologists lies in the fact that its behaviour varies from day to day and almost from minute to minute, the very reason that it has largely been abandoned in despair by physiologists. It is illogical to consider the problem of the induction of labour in lonely isolation, seeing that the physiochemical changes which then occur in and about the myometrial cells are but an extension and modification of those which occur during each menstrual cycle. The essential problem is not why nor how the uterus expels the fetus, but why it tolerates it for so many months. [Theobald, 1974, p. 341]

In this piece, from a treatise on the management of labour, 'uterus' or 'cervix' is the subject or object of the sentence forty-six times, almost twice as often as the word 'woman' or 'women'. The connections between this view and that of nineteenth-century gynaecology are not hard to see. By equating women with their wombs, obstetricians define women as pregnant patients and exclude other social and emotional considerations as irrelevant to childbearing. A pregnant woman's career as a patient begins with the medical confirmation of her pregnancy and ends shortly after the delivery of her child.[15] (Or this is where other types of medical control take over, in the form of the child health services.) During this reproductive phase, being a patient is the only relevant role in medical eyes, an aspect of the medical frame of reference that is illustrated in the following encounter between a shop assistant and a houseman:

DOCTOR: *Mrs Bates?*
PATIENT: *Yes.*
DOCTOR: *This is your first visit in this pregnancy?*
PATIENT: *Yes.*
DOCTOR: *You were on the pill?*
PATIENT: *Yes.*
DOCTOR: *Was that period in May the only period you had?*
PATIENT: *What?*
DOCTOR: *You haven't had a proper period since that one?*
PATIENT: *No, but I've had a brownish discharge since then.*
DOCTOR: *When?*

PATIENT: *Well, more or less all the time.*
DOCTOR: *Recently?*
PATIENT: *Yes.*
DOCTOR: *Do you wear a pad?*
PATIENT: *No.*
DOCTOR: *Does it itch?*
PATIENT: *No.*
DOCTOR: *Have you felt the baby move?*
PATIENT: *Oh yes.*
DOCTOR: *Why have you left it so long* [patient is about 22 weeks pregnant] *before coming here?*
PATIENT: *Well, I didn't go to the doctor for ages, I was so depressed. I didn't want the baby. I wanted an abortion.*
DOCTOR: *Have you ever had diabetes, tuberculosis, rheumatic fever, kidney diseases, high blood pressure?*
PATIENT: *No.*
DOCTOR: *Has anyone in the family ever had any of those?*
PATIENT: *No.*
DOCTOR [reading notes]: *So you've just got two babies alive – you had a couple of miscarriages?*
PATIENT: *Yes. Well, I had three.*
DOCTOR: *And you had a blood transfusion?*
PATIENT: *Yes.*
DOCTOR: *And you had twins?* [Two of the miscarriages were of twin pregnancies, one at 12 and one at 24 weeks]
PATIENT: *Yes.*
DOCTOR: *Let me have a look at you.* [Proceeds to palpate abdomen]
PATIENT: *I fell down the stairs with this one.*
DOCTOR: *Did you?* [Looks in mouth] *Are they all yours?*
PATIENT: *No, I've got dentures with six on.*
DOCTOR: *Do you go to the dentist regularly?*
PATIENT: *I do.*
DOCTOR: *When was the last time you went?*
PATIENT: *Two weeks ago.*
DOCTOR: *And you don't breastfeed your babies?*
PATIENT: *No.*
DOCTOR: *You're not going to breastfeed this one?* [Examines breasts]
PATIENT: *No.*

DOCTOR: *Have you noticed any lumps?*
PATIENT: *No.*
DOCTOR: *They just feel heavier than usual?*
PATIENT: *Yes.*
DOCTOR: *I want to have a look at this discharge of yours. Bend your knees up for me.* [Patient moves to side] *No, on your back please. That's right. Can you let your knees go floppy and just relax? This'll be a bit cold* [inserts speculum]. *Okay, just stay as you are, I've nearly finished. I just want to examine you.* [Withdraws speculum and does bimanual examination] *Okay. All finished. That's fine. Everything's alright. The brownish discharge is from a sore place you've got on the neck of the womb. That's quite common in pregnancy. You're about right for dates, but because you were on the pill, I want you to go to ultrasound.*
PATIENT: *Is that date – the third of March – right?*
DOCTOR: *When you've been to ultrasound we'll know more accurately.*
PATIENT: *Do I have to go there now?*
DOCTOR: *No, nurse will make an appointment for you.*

The patient's attitude to the pregnancy is ignored by the examining doctor, who instead focuses his and the patient's attention narrowly on its medical management.

In the main, antenatal consultations are managed so that there is no place for mention of social/emotional factors. The relevance of a woman's other roles is considered only where employment or marital status (i.e. working, being unmarried) are perceived as in conflict with the goal of the production of a live, healthy fullterm infant.[16] In other cases the intrusion of 'personal' considerations into medical decision-making transgresses the prevailing norm of reproduction as a medical process.

DOCTOR: *We want you to come into hospital today.*
PATIENT: *Today! I can't possibly come in today. I've got some furniture arriving. I can't come in till Monday at least.*
DOCTOR: *Who's at home, then?*
PATIENT: *No one. My husband's out at work.*
DOCTOR: *Well, it's time this baby was delivered. Your blood pressure's up and you've got some protein in your urine, and you need to rest in hospital until we can start you off.*

PATIENT: *But it's not due until the 27th* [two weeks' time].
DOCTOR: *I know, but we've been watching the baby's growth at ultrasound and it's quite big enough now.*
PATIENT: *There's nothing wrong with it, is there?*
DOCTOR: *No, but your blood pressure's up and there's protein in your urine and we feel that the baby ought to be delivered. If we leave it longer, the baby might be affected. I would object anyway, if I knew you were going home to have furniture shifted. That's not good for you, or the baby.*
PATIENT: *I can't get hold of my husband today.*
DOCTOR: *When will he be home, then?*
PATIENT: *Twenty past six.*
DOCTOR: *Well, could you come in this evening?*
PATIENT: *I suppose so.*

The outcome is negotiated – but only minimally so. Irritation is the typical medical reaction to patients' mentions of attitudinal factors or their other social-role obligations. Ninety-three per cent of patients' questions/statements concerning social factors met this response. In these two examples, conflict between medical and maternal frames of reference is very evident.

A registered baby minder and a senior registrar:
PATIENT: *Can you give me some sort of idea as to when my operation's* [a caesarean] *going to be done?*
DOCTOR: *Well, it's very difficult to say.*
PATIENT: *It's very diffcult for me, too. My husband's got to take time off work and I've got two kids to make arrangements for.*
DOCTOR: *Yes, I see. Well, sometime in the last week of your pregnancy, I imagine.*
PATIENT: *No.*
DOCTOR: *What?*
PATIENT: *Thirty-eight weeks, Mr Hawkins said.*
DOCTOR: *Well, I'm not Mr Hawkins.*
PATIENT: *It's a bit thick, this is. If it's not done till forty weeks, my husband'll go mad. Mr Hawkins promised faithfully it'd be done at thirty-eight weeks.*
DOCTOR: *Well, then, there's no point in asking me, is there?*
PATIENT: *I've got to ask. I've got two kids to look after.*
DOCTOR: *Well, I can't decide for Mr Hawkins. I don't know what his work commitments are.*

PATIENT: *I can't ask Mr Hawkins, can I? He's not here.*
DOCTOR: *There's plenty of time to ask him. Ask him next week.*
PATIENT: *I want to know* now. *I need to know to make arrangements.*
DOCTOR: *Why will your husband go mad?*
PATIENT: *Because of what happened last time. I'm not waiting for the selfsame thing to happen again, am I?*
DOCTOR: *What happened last time?* [Reads notes: an intrapartum haemorrhage and fresh stillbirth] *Oh, I see. Right, I'll give you a date now. Right, I'll work it out.* [Writes in notes: 'Patient very keen to know date of admission to hospital, and has many arrangements to make. Can't wait until Mr Hawkins returns . . .']

A receptionist and a senior registrar:
DOCTOR: *Mrs Carter? How are you getting on?*
PATIENT: *Horrible.*
DOCTOR: *Why?*
PATIENT: *I feel horrible.*
DOCTOR: *Have you had any more bleeding?*
PATIENT: *No.*
DOCTOR [palpates abdomen]: *Yes, that's alright.*
PATIENT: *Was the test* [urinary oestriols] *alright?*
DOCTOR: *Yes. And they're expecting you at ultrasound today.*
PATIENT: *I feel so depressed.*
DOCTOR: *Why?*
PATIENT: *I don't know.*
DOCTOR: *So, why aren't you well?*
PATIENT: *I feel it's so difficult to walk.*
DOCTOR: *You shouldn't be walking much at this stage of pregnancy.*
PATIENT: *I don't. But I have my housework to do and I've got in-laws staying.*
DOCTOR: *They should be doing your housework for you, shouldn't they? Isn't that what they're for?*
PATIENT: *They're not females. It's my father-in-law staying. Things aren't very good at home at the moment.*
[Doctor says nothing and continues to palpate abdomen]
PATIENT: *What are the chances of a caesarean?*
DOCTOR: *It's early days yet. We'll wait and see. Good-sized baby, that, isn't it! That's a good size.*

PATIENT: *It's the tightening I keep worrying about.*
DOCTOR: *It's normal in pregnancy. Your womb is supposed to tighten.*
PATIENT: *I didn't have it with the other three.*
DOCTOR: *Every pregnancy is different. Let's see you in one week.* [Reading notes] *You do seem to have put on a bit of weight.*
PATIENT: *What does that mean?*
DOCTOR: *It doesn't necessarily mean anything, but you must take things easy.*
PATIENT: *That's what my husband says. It's easy for men to say that.*
DOCTOR: *You shouldn't blame us.*
PATIENT: *I'm not blaming you, it's not your fault.*
DOCTOR: *It's your set up at home. You should have organized things better.*
PATIENT: *Well, I've got three kids to look after.*
DOCTOR: *Yes.*
[Doctor, later, to researcher: *It's her silly fault, she should have made arrangements. Now my wife, I left her without the car the other day, and she had to walk the three-year-old three miles to school, and she complained. I said ring up a friend, and she did, and they were only too delighted to help. It just takes a bit of organizing, that's all.*]

Behind this medical emphasis on clinical judgement and decision-making lies an underlying concern with social typification. Stressing the propriety of marital versus non-marital reproduction is one sign of this. Others, derived from analysis of the observational data, include a division of the patient population into 'special' and 'ordinary' cases. Whereas clinical data would predict a concentration of working-class women in the special clinic, because of their higher risk of obstetric problems (Illsley, 1967), the association in the observational data is, in fact, in the opposite direction: middle-class women were more likely to attend the special clinic ($p < .01$). Patients with any kind of medical status – being doctors, nurses, midwives or (especially) the daughters or wives of doctors – were particularly likely ($p < .001$) to be seen in the special clinic. The implications of special clinic attendance are greater privacy and more space in the examination cubicle, more doctor time and more chance of seeing a higher status doctor. In both clinics, working-class patients and white, as opposed to brown, patients were given more time by the doctor (though the differences are not statistically significant, $p<.14$ and $p<.08$ respectively).

Medical understandings of the concept of social class are limited. In one study of an obstetric unit, the researcher asked the staff how to assess social class: the replies were randomly distributed between intelligence, money, education, occupation, accent, personality, clothes and hairstyle. Most attributions in clinical practice were in terms of intelligence; in sixty-eight cases over the twelve-month study 'intellectually deficient' was written in the case notes, while in only one case was there any evidence for this statement. One obstetrician observed had two methods of conducting an examination. Either he would read the notes at length and then turn to the patient, or he would begin to talk to the patient immediately on entering the examination cubicle. The first method was reserved for patients whose notes recorded a manual occupation, and the second for those with non-manual occupations (Fish, 1966).

Of course, such discrimination against working-class, ethnic minority group and non-medical patients is not exclusive to the maternity care field. Other researchers have noted it in other areas of medical practice.[17] But so far as maternity cases are concerned, such designations are peculiarly mixed with ideological constructions of the feminine character.

(e) Medical Typifications of Women

Two paradigms of women jostle for first place in the medical model of reproduction. In the first, women are seen not only as passive patients but in a mechanistic way as manipulable reproductive machines. In the second, the mechanical model is replaced by an appeal to notions of the biologically determined 'feminine' female.

The 'reproductive machine' model has informed much of the technological innovation in obstetrics that has taken place since the colonization of reproductive care by medicine. It is no accident that this style of obstetrics is known as 'the active management of labour'. It embodies a physicalist approach to childbirth: 'To put the matter rather crudely, obstetrics treats the body like a complex machine and uses a series of interventionist techniques to repair faults that may develop in the machine' (Richards, 1975, p. 598). This approach builds on earlier definitions of the abnormality and unnaturalness of reproduction, which facilitated the medical takeover. A mechanical model directly opposes the natural model; it is 'man-made' and requires regular servicing and maintenance to function correctly. Thus antenatal care can be interpreted as maintenance and malfunction-spotting work; obstetrical intervention in delivery as repairing mechanical faults with mechanical skills. Concretely, as well as ideologically, women appear to become machines,[18] as machines are increasingly used to monitor pregnancy and labour, to initiate and terminate labour itself. One machine controls the uterine contractions, which are recorded on another machine; regional analgesia removes the woman's awareness of her contractions so that these must indeed be read off the machine; and keeping all the machines going becomes what 'looking after' a patient in labour means.

Yet, as we have seen, human and mechanical images are discordant, and conflict between maternal and medical frames of reference is intrinsic to the relations between obstetricians and their patients. Hence a need to monitor carefully the amount and type of information 'fed' to pregnant women. The mechanical metaphor sharpens into an analogy with a computer; it is only by the careful selection and coding of information that computers can be made to function correctly (to produce the desired result). The main vehicle for the programming of women as maternity patients is antenatal advice literature. The evolution of this literature in Britain in fact reflects very closely the chronology of expanding medical jurisdiction over birth.[19] Today the emphasis is on the need for women to be informed about the physiology of pregnancy and labour, and to a smaller extent to be cognizant of the rationale behind the medical management of these. Yet a very clear dividing line is drawn between desirable and undesirable information: the first two sections in Gordon Bourne's widely read *Pregnancy* (1975) are called 'Importance of Information' and 'Don't Read Medical Textbooks'. Conflict between doctor and patient in the antenatal clinic or the delivery room is interpreted as a failure in the doctor's effective communication of his intentions to the patient. Discussing the public unease about the induction of labour, a leading article in the *British Medical Journal* put it this way:

> The fact that a procedure such as induction of labour, done in good faith for the good of the mother and baby, had been so misrepresented by the media, was unlikely to be due to some malign purpose, but was more probably disquieting evidence that doctors *were not adequately communicating their intentions to their patients*. . . . The modern woman still wishes to have faith in her doctor – to believe that she can hand over to him, without anxiety, the care of herself, and, *more important*, that of her baby. ['Induction of Labour', 1976, p. 729; my italics]

For if the programme is not presented in the correct way to the computer, it will refuse to process it.

'Natural childbirth' appears to offer an antidote to this induced dependence on medicine as the proper setting for reproduction. The very notion of paradigmatic representations of women as maternity cases within medical science seems to be challenged by the idea that women can have babies naturally, by following what is 'natural' to the woman having the baby rather than what is culturally imposed on her as a feminine destiny:

> She is no longer a passive suffering instrument. She no longer hands over her body to doctor and nurses to deal with as they think best. She retains the power of self-direction, of self-control, of choice . . . [Kitzinger, 1962, p. 20]

The paradox is two-fold: in the first place, the implications of natural childbirth ideology are strictly limited by the experience of the majority of reproducers, which is that childbirth hurts; and, second, in its origins and type of cultural accommodation over the last thirty years, natural childbirth has been colonized by medicine itself. Grantly Dick-Read, the father of natural childbirth, laced the last chapter of his popular *Childbirth Without Fear* with a familiar metaphor:

> Since when have repair shops been more important than the production plant? In the early days of motoring, garages were

> full of broken-down machines, but production has been improved; the weaknesses that predisposed to unreliability were discovered and in due course rectified. Today it is only the inferior makes that require the attention of mechanics. Such models have been evolved that we almost forget the relative reliability of the modern machine if it is properly cared for . . . The mother is the factory, and by education and care she can be made more efficient in the art of motherhood. Her mind is of even greater importance than her physical state, for motherhood is of the mind . . . [1942, p. 12]

Responding to this appeal, the medical rejoinder to the natural childbirth movement has been to legitimize it by including it with the medical brief. Medical advice literature began in the 1960s to propose some form of preparation for childbirth; this consisted of relaxation or breathing exercises as an adjunct to medicalized reproduction, employing these techniques

> as ameliorative strategies to enhance the mother's experience of hospital-based and pharmacological confinement. Although ostensibly acknowledging the principle of natural childbirth, the concern with psychology and individual control is subsumed by and lost within a system of maternity care which, instead, stresses physiology and medical control. [Graham, 1977a, p. 24]

One illustration of this is the entry under 'psychoprophylaxis' in Herbert and Margaret Brant's popular *Pregnancy, Childbirth and Contraception: All You Need to Know* (a significant sub-title, this):

> Psychoprophylaxis: This is best used as a general term to cover many forms of antenatal education, prepared childbirth, etc. . . . It is obvious that the term has come to mean widely different things in different countries, cities, towns and clinics throughout the world . . . The modern tendency is for maximum emphasis on education and enlightenment of patients and a kindly supporting role by staff . . . The ideal arrangement is for a patient to attend a programme in the hospital or clinic where she is to be delivered. In this way she can be prepared for the management and experience she will have and the staff with whom she will be in contact will know what she has been taught and will be in a position to support her fully. She becomes the patient in a hospital team working together for her benefit. [1975, p. 194]

Or take the American doctor's manual *Expectant Motherhood*:

> The transcendent prerequisite [of natural childbirth] is that you have complete confidence in your doctor – confidence that he is your friend, a medically wise friend who is sincerely desirous of sparing you all the pain possible, provided that this is compatible with your welfare and that of your child. The very presence of such a friendly doctor, and the realization that he is competent to handle any situation is in itself the most effective and welcome of obstetric anodynes. [cited in Wertz and Wertz, 1977, p. 185]

Thus colonized by medicine, natural childbirth all too easily fits the old 'feminine' paradigm. The following passage from an early account by a doctor of a natural childbirth programme nicely illustrates the gender-specificity of the 'conditioning for childbirth' model:

> . . . conditioning a woman for childbirth does very much the same for her that military training does for a young soldier who must face the rigors of battle. No young man wants to die or to suffer the pain of wounds. But with military training he becomes so conditioned that he is able to face death and pain with fortitude, and to come through the experience with a sense of having proved his manhood . . . [Tupper, 1956, p. 740]

– or womanhood, in the case of women 'conditioned' to have babies.

Mechanical and feminine modes of representing women coexist in medical writing and practice. Commitment to the idea of femininity as the necessary prerequisite and consequence of successful reproduction is expressed in various ways:

> There are certainly some women who say that they have no desire to become mothers and genuinely mean it; but they are a minority. Every month a young woman is reminded that her primary role in life is to bear children and even the most ardent advocate of Women's Lib sounds unconvincing if she denies wanting to achieve motherhood at least once in her lifetime. [Newill, 1974, p. 14]

> A woman can never escape her ultimate biologic destiny, reproduction, and a goodly number of psychologic problems

encountered in the course of pregnancy are the result of conflicts concerning this biologic destiny. [Heiman, 1965, p. 473]

A woman's basic personality will not be changed during her pregnancy, but subtle and minor changes will certainly occur. All women tend to become emotionally unstable at times when their hormone levels are at their highest, such as puberty, pregnancy, the menopause and also immediately before the onset of each menstrual period. It is well known that the majority of impetuous actions and crimes committed by women occur during the week immediately before menstruation. [Bourne, 1975, p. 3]

DOCTOR: *How many babies have you got?*
PATIENT: *This is the third pregnancy.*
DOCTOR: *Doing your duty, aren't you?*[20]

In such manifestations, the model is some kind of debased psychoanalytic one, but its exact contours are not described. Its principal import is that a 'proper', i.e. truly feminine, woman wants to grow, give birth to and care for babies and regards this, along with marriage, as her main vocation in life. Such women 'adapt' or 'adjust' well to pregnancy, birth and motherhood, experience deep 'maternal' feelings for their babies and are able successfully to integrate the competing demands of motherhood and wifehood. It follows that the femininity of those women who do not achieve these goals is suspect. Either they have not attained their true feminine maturation and/or they are ridden with conflicts about the desirability of a feminine destiny.

Textbook assertions are translated into clinical dogma, as models of womanhood appear in the interaction between doctor and patient. I give below some extracts from obstetric encounters that show some important modes of feminine typification.

The necessary contentment of necessary motherhood

DOCTOR: *This is twins. They're growing well, but you need more rest. I'd advise some good books and a quiet life for three months. You're not working?*
PATIENT: *No.*
DOCTOR: *Just normal exercise – I want you to have a walk every day, but no gardening, no heavy work, postpone moving or decorat-*

ing the house. If you do rest, you'll grow yourself slightly bigger babies. After all, it's this [pats her abdomen] *that's your most important job, isn't it?*

Women, mothers, housewives

DOCTOR: *Does it make you want to wee when I press there?*
PATIENT: *It does slightly – I spend more time in the loo than anywhere else.*
DOCTOR: *Moved the cooker in there, have you?*

DOCTOR [to pupil midwife]: *She can't rest at home, and if she doesn't rest, she'll have tiny babies – like kippers. No, she can't rest at home, I wouldn't listen to arguments, not unless she's the Queen or the Duchess of Malborough. There's a good case for telling her that now, so she can get granny over from Limerick or wherever.*

The marriage symbol

PATIENT: *When I wake up my fingers and ankles are so swollen.*
DOCTOR: *And I see you haven't got your wedding ring on.*
DOCTOR [to researcher]: *And she's got some oedema – fluid retention.* [To patient] *Is your ring tight?*
PATIENT: *I don't wear it.*
DOCTOR: *Why don't you wear it?*
PATIENT: *It's tight.*
DOCTOR [to researcher]: *You see, when they get embarrassed not wearing a ring in pregnancy, they borrow someone's – their mother's or grandmother's.*
PATIENT: *I'm not embarrassed.*

A proper family

DOCTOR [palpating abdomen]: *Ah, a nice-sized baby.*
PATIENT'S TWO-YEAR-OLD SON: *Yes.*
DOCTOR: *So you want a little girl, I suppose?*
PATIENT: *No.*

Women never know, do they?

DOCTOR [to researcher]: *Mrs Connell hasn't got a clue about her dates. I bet you don't know when your last period was?*
RESEARCHER: *Yes, I do.*
DOCTOR: *I don't believe you. Women never know.*

DOCTOR: *Have you felt movements, yet?*
PATIENT: *Yes.*

DOCTOR: *When?*
PATIENT: *They started on March 18th.*
DOCTOR: *That's a good girl, a very good girl, that's what we like to see, someone who knows the date.*

DOCTOR [reading case notes]: *Ah, I see you've got a boy and a girl.*
PATIENT: *No, two girls.*
DOCTOR: *Really, are you sure? I thought it said . . .* [checks in case notes] *oh no, you're quite right, two girls.*

Doing what comes naturally, or you shouldn't believe all that

DOCTOR [to audience of pupil midwives]: *I don't agree with husbands being there when women are in labour. After all cows and bitches kick the stallion away.*
PUPIL MIDWIFE: *Yes, but women aren't cows, are they?*

DOCTOR: *How old are you?*
PATIENT: *Eighteen.*
DOCTOR: *Do you want an epidural, dear?*
PATIENT: *What?*
DOCTOR: *Do you want an injection to take the pains away?*
PATIENT: *No, it's dangerous.*[21]
DOCTOR: *There's nothing dangerous about it. You mustn't believe all you hear, you know. I've just done an epidural for a friend's wife, and he's an anaesthetist.*

PATIENT: *Last week Mr Mitchell said he'd have me in at term to be induced. I'd rather not be induced – unless there's a reason.*
DOCTOR: *Well, we won't induce you if there's no indication. We don't do social inductions.*
PATIENT: *Okay, fine. The other thing was, I've heard you do routine epidurals.*
DOCTOR: *Yes, on request.*
PATIENT: *Do you have to have them?*
DOCTOR: *Oh no.*
PATIENT: *That's alright then.*
DOCTOR: *You want it* au naturel*?*

Now then, sweetie

DOCTOR: *Have you had a smear test from the neck of the womb recently?*
PATIENT: *No.*
DOCTOR: *Well, I want to do one today. Could you turn over and face*

the wall, move your bottom over, and put your feet forward, so you don't kick me in the chops. I'll just go and get the equipment I need, I'll be back in a tick. [Leaves cubicle, returns with speculum] *Now then, sweetie, I have warmed it for you under the tap, so that's nice of me, isn't it?*
PATIENT: *Thank you, doctor.*

This feminine paradigm of women is presented in parallel with two other ideological tendencies: a hostility to female culture, and an identification with masculine interests. The first point is best explained through quotation:

> Another hidden anxiety is a fear of the pain of childbirth. All too often the young mother is told of the gruesome imagined experiences of older women ... [Llewellyn-Jones, 1965, p. 65]

> ... an effort should be made to restrain or rebuke the parous women who relate their unpleasant experiences to the unsuspecting primigravidae. [Matthews, 1961, p. 874]

> Why do women have to recount such stories to one another, especially when the majority of them are so blatantly untrue? ... Probably more is done by wicked women with their malicious lying tongues to harm the confidence and happiness of pregnant women than by any other single factor ... Perhaps it is some form of sadism ... [Bourne, 1975, p. 7]

There is an obvious conflict between the obstetrician's 'knowledge' about reproduction and the received wisdom of women who have actually given birth.

On the second point, Diana Scully and Pauline Bart carried out a study of women in gynaecology textbooks and found that they 'revealed a persistent bias toward greater concern with the patient's husband than with the patient herself' (1973, p. 1045). The same tendency is evident in obstetrics, where, for example, concern with the role of husbands in labour is associated with the promotion of types of analgesia that make the *husband's* experience of childbirth more pleasant.[22] In one development, that of 'husband-coached childbirth' (Bradley, 1964), the husband *becomes* the doctor – that is, he adopts the doctor's role of programming the patient for birth. Or the doctor becomes the husband: a well-known popular treatise on the treatment of infertility proposes medical students as the ideal donors of sperm to women with unfertile husbands:

> Who are the donors? . . . My own preference is for medical students, and other doctors who engage in AID tend to use the same source. Medical students are generally acceptable to the recipients as being intelligent young men who have gained a place in a medical school. They generally are emotionally stable people and are frequently good all-rounders who take part in the sporting and social activities of their hospitals. [Newill, 1974, p. 165]

The merging of doctor and husband roles through the identification of doctors with husbands is one device used to 'desexualize' the intimacy of the obstetrical encounter. The registrar in the following case was seeing a childless woman in her late twenties for a follow-up appointment after an emergency hysterectomy. This was preceded by an emergency caesarean section for foetal distress in premature labour: the baby was stillborn and in the early puerperium the patient sustained an uncontrollable haemorrhage and was admitted to hospital in acute shock.

DOCTOR: *Hello, how are you?* [Reading case notes] *You came to see Mr Mitchell again?*
PATIENT: *Yes* [smiles] *but it's proving rather difficult to see him.* [The consultant failed to turn up to take his clinic.] *You took some urine tests because it hurts a bit when I go to the toilet, and they thought there might be an infection there.*
DOCTOR: *I can't find the result* [looks in notes]. *You brought some urine in today, did you?*
PATIENT: *Yes.*
DOCTOR: *Ah, here it is; no, there doesn't seem to be an infection.*
PATIENT: *Do you know if it's healed up inside?*
DOCTOR [obviously reluctant to examine patient]: *I thought Mr Mitchell had done all that.*
PATIENT: *He did, but he said it wasn't quite healed and he'd like to look again.*
DOCTOR: *Turn on your left side, will you, and I'll have a look. How long has it been now?*
PATIENT: *Six weeks.*
DOCTOR [inserting speculum]: *And how is your poor husband bearing up all this time?*

PATIENT: *Alright. I don't think it worries him, really. He's more worried about how I am.*
DOCTOR [looking inside the vagina]: *Poor chap. How long altogether has he been without his rights?*
PATIENT: *I don't think he minds. I think he's worried something else might happen to me – all that bleeding upset him.*

The doctor's concern for what he sees as her husband's sexual deprivation, a concern expressed significantly at the exact moment he inserts a speculum into her vagina, contrasts with the patient's calm insistence that lack of intercourse is not a problem for her husband. She refers to the trauma of what happened to her medically – after all, her husband saw her nearly die. The doctor repeats the same point: 'poor chap . . .'.

Medical work in obstetrics and gynaecology is characterized by these two themes of sexuality and gender. The manner in which these themes are handled and absorbed into the medical frame of reference has considerable implications for the role of women as maternity cases.

Most obstetricians are men. Of the NHS hospital medical staff listed under the heading 'Obstetrics and Gynaecology' in 1977, 75 per cent were male, and in the upper reaches of the profession this rises to 88 per cent. Overall, the proportion of NHS hospital doctors who are women is 18 per cent; of consultants, 10 per cent (DHSS, 1978). Bias against women achieving on equal terms with men in medicine is a mixture of direct discrimination and domestic oppression. There is a cultural incompatibility between the domestic structure of women's lives and the career-structure of medicine, which is geared to the masculine pattern of permanent full-time promotion-oriented work (Bewley and Bewley, 1975). As the *British Medical Journal* recently pronounced the moral verdict: 'Those [women] who opt for two careers cannot normally expect to reach the highest points in medicine. They must be satisfied with achieving less . . .' ('Women in medicine', 1974, p. 591) – a dictum that is hardly applied to male doctors who combine marriage and parenthood with work.

Despite recent increases in the proportion of medical students and doctors who are female, the typical image of doctors associates them with masculinity. In one American survey of patient attitudes, the exception to this was obstetrics and gynaecology, which was viewed as a field where women ought to be prominent (Engleman, 1974). And yet neither in America nor in Britain is obstetrics and gynaecology an especially female health care specialty. Since it was originally developed as a challenge to female modes of reproductive care, its ideology has historical roots in anti-feminism, in the creation of a mythology of women that represents them as a marginal group. Combined with women's minority position within obstetrics and gynaecology, this means that medical styles of relating to maternity patients are predominantly masculine: they typify women as a special category of patients. Such categorization hinges on the perception of women as especially 'troublesome' patients who must be 'adjusted' to their domestic roles (Stimson, 1976a; Barrett and Roberts, 1978). Through these stereotypical visions of female patienthood, doctors exercise a social control function over women's lives that has little to do with the ostensible medical rationale of disease diagnosis and treatment.

DOCTOR [to researcher, discussing second doctor]: *How do you rate him, then?*
RESEARCHER: *What do you mean?*
DOCTOR: *I don't think he'll ever have any sexual impact on the patients, that chap.*

The typical obstetrical encounter is between a man and a woman. Moreover, through the intimacy of the 'clinical' procedures that are medically defined as necessary, the encounter has strong sexual connotations. These provide a base for many of the communicative patterns characterizing doctor–patient interaction as, for example, in the following episodes:

DOCTOR: *Hello, how are you?*
PATIENT: *Alright.*
DOCTOR [reading case notes]: *This isn't our first rendezvous, is it? We can't go on meeting like this, you know.*

DOCTOR: *I think you'd better go to ultrasound – it might be twins. I'm sure they'll tell us the answer one way or the other.*
PATIENT: *There aren't any twins in the family. But I'd like it.*
DOCTOR: *There's a first time for everything, as the archbishop said to the actress.*

DOCTOR: *Hello.*
PATIENT [taking pants off]: *Sorry.*
DOCTOR: *Touting for business?*
PATIENT [smiling]: *Yes.*

DOCTOR: *I'll give you some tablets for the tingling – the only thing is, you shouldn't take them too late or they'll make you pee all night: they increase the water flow, you see. What time do you go to bed?*
PATIENT: *Oh luxuriously early – about 9 o'clock, and I have an orgy of* TV *watching.*
DOCTOR: *An orgy of what?*
PATIENT: TV.
DOCTOR: *Oh yes, well* [exiting from cubicle, talking loudly], *I should cut out the orgies at this stage, if I were you.*

Significantly, sexual joking of this type is restricted to the beginning (first and third examples) and ends (second and fourth examples) of the encounter. Examination of the patient's body, especially a vaginal examination, brings doctor and patient into greater intimacy, which must be denied if the encounter is to retain its overtly clinical purpose. Many manoeuvres are used to achieve this end, but the main one is making sure a nurse is there to 'chaperone'. Every doctor in the series of antenatal encounters observed was selective about this procedure, for instance: 'It isn't the youngsters I worry about, but the thirty to forty year old woman: I always insist on a chaperone' (Registrar, early forties). Talking about something else is also a mode of distracting attention from the sexual embarrassment of the situation:

DOCTOR: *I'd like to examine you down below to do what we call pelvic assessment, to see if the pelvis is the right size.*
PATIENT: *Okay.*
DOCTOR: *Can you bring your knees up for me?* [Inserts gloved hand into vagina] *Right now, we don't have a clinic next week, because of Easter, so you'd better come next in a fortnight's time.*

And the sexual embarrassment itself is occasionally given overt recognition:

DOCTOR: *Right, could you turn on your side, put your bottom over here, and pull your legs up?*
PATIENT [doing so]: *I'm sure I didn't have this last time.*

DOCTOR: *Did you have it on your back?*
PATIENT: *Yes, I think so. Is it better this way?*
DOCTOR: *Well it is, because I don't have to stare you in the face.*
PATIENT: *Oh, I see. It's better for you, not for me.*[23]

Technical words for the woman's genitals are significantly not used, 'down below' being the most common euphemism, though 'inside' and 'tail' are also prominent. Such parlance contrasts with doctors' tendencies to 'technicalize' during other parts of the consultation. Both manoeuvres are distancing techniques, the requirement of keeping the patient in her place and of desexualizing the episode calling for different strategies on the doctor's part (see also, Emerson, 1970).

Male motives for entering obstetrics and gynaecology have never been systematically studied. It is not, however, highly regarded within medicine, ranking with paediatrics and dermatology in Becker *et al.*'s *Boys in White: Student Culture in Medical School* (1961) as possessing low prestige. A survey of eminent British physicians' backgrounds in relation to their chosen specialisms compared those from public schools with those from grammar schools, and found that pupils from the former 'were more likely than others to work on living bodies rather than dead bodies or parts of bodies, on the head rather than on the lower trunk, on male bodies rather than female bodies and on the body's surface rather than its inside' (Hudson and Jacot, 1971, p. 162). Only 39 per cent of eminent obstetricians had attended public schools, compared with 100 per cent of those in plastic surgery, 89 per cent in ophthalmic surgery and 71 per cent in cardiology. Obstetrics and gynaecology may have this stereotype partly because of its demanding work routines, but it is also seen as intrinsically boring because of the restricted range of problems (women's) with which it deals (Becker *et al.*, 1961, p. 411).

If motivations for becoming an obstetrician are unresearched, so also are obstetricians' attitudes to women. There is no doubt that clinical behaviour is shaped by moral judgements in which culturally normative paradigms of femininity abound: such investigations of physicians' beliefs as J. Aitken-Swan's *Fertility Control and the Medical Profession* (1977) give ample evidence of the interaction between attitude and practice. A truly horrific and terrifying revelation of how medical behaviour can exemplify the most 'criminally negligent' aspects of social ideologies that degrade women is Ian Young's *The Private Life of Islam* (1974), an account of a London medical student's midwifery training in Algeria, where obstetricians are 'unhappy executioners, working in the blood, excrement and death of the most respected attitudes' (p. vi).

In the less overtly sexist tableau of modern industrialized society, the feminine paradigm has been clothed in a more subtle veil. The ideological appeal is to sexual *difference* rather than sexual inferiority. Paradigmatically, women are just different sorts of people from men, and the matrix of the argument is that their reproductive behaviour and attitudes can only be understood against this background of cultural femininity. Aside from its influence on clinical theory and behaviour, the feminine paradigm has stimulated an enormous amount of medical research on feminine status and reproductive outcome – measured physiologically in terms of abortion, stillbirth, foetal deformity, labour and delivery difficulties, pregnancy complications, and so forth. For example, infertility, habitual abortion and premature delivery have all been analysed as psychosomatic defences, as a result of hostile identification with a woman's mother, as rejection of the feminine role, as failure to achieve feminine maturity and as evidence of disturbed sexual relationships with husbands/boyfriends. (Some such studies are Rubenstein, 1950; Ford *et al.*, 1953; Mandy and Mandy, 1959; Mann and Grimm, 1962; Tupper and Weil, 1962; Blau *et al.*, 1963.) Much the same hypotheses have been applied to the study of other complications of pregnancy and labour (e.g. nausea and vomiting, toxaemia, uterine 'dysfunction' in labour) and to the status of the child (its physical condition and behaviour) after birth (for instance, Kroger and DeLee, 1946; Harvey and Sherfey, 1954; Coppen, 1958; Crammond, 1954; Stott, 1957). Elaine Grimm (1967) has described much of this research and has pointed out its many methodological flaws. A great many studies are retrospective, taking a group of women in whom some pathology of physiology has been identified and investigating these in isolation from any control group of 'normal' women. Prospective research on 'normal' women (those without identifiable physiological pathology) itself suffers from a failure to assess personality variables *before* pregnancy (a woman who is ambivalent about her pregnancy may already be reacting to uncomfortable physical experiences, for instance). Grimm concludes:

> The most salient criticism applicable to all the studies, whether of normal women or of women with a pathological condition, is that none of them can be said to contribute any data about cause and effect . . . it is impossible to tell whether the psychological reactions are the cause, accompaniment or consequence of physiological reactions. [1967, p. 37]

The psychological variables themselves have a dubious status. How reliable and how valid are the measures employed? What constitutes 'rejection' of the feminine role? What, indeed, is 'the feminine role'? How, and from whose viewpoint, are these assessed? For the precise contours of the paradigm and the logic of its operationalization in reproductive research, it is necessary next to turn to psychology as the domain in which pre-formed notions of reproducers' feminine status have found their fullest expression.

CHAPTER 2

Psychological Constructs

Like all science and all valuations, the psychology of women has hitherto been considered only from the point of view of men . . . An additional and very important factor in the situation is that women have adapted themselves to the wishes of men and felt as if their adaptation were their true nature.

[Horney, 1974, p. 7]

Cultural femininity and biological reproduction are curiously synonymous in the proclamations of medical science about women. In this, as well as other senses, the task of reformers must be, as John Ehrenreich (1978) has said, not to overthrow scientific medicine, but to answer the question how (or whether) medicine may *become* scientific. Yet it is not only in medical science that the character of women as reproducers is mythologized: 'social' science is no less culpable. Psychology and sociology ape the customs of medicine, and built into their universe of discourse are images that masquerade as facts, guises in which female persons are clothed in the habits of femininity for the performance of that most biologically female of all activities, the bearing of children.

In the next chapter I look at signs of the feminine paradigm in sociology. In this chapter I want briefly to outline (and it *is* a brief outline – the subject is enormous) the kind of constructs that have labelled women's roles as reproducers in psychiatry and in clinical and academic psychology. I am concerned throughout chiefly with child*bearing* rather than child*rearing*, for women's functions as mothers have constituted a vast topic that it would be out of place to tackle here.[1]

Psychological characterizations of women as reproducers replicate three weaknesses of the medical model: they persistently confuse the individual and the social, blurring the distinction between what Rich (1977) has called motherhood as 'experience' and motherhood as 'institution'; they assume a crude causal paradigm of psychological states as epiphenomena of physiological ones; and they treat women in an *a priori* fashion as representatives of femininity rather than of humanity.

This is true both of the medical–psychiatric literature and of academic psychologically oriented research and writing on women and reproduction. The two fields are symbiotically connected: medical–psychiatric literature is the main repository of psychological research on women, and a cultural reduction of women to the status of a medical problem (people who need treatment to adjust them to their social roles) has been influential in shaping women's status as psychology's subject matter. The two covert premises are that women's mental/emotional lives are governed by their bodies and so, therefore, is their place in society. Social and biological roles are, in other words, concordant in precisely the same way as they are in the cultural consensus about gender identity and relations that flourishes in the particular historical mode of advanced industrial capitalism. Not surprisingly, the other area within psychology that has attended to women is the corpus of literature concerned with sex 'differences', much of which is designed to provide a 'scientific' pedestal on which our cultural ideology of gender differentiation can be construed to rest.[2] It is not coincidental that men have predominated in the psychiatric field, just as they have in obstetrics and gynaecology. NHS hospital medical staff figures for 1977 (DHSS, 1978, Table 7A)[3] show that 94 per cent of psychotherapists are male, as are 89 per cent of those who specialize in mental illness and 67 per cent of those whose field is child and adolescent psychiatry – this latter figure illustrating the common tendency for professional women to work in areas that can be construed as feminine interests.

Feminist psychologists have sketched out the place of women in psychology as a mirror image of their ideological, social and economic location:

> How are women characterized in our culture and in psychology? They are inconsistent, emotionally unstable, lacking in

> strong conscience or superego, weaker, 'nurturant' rather than productive, 'intuitive' rather than intelligent, and, if they are at all 'normal', suited to the home and the family. In short, the list adds up to a typical minority-group stereotype of inferiority: if they know their place, which is in the home, they are really quite lovable, happy, childlike, loving creatures. [Weisstein, 1970, p. 219][4]

These statements are supported by evidence, whereas most psychological theories about women usually are not. The point is that a mythology of women that decrees them inferior for biologically determined reasons is built into the terms of the 'scientific' debate. Since such a mythology is embedded in the language of 'science', it is inseparable from the generality of 'scientific' findings. One important consequence of this is that the social context of reproduction is not quantifiable as an independent variable. It is, instead, part of the conceptual armoury with which any investigation or discussion is conducted, being represented within the term 'femininity' itself. A second consequence is that psychological work on reproductive behaviour has been chiefly concerned not with the subjective experiences of reproducers as shaped by their own frame of reference, but with the outcome of reproduction as defined by 'successful' childbirth and unproblematic 'adaptation' to the social role of mother. Although 'successful' reproduction in this sense shares some features of the medical definition commented on in the last chapter, one strictly non-medical idea is important in the psychological model. This is the idea that femininity is coterminous with 'normal' reproduction – the growing and bearing of a baby without illness symptoms, devoid of medical complications and free of the necessity for medical intervention. Such a notion is a very particular interpretation of the term 'normal'. Since it is used independently of any particular historical context, there is no appeal to the idea of statistical normality, and no account is taken of how childbirth is handled in the sense of whether or to what extent it is medicalized. One can only conclude that the psychological construction of women's functions as reproducers gives rise to a fundamental double-bind situation: women are only proper women if they don't need doctors, and yet, according to the medical paradigm, proper women must be dependent on, and deferential to, medical management and control.

These weaknesses, paradoxes and dilemmas of the psychological approach are illustrated especially clearly in the literature on postnatal depression. The term itself is of primary ideological importance, since it is the main psychological construct expressing an assessment of 'poor' outcome, a failure on the part of women to achieve reproductive and feminine normality. It is, of course, essential that postnatal depression should *appear* to be a technical concept – a clinical term evolved by experts to describe a clinical syndrome: the covert ideological function of 'science' is exactly expressed in the hidden character of such 'technical' evaluations.

Even as an overtly technical term, postnatal depression is extremely ill-defined in the medical–psychiatric literature. As Brown Parlee (n.d.) has pointed out, at least three phenomena are discussed under the same heading: the postpartum blues, a transient syndrome of 'weepiness' in the early puerperium; acute psychosis akin to other psychoses, except that it is preceded by childbirth; and depression – though this is itself an 'umbrella' term, psychiatric consensus acknowledging only that it involves more than just simply a depressed mood. Though neither the blues nor psychosis constitutes depression in either psychiatric or lay understandings of this word, 'true' depression has never been adequately defined. Its definition and classification have been accomplished only by using certain aetiological assumptions, for example, that depressions fall into two groups: 'endogenous' depressions, which arise autonomously, and 'reactive' depressions, which represent a response to environmental circumstances. The primary differentiation according to the manual of the *International Classification of Diseases* is not symptomatology but aetiology – a claim that is either self-validating or incapable of validation.

Postnatal depression (in any of its meanings) is a form of 'reactive' depression, the prior circumstance in this case being childbirth. Two main psychiatric theories describe its aetiology as (a) hormones and (b) some disturbance of, or in, femininity. Katherina Dalton is one modern protagonist of the hormone theory, and she sums up her work on puerperal depression thus:

> After the birth of the baby the placenta comes away from the womb ... The additional source of progesterone has therefore been removed ... the woman's body adjusts to a normal

> progesterone level, which is a hundred times lower than the level she experienced during late pregnancy. This is responsible for the 'puerperal blues' or tearfulness so frequent among women during those few days after the baby's birth. The woman . . . may be upset by this sudden decrease in her progesterone level and may develop a more severe puerperal depression in which she becomes apathetic and tearful, losing appetite, interest, energy and initiative; she may also become sexually frigid. [1969, pp. 105–6][5]

The theory is not based on empirical evidence of the relationship between different levels of progesterone in the puerperium and a linked different incidence of depression. In fact, there has been very little work indeed in this field. A few studies have examined such aspects of puerperal biochemistry as electrolyte pattern (Coppen and Shaw, 1963), plasma cortisol concentration (Gibbons and McHugh, 1962), glucose tolerance (McGowan and Quastel, 1931), progesterone/oestrogen levels (Nott *et al.*, 1976), and tryptophan metabolism (Handley *et al.*, 1977), but in relation to early postpartum mood only. With the exception of tryptophan metabolism, which shows a possible relationship with the blues (how such a relationship might be interpreted is far from clear), the findings of these investigations have been negative or inconclusive. Despite the inadequacy of research, the 'hormonal' explanation has a wide currency in medical practice, and is often simply asserted as the cause of postnatal depression. What causes weeping four or five days post partum is also held to bring about more severe depression occurring later in the puerperium (how much later – two months? nine months?); the association is, again, not derived from empirical surveys (nor from randomized controlled trials of administered progesterone) and is actually counter to evidence that mothers who experience the blues are not especially likely to suffer from later depression (Kaij and Nilsson, 1972).[6]

Other hormonal theorists invite similar criticism. For instance, Hamilton's (1962) contention that acute postpartum psychoses occur within a fixed time period of birth and thus must be biologically, i.e. hormonally, caused, is not validated either by evidence about the timing of onset of psychoses after childbirth or by physiological data showing some particular hormonal deficiency in psychotic women (Parlee, n.d.). The hormonal aetiology of postpartum mental disorder is part of a received medical wisdom, which in turn is imported into the domain of commonsense understandings:

> The subsequent three or four days [after birth] are characterized by extreme emotional lability. To the observer, the mother appears slightly euphoric, unrealistic, 'whimsical' ... The slight euphoria, the irritability, the emotional lability, the stereotyped crying behaviour and the impression of slight confusion are all, *in our opinion*, characteristic of the early postpartum period. *We are inclined* to interpret these symptoms as physiological, rather than psychological reaction, perhaps due to an increased secretion of corticosteroids. [Kaij and Nilsson, 1972, p. 371; italics added]

And from Herbert and Margaret Brant's already quoted dictionary of *Pregnancy, Childbirth and Contraception*:

> Depression: see Moods. . . . Moods. . . . In the puerperium a husband may visit his wife one evening and leave her feeling sublimely happy; but the next night when he arrives a few minutes late or forgets to bring flowers, he will meet an unwarranted storm of protest and then tears. It is a sudden withdrawal of hormones with the delivery of the placenta which has this upsetting influence. [1975, pp. 81, 151]

Most strangely, hormones are also counted responsible for depression in pregnancy, when the placental effect is in full swing: thus both the presence and absence of high levels of progesterone apparently have the same mental effect. And these effects of a woman's biology on her reproductive behaviour are then characterized as 'normal': '. . . every mother should experience "the blues" . . . Most midwives and doctors consider that an attack of "the blues" is almost essential to relieve tension after delivery' (Bourne, 1975, p. 422) – the implication being, obviously, a dual one: (a) that normal women are at the mercy of their hormones and (b) that the characteristic state of women is emotional lability, weepiness, 'whimsicality' and so forth. (Consider the application of such terminology to men suffering from mild depression following surgery. Would they be described as exhibiting 'whimsical' tendencies, and 'stereotyped crying behaviour'?)

But perhaps the most striking feature of the hormonal explanation is that it is regarded as being totally incompatible with and, as it were, virtually disproving, any *social* influence on reproductive feelings and behaviour. Thus, for example, Kaij and Nilsson, the authors who favoured the idea of corticosteroids, continue:

> In the second half of the first postpartum month the picture changes again ... Many women ... become more easily fatigued, need much more sleep than usual, feel tired, irritable and complain of a number of psychosomatic symptoms. These complaints are often explained as a consequence of caring for the child. The fact that some overburdened women do not complain, while others who lead an easy life experience an abundance of symptoms, suggests, however, that exogenous factors are relatively unimportant. We feel that the main cause of this postpartum 'hang-over' is to be found in physiological factors, perhaps in the hormonal readjustment. [1972, pp. 371–2]

The language ('suggest', 'we feel', etc.) belies the importance of judgmental perceptions about the relationship between women's bodies and their minds. No figures are compiled to illustrate the non-association between domestic burden and postnatal depression: the 'social' explanation is discounted on what are almost moral grounds – or at least in total accordance with the mechanical charter of womanhood described in the previous chapter. A woman is a machine and maternity is a cause of mechanical breakdown, the very frequency of this being held to confirm women's inherent fragility and unreliability (women are not even very good machines). Quite clearly such social items as having too much housework to do, having inadequate housing, having to deal unaided and quite unprepared with a difficult and demanding baby, confronting a resentful and equally demanding husband, not having more than three hours' sequential sleep, experiencing a total inability to go out of the house without the baby, and having to put up with the physical aftermath of birth (haemorrhoids, engorged breasts, an unhealed perineum, etc.) have no capacity to influence the functioning of reproductive machines.[7] These contextual variants have thus received almost no research interest – even such a simple question whether the incidence of postnatal depression (however defined) is related to place of confinement remains without an answer.[8]

The medical–mechanical model of women as reproducers is

applied in two ways to psychological constructions of their reproductive role. In the first place physiological changes are seen to cause psychological problems directly, as in the hormonal interpretation. But, secondly, psychological problems are viewed as resulting from intrapsychic conflict in the individual as she reacts to the stresses of reproduction. Thus, recourse is had to the feminine paradigm as a tool that must be used to diagnose faults in the reproductive process. It is this latter interpretation that is the most popular in the psychological literature – though, of course, whichever way you look at it women are at the mercy of their bodies. Whether controlled by hormones or by the psychic representation of reproductive events, the shaping of female destiny by anatomy is the message.

In the intrapsychic conflict model, each individual enactment of pregnancy, birth and motherhood is part of the great drama of femininity. Menstrual problems, not conceiving, aborting, giving birth prematurely, experiencing nausea and vomiting, having toxaemia, bearing a deformed infant, having a prolonged labour and being postnatally depressed are disturbances of 'normal' reproductive function and are evidence of a woman's inability to achieve mature femininity. This, as we saw in the last chapter, has been a dominant mode of medical research on reproductive behaviour. But the other version of the feminine paradigm is the converse of this: all mental/emotional behaviour during reproduction is essentially reactive. The stimulus is biological, but it is manifested psychologically and socially via the operation of a code of preselected meanings. Individual reproductive histories call forth different translations of the 'femininity' code, and it is these that are held to account for variations in personal reactions to childbearing.

There is a veritable armada of studies that take this line on reproductive womanhood.[9] To regard them seriously as scientific investigations demands a suspension of belief in even the most basic credentials of science, for the central problem is elementary: 'femininity' is a chameleon concept. As a personality constellation it is defined deductively, i.e. symptomatically, according to the investigator's own preferred schema. Thus pregnancy nausea may constitute evidence of lack of femininity ('unconscious rejection' of pregnancy – Kroger and DeLee, 1946, p. 544) or of its presence: Nilsson, in a survey of 'Paranatal Emotional Adjustment' reports that women with postpartum adaptational difficulties displayed a tendency towards 'denial of their reproductive functions' as measured by the presence of 'symptoms from the genital sphere' (for instance dysmenorrhoea) and other relevant symptoms, including late antenatal clinic booking and *absence* of pregnancy sickness (1972, p. 159). Labour pain is another symptom with a dual identity, as a proof of feminine personality: '... pain enhances the mother–child relationship ... a certain amount of pain experienced by the woman may be useful' (Heiman, 1965, p. 487); and as its negation: 'In some women, we even note behavior in labor that is decidedly content and even colored with joy ... These are not women whose image of womanhood revolves exclusively around motherhood' (Molinski, 1975, p. 341). And so on – many instances can be found of such contradictory interpretations.

The reason why the meaning of 'femininity' in the psychological studies is so highly contextual is because it can have no fixed referent. It is a specific cultural product, a symptom of a particular kind of thinking about women that has arisen in one cultural–historical milieu (see Oakley, 1972). As a research variable femininity cannot be defined in terms of its lowest common denominator because it has none. Or, rather, the core of any agreement people are able to reach concerning it reflects their own participation in the same feminine paradigm. To most psychological researchers this fact about 'femininity' has not been evident, or else it has been overridden by an attachment to paradigmatic interpretations of female reproductive behaviour. Such a triumph of dogma over deductive logic is exemplified once again by Nilsson's study (1972). He used a Masculinity–Femininity Scale to assess the orientation of his sample women. This consisted of ten 'masculine' and ten 'feminine' adjectives from which each woman was invited to choose the five that best, and the five that least, described herself. He found that those women who came out as more 'masculine' than the others reported fewer symptoms during pregnancy and fewer 'life history' symptoms, and concludes that 'masculine' women wish to appear healthy and so *deny* their symptoms. (In other words, considerable distortions are needed to avoid the conclusion that 'femininity' militates *against* problem-free reproduction.)

A common label in psychological studies is that of a 'confused sexual identity'. Maturity in a mother is equated with femininity: mature mothers are

> ... women whose feminine identification and capacity for relating closely to the important people in their lives have led to a marriage based on reason, tenderness and sexual compatibility; whose desire it is to have a home and children, with moderate ambitions to improve their situation in life ... whose organization evidenced in the past by competence, by adequate performance at school and at work, will now be evident in sound planning for their home and their husbands' comfort ... [Chertok, 1969, p. 64–5][10]

Conversely, immature mothers are women in whom sexual identity is not clear, women 'for whom marriage and motherhood are states that they accept, but with varying degrees of trepidation', making it possible that they 'will remain extremely demanding and dependent and will be unwilling or unable to enter into marriage or to contemplate the arrival of an offspring with the necessary selflessness; they will feel abused' (Chertok, 1969, pp. 65–6). All sorts of signs and symptoms point to failures in femininity development that prognosticate poorly for unproblematic childbirth and adjustment to motherhood. Chertok (1969), using the concept of a 'negativity grid' as an instrument predicting ease or difficulty with childbirth, lists under 'womanhood' a profusion of diverse factors, including miscarriage, breaking off of a love affair, playing boys' games in childhood, 'negative' valuation of sex; and under 'abnormal attitudes to motherhood' are included fear of not knowing how to care for the child, and problems with sexual intercourse. Why all these factors should be considered to have such an intense relevance to the experience of childbirth, when they clearly can have entirely different origins, associations and consequences, could be said to constitute a research problem in itself.

Chertok includes 'enforced interruption of highly valued employment' as a negative factor. Evidently, though rarely explicitly, rejection of femininity entails and is entailed by, working or wanting to work outside the home:

> In modern western society the rejection of motherhood is in turn reinforced by a demand on the woman to be economically productive. . . . There is no doubt that the emancipation of woman has increased her difficulties. . . [Kaij and Nilsson, 1972, p. 381]

Freud may not have said that anatomy is destiny, but this claim is embedded in much of the psychological research on motherhood. Any distraction from devotion to a career as housewife–mother, any attempt to 'emulate' the role of men, is taken as a proof of deflection from the proper feminine path. Women are a sum of their biological attributes and the cultural complexity that surrounds and informs the translation of biological potentiality into cultural possibility is discounted. This has the effect of reducing maternity to a mere symbol of the extent to which women are, or are not, enmeshed in a cultural nexus of femininity.

This is only one meaning – one way to analyse – becoming a mother. The predominance of 'adaptation' or 'adjustment' as terms indicating successful reproductive outcome raises the persistent question: adjustment to what? The notion that in becoming mothers women must adjust to something is inseparable from the conclusion that what has to be adjusted to is external to the self, i.e. is a socially coded formula for the production of personalities appropriate to the social and economic exigencies of institutionalized female domesticity. The question that needs to be asked is why, in psychological research on reproduction to date, it should have been considered so crucial to demonstrate the associations between reproduction and cultural femininity, between having a baby and having acquired, or failed to acquire, the particular psychodynamic structure that expresses the socially secondary meaning of womanhood. Research with this methodological focus is programmed to parallel, and not to challenge, the existing social order; the data 'produced' in the research enterprise will persistently confirm traditional social practice. This, in itself, as Myrdal (1969) and others have noted, should raise suspicions about the procedures behind the generation of the data. Such data have the character of an ideological representation. The rate at which maladaptation (however measured) to maternity occurs does not necessarily reflect women's problems in becoming mothers. The behaviour-producing process and the rate-producing process are, as Kitsuse and Cicourel (1963) have pointed out, two differing social facts.

The notion that maladaptation to maternity occurs when women reject their feminine role can be 'unpacked' into the following components; i.e. the following are some of the meanings this notion is given in psychological research:

women dislike menstruation;
women dislike pregnancy;
women dislike childbirth;
women dislike breastfeeding;
women dislike (hetero)sexual intercourse;
women dislike their status as wives;
women dislike husband-servicing work;
women dislike their husbands;
women dislike their status as housewives;
women dislike housework;
women dislike their status as mothers;
women dislike childcare work;
women dislike their children.

It can be seen from these different meanings of 'femininity rejection' that its investigation is operationally much more complex than any existing psychological research has acknowledged. The use of the word 'dislike' as opposed to the emotionally laden 'reject' or 'deny' exposes, moreover, the morally condemnatory way in which perfectly reasonable, i.e. socially explicable, negative attitudes to specific roles/processes/activities has been interpreted. Approaching these matters with commonsense rather than with prejudged normative values about what constitutes feminine womanhood, one might ask, for example, why women should enjoy menstruation (which entails blood loss, fatigue, perhaps pain and/or premenstrual irritability and discomfort, a restriction on normal activity, the financial and social nuisance of sanitary 'protection'[11]) or childcare work (4000–5000 wet/dirty nappies per child, months or years of disturbed nights, loss of personal freedom, many extra hours of domestic work per week per child,[12] an economic burden of £64,500 from birth to age twenty-one[13]) – the dilemma can be posed in this way for every item on the 'femininity rejection' list. Indeed, it is clear that the main reason why women should enjoy or accept these aspects of biological womanhood and cultural femininity is because they are supposed to. Cultural norms conspire to identify them with their biological and social status, and social and economic institutions depend on their acceptance of them. (The fact that these institutions may militate against women's happiness in the acting out of female biological and feminine cultural destinies is, of course, not apparent in much psychological research because only certain questions are seen as important.)

Dana Breen (1975) has singled out two alternative perspectives within the psychological literature on motherhood. In the first, reproduction is a hurdle to be overcome: pregnancy is a pathological condition, birth a trial, and a woman's task in becoming a mother is to overcome these obstacles without permanent impairment to her mental health. The second perspective gives a slightly more positive picture, in which birth represents growth and offers possibilities for personal integration. The model here is not purely medical but developmental. Yet despite its welcome emphasis on birth as an achievement (a 'degree in femininity'[14]) rather than a handicap, the framework within which reproduction is analysed is once again rooted in a psychoanalytic ideology of femininity.

For Grete Bibring, one of the most influential proponents of this model, pregnancy is a 'normal crisis' in a woman's psychological development:

> Pregnancy, like puberty or menopause, is regarded as a period of crisis involving profound endocrine and general somatic as well as psychological changes. The crisis of pregnancy is basically a normal occurrence and indeed even an essential part of growth, which must precede and prepare maturational integration ... The woman moves through a phase of enhanced narcissism early in the pregnancy, until quickening undeniably introduces the baby as the new object within the self. The mother's relationship to her child, if it finally fulfils the maturational requirements, will have the distinctive characteristics of a freely changeable fusion

> ... of narcissistic and object-libidinal strivings so that the child will always remain part of herself, and at the same time will always have to remain an object that is part of the outside world, and part of her sexual mate. [Bibring *et al.*, 1961, p. 22]

The notion of a 'normal crisis' is, as Rossi (1968) has noted, uncomfortably incongruous. To restrict attention to 'normal crises' entails an exclusive concern with successful outcome. Those instances in which successful integration of personality does not occur are failures – and to ask what they are failures of is, once more, a political question. Maturational integration of femininity is one response to the stresses of reproduction, but becoming a mother could, conversely, be viewed as a 'turning point', a 'point of no return', in which there is no consolidation of femininity; instead there are more varied changes in personality structure, in self-concept and in relational identities that establish motherhood as decisively different from non-motherhood.

Two recent psychological studies of the birth of a first child both attempt to revitalize the developmental model. Breen, in her study of fifty primigravidae (1975), considers that much previous psychological research on motherhood is unhelpful, conceptually confused, methodologically inadequate and over-determined in the use it makes of normative notions of femininity. She makes the analytical distinction between the female biological role and the female cultural role that is missing from most previous work. The focus of Breen's own research is the changes in a woman's self-concept that occur with the onset of motherhood. Using a combination of interviewing and psychological testing, she compared adaptational processes over time in a group of pregnant women with those in a non-pregnant group. Her findings are interesting, not least that she is able to show the falsity of the assumed link between traditional femininity and adjustment to motherhood. The most feminine women in her sample were those who encountered problems most often:

> In sum, those women who are most adjusted to childbearing are those who are less enslaved by the experience, have more differentiated, more open appraisals of themselves and other

> people, do not aspire to be the perfect selfless mother . . . and do not experience themselves as passive, the cultural stereotype of femininity. [p. 193]

Since the least 'adjusted' women had difficulties with the split between ideal and reality – the mothers they felt they were, as opposed to the mothers they thought they ought to be – one interpretation of Breen's material is precisely that it is the cultural idealization of motherhood/femininity that poses the greatest dilemma for women in becoming mothers. Because their experiences of reproduction and motherhood conflict with the cultural paradigm they have been socialized to hold, what is experienced is a disintegration of previous identity, a debilitating lowering of self-esteem. Those women who are able to see the ideological character of the association between perfect and actual motherhood are more likely to accept their own experiences in becoming mothers as valid (self-validating). Hence mothers in the women's movement, who are often stereotyped by the media as 'rejecting' femininity, in fact may espouse both 'natural' childbirth and breastfeeding: the cultural role is rejected, a manoeuvre that allows the biological role to be enjoyed more completely. (See chapter 11 for more on the idealization of motherhood.)

Breen, however, ultimately sees no alternative but to ground definitions of femininity and masculinity in their biological substratum of sex differences.

> Femininity is the 'nature of the female sex'; the female sex is the one 'that bears young or produces eggs'. We must start by looking at this childbearing aspect if we are to define femininity . . . femininity refers to those qualities which make for a good adjustment to the biological female reproductive role. [p. 14]

Her criteria of 'adjustment' to motherhood are: lack of negative physical symptoms in pregnancy, labour and delivery and the baby's condition after birth; no postpartum depression; and no difficulties with the baby or mother–baby relationship. The first criterion was rated by the obstetrician (a golden opportunity for the replication of medical notions of 'normal' femininity), the second two by self-report in response to questionnaires and psychological testing procedures. Thus, underlying

Breen's idea of adjustment is the classic psychoanalytic assumption that unproblematic reproduction and unproblematic motherhood are equivalent states, with identical aetiologies. The physical/medical experience of childbirth is confused with the social/emotional experience of looking after and loving a baby. Thus, the possible effects of the medical management of birth on maternal outcome cannot be studied. While the attempt to rescue the idea of femininity from the conceptual morass into which many psychological researchers have plunged it is laudable, the problem is that Breen retains 'adjustment' as the defining characteristic of feminine women.

The same criticism could be levelled at the other recent study of first childbirth, Pauline Shereshefsky and Leon Yarrow's *Psychological Aspects of a First Pregnancy and Early Postnatal Adaptation* (1973). Like many other studies that use the terminology of 'adaptation', this one is notably unclear about what it is that mothers are supposed to adapt to, but the implicit, and at times explicit, equation informing Shereshefsky and Yarrow's work is between acceptance of the motherhood role and acceptance of the baby. This equation of course begs the question of which dimensions of the motherhood role are (a) considered relevant in the study, and (b) experienced as relevant by women who are actually having babies. As in Breen's work, the data – on sixty middle-class urban couples – were collected by means of interviews and psychological testing procedures. And as is the case with Breen's findings, many of the conclusions Shereshefsky and Yarrow are able to draw out of their material pose a challenge to the older psychological formulae describing women's experiences of reproduction. For example, the role of husbands in taking over a portion of the childcare work proved crucial to the women's adaptation, and women's own previous experiences with children proved the only 'life history' factor of relevance to the outcome of adaptation.

Shereshefsky and Yarrow devote one chapter to maternal personality and adaptation in relation to infantile colic. The social responsibility women are allocated for children's behaviour is, as they observe, reflected in the brand of psychological research that investigates the correlations between the way the mother is and the way the infant behaves and then imputes a cause and effect relationship between the two. Shereshefsky and Yarrow found no link between anxiety in the mother and colic in the infant, although they did find that mothers of colicky infants became temporarily less confident and less accepting (of the baby) in response to the infant's behaviour. The labelling of maternal personality and behaviour as causal factors in the provocation of certain infant conditions is one theme that flows from the use of traditional feminine paradigms in psychological research. It has had a longevity within such research that can only be accounted for in terms of its cultural normativeness, but it is now beginning to be diluted by an awareness that infants constitute in some important ways independent variables. What they are and how they behave can affect a woman's experience of the role of mother, her ideas about herself as a mother and a person (see Lewis and Rosenblum, 1974).

To sum up, then, psychological constructions of women as childbearers have suffered from three main and related weaknesses. First, they have been embedded in mainstream psychology's identification of a 'psychology of women', which 'implies the need for a special set of laws and theories to account for the behaviour and experience of females' (Parlee, 1975, p. 120). Second, they have been asocial, displaying an almost total disregard for social–contextual influences on all facets of reproductive behaviour. And, third, they have echoed a psychoanalytic ideology of femininity in a confused and confusing fashion, losing the internal coherence of the Freudian psychological model in the pursuit of dogmatic connections between reproductive physiology and female psychology.

These three faces of psychological representations are closely linked. *Because* the psychology of reproduction has been a sub-unit of the psychology of women, the main task has been seen as interpreting the former in terms of the latter, placing the mental phenomena of childbearing within the category of those pertaining to femininity. The social location of reproduction has not been considered important and social influences on psychic health and illness have been disregarded. Commitment to some kind of psychoanalytic ideology has reinforced both these tendencies, insisting on the powerful primacy of hidden psychic structures as the stage on which individual interpretations of reproduction are enacted.

Freud's analysis of the role reproduction plays in a woman's life has greatly influenced the whole corpus of psychological literature on reproduction in this sense. I do not propose to enter into a discussion of the Freudian model here – this has been done well by other critics, from Karen Horney (1967) and Clara Thompson (1941) to Kate Millett's spirited dissection in *Sexual Politics* (1971). But I want to note in passing that several aspects of Freud's thinking on reproduction have particularly shaped psychological constructs of women as mothers. These are: his assumption that sexuality includes both eroticism and gender; his view that having a baby is an expression of penis envy; and his interpretation of postpartum problems as overt manifestations of underlying personality defects.

Freud's unitary definition of human sexuality as combining both the development of gender identity and the arbitration of correct (hetero)sexual object choice, has imposed the additional obligation on psychological investigators of matching sexual and reproductive behaviour. How a woman behaves in the (usually) marital bed is seen to have a necessary connection with how she behaves when she grows and gives birth to and looks after a baby. An elusive quest for disturbed sexual functioning has thus characterized many studies, but has proved disappointing, since, as the work of Stoller (1968) and Money and Erhardt (1972) on abnormalities of sex- and gender-development has shown, biological sex status, eroticism/sexual object choice and gender identity are to a considerable extent independent variables. In 'normal' individuals, sex and gender are equated and heterosexuality achieved through socialization; but this is not always so, and it cannot be assumed that, because it often is, sex, gender and sexuality are equivalent states.

A further point is that the physical dimensions of pregnancy, birth and breastfeeding are subsumed under the general heading 'sexuality', but their subjective experience (which may not be 'sexual') has lacked documentation (Rossi, 1973). As Karen Horney observes in her objections to Freud's conceptualization of womanhood, it is the genital difference between the sexes around which the analytical conception of femininity and masculinity has been organized. The sexes' different reproductive roles have been treated within the framework that results from this starting point, namely in terms of female inferiority:

> At this point I, as a woman, ask in amazement, and what about motherhood? And the blissful consciousness of bearing a new life within oneself? And the ineffable happiness of the increasing expectation of the appearance of this new being? And the joy when it finally makes its appearance and one holds it for the first time in one's arms? And the deep pleasurable feeling of satisfaction in suckling it. . . . [1974, p. 10]

Horney goes on to note that motherhood is only *necessarily* a handicap within an ideology that valorizes the penis and demotes the womb and vagina from their position of biological and social uniqueness. Another way to put this is to say that the only thing a woman wants more than a penis is a vagina (a point made by Stoller, 1974, p. 260).

Whether women see babies as equivalent to penises, or feel that motherhood compensates for female inadequacy and accomplishes feminine maturation, has never been the issue. Reproduction has a certain predetermined status in the Freudian model that cannot be tested by *any* kind of research data. (This is demonstrated by the challenge presented to the oedipal theory of gender development by gender identity research, which shows that convictions of femininity or masculinity are irreversibly fixed by the age of two. So far as I know this has not met with any major attitude of rapprochement on the part of psychoanalysts – Money and Erhardt, 1972.[15])

The third way in which psychoanalytic ideology has particularly handicapped the psychology of reproduction is through the view that individual psychodynamics are the main determinant of responses to reproduction. The dominant orientation is towards 'blaming the victim'. Problems in pregnancy, birth and the postpartum period are interpreted as arising from personal failure or personality 'defect',[16] a methodological feature that follows from the *en masse* treatment of women as residing in a psychology of their own. For, by implication, problems with motherhood cannot be traced to the *human* condition and must therefore be located in the feminine psyche. A further corollary is that it is the 'difficult' cases that need to be studied, without recourse to a control group of 'normal' individuals (since we already know what the feminine personality structure is and ought to be). Markham demonstrates this methodological fallacy in her study of postpartum reactions. She followed up a study of eleven patients with postnatal depression by taking a second group of women who had not been classified as suffering from postnatal depression, and found that they all gave evidence of a depressive reaction too. She concludes:

> The important distinction between the normal and pathological women was not the fact that both were experiencing depressive reactions but that the normal mothers were able to draw upon a vast arsenal of defenses to ward off or alleviate their depressive feelings. [Markham, 1965, pp. 500–1]

Although she concentrates on psychodynamic defences, one might reasonably ask about the role of social supports in preventing a diagnosis of postnatal depression. Some of these are discussed later in this book (pp. 172–8).

In short, the assessment of psychological work on reproduction introduces a major caveat:

> The question of what we may actually know (in the scientific sense) about women's behaviour and experience seems less important at this stage than knowing what investigators have tried to find out, what questions they have not asked, and how their methods and procedures have helped or hindered the development of a psychology that is relevant to women. [Parlee, 1975, p. 121]

Women's psychology has been encapsulated within the two fields of 'sex differences' and reproduction. This is in itself ample testimony to the concealed evaluative character of 'science'.

CHAPTER 3

The Sociological Unimagination[1]

> *The inattention to women derives from understandings about social science commitments to 'important' topics. Male scientists assign priorities for study and then assume that the pictures of lives, events and relationships presented are of universal importance.* [Daniels, 1975, p. 346]

'Science' as a human enterprise pretends to disassociate itself from specific cultural themes, instead focusing objectively on universal problems. But, as we have seen, its hidden stances exemplify social preoccupations. The particular instance of how women as reproducers have been seen, treated and researched within medical and psychological science displays the importance of such concealed curricula. By and large, what both medicine and psychology do is try to return reproduction and the character of women to the domain of nature. The childbearing function, and women through their natural association with it, are given a basic biological categorization, so that every aspect of reproductive and female behaviour can be referred to underlying biological constructs. Thus labelled, the problem of maternity is disposed of, the threat women's reproductivity poses to cultural organization is diminished, and women themselves become unequal actors in it.

Is it, then, to 'social' science that we must look for a more ingenuous treatment of reproduction? Self-conscious of its participation in the human social world, is sociology thus enabled to view women's reproductive activities through less blinkered eyes? Although there is currently no single agreed sociological method, objectivity has traditionally been cited as one of its most important canons. Sociologists have said they must claim to be scientists, or else they are merely commentators, rapporteurs, voyeurs. Moreover, in studying the 'social', surely sociology has a predisposition to detach reproduction from its biological location and examine it in its cultural guises?

Unfortunately, as Hobhouse said, sociology is 'a science which has the whole social life of *man* as its sphere' (cited in Bottomore, 1962, p. 17). We assume he meant the noun in its gender-inclusive sense, but it is unhappily true that those who think in a masculine language are likely to come up with masculine interpretations. More broadly, sociology has been in its modes of thinking, methodologies, conceptual organization and subjects of inquiry, one of the most sexist of academic disciplines, embodying in largely uncritical fashion the structure and values of the existing social order. 'Indeed "man" and "adult" are presumed as the norm in concept formation and the language used in description and in methodology. To study people is to study adult men . . .' (Barker, 1978, p. ii). Public, formal and official aspects of the social order have been investigated to the detriment of interpersonal, private and informal life (there is a large sociology of politics, but no sociology of feeling),[2] repeating and reinforcing the patterns of gender differentiation in society at large. The male's social world has constituted the world of male sociology. Women's relative social invisibility in public and formal life is not simply replicated but telescoped in the sociological view: they hardly exist at all. To compensate for this negation, women reign supreme in the field of marriage and family relations – though not without a chaining of their talents to the quasi-biological justification of an 'expressive' role. As Epstein (1974) has observed, an emphasis within mainstream sociology on the overwhelming importance of early socialization (as the process that produces adult human personality) deflects attention from those forms of social control that regulate adult gender relations and ensure feminine inferiority. Millett summarizes these chauvinistic sociological tendencies as an integral part of the mid-twentieth century counter-revolution in sexual politics:

> Thus sociology examines the status quo, calls it phenomena, and pretends to take no stand on it, thereby avoiding the

> necessity to comment on the invidious character of the relationship between the sex groups it studies. Yet by slow degrees of converting statistic to fact, function to prescription, bias to biology (or some other indeterminate), it comes to ratify and rationalize what has been socially enjoined or imposed into what is and ought to be. And through its pose of objectivity, it gains a special efficacy in reinforcing stereotypes. [1971, p. 232]

Since about 1970 sexism in sociology has begun to be documented and revised notions of women's place have led to the channelling of theoretical and research interests into new female fields. But while, looking forward, we may hope for better things, the task of this chapter is to explain the way in which sociology has described and defined the role of women as childbearers; this requires a backward look.

Sociological paradigms of women as reproducers have flourished in two specialisms: the sociology of marriage and the family and medical sociology – this last being a recent but rapidly expanding addition. However medical sociology is defined (sociology *of* medicine? sociology *in* medicine?), it is easy to see its relevance as a context for the examination of reproduction. Marriage and the family seem an obvious area too, but for different, and rather more invidious, reasons.

CAPTIVE WIVES

If, in psychology, the psychodynamic structure of the individual is seen as the main context that interprets the meaning of reproduction, in sociology the relevant psychodynamic structure is that of the marital relationship. Marriage replaces (or joins) femininity as the locus of reproduction. This perspective has had four main consequences for sociological representations of women as reproducers:

(1) Research on reproductive intentions and motivations and on contraceptive attitudes and techniques has been undertaken almost exclusively with samples of *married* women;
(2) Single women's sexual, contraceptive and reproductive behaviour has been conceptualized as a 'social problem' and studied from the perspective of deviancy;

(3) Maternity has had an exclusively marital meaning: what women feel about having babies has not been seen as a valid research/analytic concern, whereas the contribution (or otherwise) of reproduction to marriage has;
(4) The examination of motherhood has been child-centred and not woman-focused, echoing a concern with children's 'needs' rather than with the physical and psychic health of women as individuals.

Point (1) is self-explanatory, and can be gauged by a brief look through the 'methods' chapters of 'family intentions', and 'family planning' surveys. Three representative ones are Ann Cartwright's *Parents and Family Planning Services* (1970), John Peel and Griselda Carr's *Contraception and Family Design* (1975), and Joan Busfield and Michael Paddon's *Thinking About Children* (1977). Cartwright's survey uses a sample of 1495 married mothers (and 257 married fathers); Peel and Carr's 1678 'wives' (thus designated). Busfield and Paddon's account of a research project on 'the social determinants of fertility' draws its data from some 350 married women, and the authors say their research model

> ... was designed primarily to cover the 'normal' situation in which a man and a woman marry, then have children. Those who had children outside marriage, or those who neither married nor had children did not readily fit into our explanatory framework, and we did not intend to study these 'deviants' ... [1977, p. 67][3]

It is perhaps somewhat unfair to criticize the marital bias of these samples, given the self-professed goal of such surveys – to elaborate family-building patterns. The basic question is, of course, a prior one: why sociological researchers should have regarded it as so important to study the logistics of marital and family-oriented reproduction in the first place.

Point (2) follows. The behaviour of those who do not conform to the norm requires special explanation (irrespective, really, of the numbers involved: the 'illegitimacy' of 20 per cent (Macintyre, 1977a, p. 9) of all conceptions is a minority figure, but so, probably, would 70 per cent be). Again the literature illustrates the 'social problem' approach. Like sociological sexism in general, this could be regarded as a realistic and reasonable response to a set of social practices that define certain kinds of behaviour as abnormal. But sociologists' involvement in practical social problems can act to magnify the stigma. This is particularly true of those approaches that use deviancy theory to 'explain' non-marital sex and reproduction. In Reiss's textbook *The Family System in America* (1971), Part 3 'The Sociology of Marriage and Family Institutions' is followed by Part 4 'Deviant Behaviour in the Family System', which lists divorce, premarital pregnancy, homosexuality and delinquency as the main areas. Such meanings are imposed on all non-marital reproductions regardless of how mothers themselves see them.[4] Macintyre has shown how in many cases the presumption of deviancy does not apply; unmarried mothers-to-be may assume 'acceptance of the natural course of events, continuing the pregnancy to term and keeping the baby' (1977a, p. 177). Taking the focus one step further back, Kristin Luker (1975) has re-examined traditional assumptions of rationality in studies of contraceptive behaviour, which include the idea that single women who engage in sex without contraception are behaving irrationally. She has exposed an alternative reproducer-centred meaning, in which women balance the costs of contraception against the benefits of pregnancy; for some the result is a rational decision not to take the risk of using contraception.

The presumption of deviancy attached to such contexts of reproduction is rarely statistically defined and tends to be moral in character. It is probably for this reason that deviancy explanations often appear to explain so little of the subjective meaning reproductive behaviour has for women themselves. The broader significance of deviancy as the chosen perspective is that deviancy is the opposite face of the coin of socialization. Moving into point (3) above, since the family is socialization's sacred vessel, it is not surprising to find that in sociology reproduction has a particular significance as a theme in the evolution of marriage. Rather than representing individual feminine maturation, as in the psychological approach, reproduction in the sociological scheme signals the maturation of a marriage.

Dividing life into cycles or stages, courtship precedes marriage and the 'honeymoon' period of marriage gives way after an interval to the anticipation of parenthood (Rapoport, 1967;

Rapoport and Rapoport, 1964). Parenthood is important, not by virtue of what it does to husbands and wives as people, but because it transforms a marriage into a family. 'Having' a family is what marriage is all about in commonsense understandings of this institution and in sociological analyses of its aetiology:

> INTERVIEWER: *Why did you want a baby?*
> MAUREEN PATERSON:[5] *Just to make a family, really ... being married and having children go together, really.*

> Another point of great importance is that the family is not rooted in marriage, but marriage is an institution rooted in the family. ... Marriage does not exist in and for itself, but is an institution whose raison d'etre is the foundation and maintenance of the family. ... The central consideration in this establishment of a mating relationship is the having and rearing of children. ... [Fletcher, 1962, pp. 22–5]

Getting married is a prelude: the main drama is having children. Tied to this characterization of marriage are the normative adult roles of men and women for whom parenthood gives differing but equally important credentials: a pass to proper femininity for women, the confirmation of heterosexual identity for men. Meyerowitz and Feldman, in their paper on the 'Transition to Parenthood' sum up these points when they say the crisis of first childbirth is a 'significant transitional point in the maturation of the marital relationship – transition from the dyadic state to a more *mature* and *rewarding* triadic system' (1968, p. 94; my italics). The outcome variable that their interviews with 400 primiparous couples was designed to measure was husbands' and wives' satisfaction with the marital relationship, the emphasis being on sexual satisfaction. More satisfaction was expressed during the pregnancy interview than at five weeks or five months postpartum, though there were discrepancies between husbands' and wives' accounts – women, for example, reported sex as more important in the success of a marriage than husbands, a finding that Meyerowitz and Feldman are unable to handle within the prevailing cultural paradigm; they therefore conclude that when women refer to 'sex' they mean the entire female–male relationship.

As this work shows, the 'rewarding' nature of parenthood is a hypothesis that the actual experience of childbearing and childrearing may confirm or reject. Even within the marital paradigm, it appears that for many people parenthood has the opposite effect, according to the formula time + children = disenchantment (Reiss, 1971, p. 217). Couples without children experience a drop in marital satisfaction with time, but for those with children the descent is more profound.[6] In other words, 'marital' satisfaction and 'family' satisfaction are not the same thing, suggesting a certain cultural conspiracy of silence about what the *realization* of parenthood means.

It was LeMasters who, in 1957, first proposed the idea that marriages are disrupted by childbirth and that the cultural treatment of parenthood as a romantic complex far exceeds the romanticization of marriage (LeMasters, 1957). Reporting a study of urban middle-class couples, LeMasters delineated the problems mothers and fathers experienced with the onset of parenthood. Eighty-three per cent of his respondents described first childbirth as a severe crisis of adjustment. Comparison of this figure with Hobbs' findings (1965) suggests that a parental perception of crisis is less likely shortly after the birth than some months or years later.

In LeMasters' survey, the mothers' adjustment problems (exhaustion, social isolation and restriction, loss of paid work, more housework, guilt over mothering behaviour, worry over the loss of 'feminine' appearance) are conceptualized as posing problems for marital harmony and stability rather than for the women's own health and satisfaction, self-esteem and relational identities. This is the general orientation of the bulk of the marriage and family literature, despite the fact that various studies point to the concentration of problems among wives rather than husbands. Meyerowitz and Feldman's study reported that husbands more often complained about the decline in the quality of the marital relationship than wives, but wives more often than husbands agreed with the statement that 'it is harder to be a parent than I imagined'. Another American excursion into the territory of marital satisfaction found, again with a sample of middle-class families, a much more marked decline in happiness among women than men from the beginning of marriage through the pre-school children stage (Rollins and Feldman, 1970). As Jessie Bernard (1973) has argued, the institution of marriage is not one, but two – his and hers. Any objective reality that is described has to take account of the discrepancy between the two subjective realities of husband and wife, differently socialized as to gender, and differently encumbered with the reproduction and maintenance of family life.

'Transition to parenthood' as a sociological concept has, then, had a limited meaning. Applied narrowly to marriage as the culturally approved context for reproduction, it has been interpreted in a divisively gender-differentiated way. The tasks men and women confront in 'adjusting' as husbands and wives to parenthood have been regarded as different, both explicitly in the framework and conclusions of particular studies, and implicitly in the instruments of inquiry (methodology, interviewing techniques, interview questions) selected for the generation of data. Transition to parenthood has meant transition to the normative roles of mother-at-home and father-at-work, so that the 'adaptational' tasks of each have been seen as different *a priori*, instead of as contingent on individual orientation and circumstances. (Some women, for instance, decide to continue with employment after childbirth, and the 'adjustment' task for them is to this combination of employment and motherhood, rather than to the primacy of motherhood itself.) It follows, therefore, that in sociological studies of the transition to parenthood, *only* those 'adaptational' tasks relevant to the traditional gender-differentiated model constitute the research enterprise (are taken as the research problem).[7]

Alice Rossi discussed some of these biases in a timely paper published in 1968. She revised the focus of research interest from 'how do married couples adjust to parenthood?' to 'what is the effect of parenthood on the adult – particularly on women?' 'in what ways do they change in response to their parental experiences?' By locating the transition to motherhood in the cultural relativity of the Western family system, she is able to translate the conventional sociological interest in parenthood into the more radical and certainly more illuminating question: what does maternity deprive a woman of? Through a review of some of the relevant literature, she concludes that the major effect of maternity is probably 'the negative outcome of a depressed sense of self worth' (1968, p. 34). Exploring the traditional model of 'instrumental' and 'expressive' roles, she suggests that the parental role for women contains a very high proportion of 'instrumental' components. This conclusion is at odds with social and sociological representations of maternity, which both serve to stress the function of maternity as emotional gratification for the 'feminine' character.

The sociological paradigm of reproduction as a marital affair has distanced women from their reproductive experiences just as medical appeals to biology or psychological constructions of femininity have done. I am not suggesting that this has been a deliberate strategy; rather, it seems to have occurred by default, as sociologists have not detached themselves sufficiently from prevailing cultural norms about reproduction. The net effect has certainly been that maternity is annexed to wifehood, a procedure akin to the identification of obstetricians with husbands described in chapter 1. A further consequence has been that the physical dimensions of motherhood become the sexual components of wifehood, and their satisfactions are overcast by the dominance of male heterosexual needs:

> There is a tendency in our society to place special emphasis on the types of female sexual behavior that are of particular pertinence to adult men. Thus women's responses in coitus are singled out for considerable attention, while discussion and research on the psychophysiologic aspects of their other reproductive behavior tends to be muted. [Newton, 1973, p. 77; see also Rossi, 1973]

The sexual meaning and satisfaction to women of birth and lactation are neglected by this stress on the contribution (or otherwise) reproduction makes to the development of marriage. Few people have thought to ask women what it feels like to be pregnant, give birth to a baby and breastfeed, nor has the iconoclastic inquiry been put as to how these experiences compare with heterosexual coitus as sources of physical gratification.

Since the focus of the sociological perspective is on the *advent* of parenthood, most of the literature is concerned only with first childbirth. Subsequent births are usually relegated to a position of minor importance – irrespective of their impact on a woman's identity, satisfactions and life-style.[8]

Sociological literature on the development of the parental role and on parent–child relationships follows this theme through, and displays a lack of concern with the impact of parenthood on women. For just as reproduction is attributed a primary meaning within the marital framework, so motherhood becomes the child's, and not the woman's, experience. Mothers exist to serve children's needs, amorphously but normatively defined, and whatever children become is traced to the character of their mothering.[9] (The intransigence of mothers in allowing themselves to be affected by their children is another story.)

The sociology of the family has often not distinguished between the biological and the social, between having a baby and bringing it up. Furthermore, the language of roles that has dominated sociology permits only role-incumbents to enter the discussion: mother, meaning 'social childrearer', qualifies whereas 'person who gives birth to a baby' does not. Functionalism, the major paradigm of 'normal' sociology (Morgan, 1975, p. 26), has constituted *the* sociological theory of the family, and has been a main target of feminist attack for its conversion of conventional un-wisdom on the subject of femininity to the status of social and theoretical necessity.[10] Women are accorded an expressive responsibility in the family that is functional to its maintenance, child-socialization and the family's role vis-à-vis the economic system. Women manage internal family affairs and regulate intra-family tension so that home is truly a haven (but for men and children only) from the harshness of the outside world. The gender division is presented as unevidenced and self-evident efficiency of fit between economic and personality production.[11] Ultimately, functionalism is addressed to the (suitably misconstrued) 'problem' of the universality of the family and of gender differentiation in human culture, and so tendentiously calls upon biology to explain the patterning of family roles – in the form of 'biosocial' factors (a term used widely by Blood and Wolfe, 1960) or 'the division of organisms into lactating and nonlactating classes' (Zelditch, 1956).

Gender differentiation between parental roles is regarded in the functionalist paradigm as the axis of family structure. For the subjective importance of bearing children is substituted the social convenience of bringing them up.

> . . . the arrival of the first child, in particular, marks not only the beginning of a new generation, but also a radical change

> in social commitments. . . . The incorporation of the position of mother alongside that of wife clearly amounts to a substantial modification in the structure of household relationships. The restrictions of pregnancy, and subsequent recurrent needs of the new infant during the first few months after birth, serve to curtail the mother's activities outside the home. The working wife normally gives up her job, and finds her freedom to engage in leisure activities severely circumscribed. The new mother–child relationship is intensified by the obvious dependency of the infant, and the period . . . is one of considerable emotional involvement for the mother. . . . The development of the relationship between father and child tends to be somewhat detached from the immediate circumstances of gestation, birth and early physical dependency. [Turner, 1969, p. 64]

These thoughts on the impact of childbirth from Christopher Turner's *Family and Kinship in Modern Britain* are a cameo of normative expectations. The epithets 'recurrent needs' and 'considerable emotional involvement' describe the two main social conventions of the mother–child relationship; the domestic diagram is functionalist and non-empirical. Absent or peripheral fathers maintain the national economy. Ever-present and ever-nurturant mothers make up for missing fathers. The arrangement suits everyone – which is why such statements never refer to the evidence of female unease with domesticity, not to mention the strains of ever-provident masculinity and the profound vulnerability of little children to parental resentment and violence.[12]

Through the encapsulation of reproduction within the social domestic structure, sociology thus separates women from the personal meaning of reproduction. By its confusion of the unique female capacity to give birth with the cultural preference for maternal childrearing, sociological paradigms demarcate reproduction as a *social* activity in contrast to those of medicine and psychology. But they do so by a deceit, a faulty syllogism:

> only women can give birth
> only women look after children
> therefore only women can look after children

– and by further deduction, if we study women in their

child-socializing roles, we will also be studying what it means to them to give birth. It is not necessary to say that these arguments do no more than bolster an image of gender relations in post-capitalist society. The point is not what biological basis the functionalist paradigm of gender can be contended to have, but the depth of the influence it has exerted on the whole field of marriage and family sociology, and the misrepresentations it has created of the biology of motherhood.

A SOCIOLOGY OF REPRODUCTION?

Opposing this general sociological consensus about maternity, one sub-area does take reproductive experiences as valid subject matter: the infant but thriving discipline of medical sociology. In Britain the medical sociology group is the largest study group within the British Sociological Association. At the medical sociology conference in 1975, a separate study group, 'The Sociology of Human Reproduction', was set up.

Medical sociology as it has developed in the last thirty years has represented medicine as a control agency akin to education or religion; it has undermined medicine's stance of value-neutrality, and has thus opened its territory to sociological inquiry. The initial development of medical sociology in Britain, as Stacey and Homans (1978) show in a recent review of its origins and prospects, was in response to practical rather than theoretical concerns. The medical specialty of social medicine in the post-war years expounded on the importance of social factors in disease, and this emphasis became increasingly relevant as the balance between acute and chronic illness has shifted: multicausal models relevant to explanations of chronic illness entail the input of social factors. Administrators and patients have recognized the importance of sociological variables, especially that of patients' attitudes. The influence of feminist critiques of health care has been important, and these have both stemmed from, and articulated, the special stringency with which medicine manages women. Obstetrics and gynaecology have received a disproportionate share of medical sociologists' attention, and the medical colonization of reproductive care has ceased to be a taken-for-granted aspect of relations between medicine and society and become instead an area meriting critical evaluation.

Until this recent expansion of interest, the main theoretical attraction of reproduction to sociologists was the relationship between pregnancy and illness as distinct social roles. The historical antecedent of this concern was Parsons' account of illness as constituting a distinct social position, a role with its own rights and obligations (1963; 1964). Parsons was, in fact, the first sociological theorist to recognize the importance of medicine for society as a whole. He drew attention to illness as a form of deviance and to the sick role as a mechanism of social control. As defined by him, the two main rights of the 'sick role' are exemption from normal social-role obligations and from responsibility for one's own state: the two corresponding obligations are a motivation to get well as soon as possible and a duty to seek technically competent help and to cooperate with medical authority. In the Parsonian functionalist view, the object of this social phasing of illness is to ensure that ill people get better and that not too many people define themselves as ill at the same time.

Since Parsons set out these ideas, sociologists have challenged most of them, pointing out their heuristic base (see, for example, Stimson and Webb, 1975; Davis and Horobin, 1977). As a tributary of this debate, various investigators devoted themselves to the notion that pregnancy is particularly 'interesting' because it challenges the customary parameters of health and illness. Its medicalization has provoked the paradox of large numbers of healthy people being subjected to medical control: 'The state of pregnancy is intriguing to sociologists precisely because the attached role is so ill-defined' (McKinlay, 1972, p. 569). As McKinlay observes, pregnancy is not equivalent to 'ordinary' illness – pregnant women are not, for example, generally exempted from their normal social-role obligations, and on the whole the 'curing' of pregnancy is not their, nor their doctors' aim. While it may not be possible to describe a particular and unambiguous pregnancy 'role' that mothers-to-be perform, there is, on the other hand, clearly *something* special about pregnancy.

This theoretical concern provided a genus of somewhat barren accounts of just where childbearing may be considered to stand in relation to illness, and has stimulated limited empirical investigations of the conditions under which pregnancy most resembles, or most fails to resemble, other reasons for receiving medical treatment. William Rosengren, who has pursued this line of investigation in the United States, has produced various conclusions relating to the sick role hypothesis: that socially mobile women are more sick role oriented during pregnancy than others (1961a); that sick role oriented women have longer labours than other women (1961b); that middle-class women have higher sick role expectations in pregnancy than lower class women (1962a); that women who regard pregnancy as an illness tend to express highly 'retaliatory' attitudes to childrearing (1962b). Rosengren's findings are unimpressive, both because they propose what could equally well be spurious connections (other variables could account both for sick role attitudes and so-called retaliatory attitudes to childrearing, for example) and because the exercise of producing the data entails the imposition of certain prejudged values. The general tenor of Rosengren's work imputes an unfortunate moral accountability to women, for they are seen as potentially causing their own reproductive difficulties by maintaining a false image of themselves – as ill rather than well. Moreover, forcing a match between the attitudes of childbearing women and some abstract (male-devised) theoretical paradigm is not likely to be an enlightening exercise.

A thorough survey by Illsley in 1967 of 'The Sociological Study of Reproduction and Its Outcome' reveals the (then) general nature of the medical sociologist's interest in reproduction. Illsley bemoans the lack of concern shown by sociologists about the influence of social conditions on the course of pregnancy, labour and delivery. He contends that 'The events of reproduction are explicable only against a knowledge of the woman's life experience'. He divides his review into five sections: (1) the influence of general social factors on reproductive outcome; (2) the effect of biological variables (e.g. maternal health) on social factors; (3) the relationship between particular factors (e.g. smoking, diet) and reproductive outcome; (4) the interaction between social and biological influences; (5) the relevance of social differences in reproduction on foetal and child health.

In this kind of endeavour, the sociologist regards herself/

himself as a kind of medical statistician, dealing in a one-sided way with the impact of social facts on reproductive outcome. The definition of outcome is exclusively medical, however. The paradigm is borrowed from the medical model, so that the assessment of outcome is carried out in terms of mortality and physical morbidity rates, or in terms of other clinical parameters. The sociologist's contribution here is not to the description, understanding or analysis of women's reproductive experiences, but rather to a limited extension of the medical model, a more elastic conception of the variables that can influence the biological outcome of maternity.

To point out these limitations of the epidemiological approach is not to criticize its practitioners, but rather to observe how far medical sociology has moved from this position in the period since Illsley wrote. While Illsley entitled his review 'The Sociological Study of Reproduction and Its Outcome', Sally Macintyre, surveying sociological research in this field more recently (1977b), entitled hers 'The Management of Childbirth: Review of Sociological Research Issues'. The juxtaposition of these two titles suggests the nature of the transformation in sociological interest in the intervening decade: the medical model, and medical paradigms of women, from being uncritically embedded in the sociological enterprise, have been extracted from it to become objects of study in themselves.

Macintyre distinguishes four types of sociological approach to the management of childbirth. The first is *historical/professional*, a perspective in which the managers and practitioners of childbirth are studied in a historical context, using a sociology of science, social policy or sociology of professions framework. Second, there is the *anthropological* approach, which focuses on the relation between the management of childbirth and prevailing belief systems in different cultures. Third, *patient-oriented* studies articulate the perspective of the consumers/users of the maternity services. Fourth, studies of *patient–services interaction* provide a synthesis of approaches (1) and (3) by examining the interplay between service-providers and service-users.

In the last five years there has been an expansion of studies using all four of these approaches. Renewed efforts to combine historical and sociological perspectives are producing some interesting work on the evolution of obstetrics and its ideological charter of womanhood. Richard and Dorothy Wertz (1977) have examined the evolution of modern technological childbirth in the American setting and have accounted for its emphasis on medical intervention in terms of an especially strong tradition of faith in the benefits of practical science. Only against such a background, they argue, could such a collusion between doctors and reproducers in the portrayal of birth as pathology have taken place. In Britain, Margaret Versluysen (1977) has traced the medical colonization of childbirth back to the creation of the first lying-in hospitals in London in the mid-eighteenth century; she points out that no satisfactory explanation for the establishment of these institutions exists. She provides an analysis whereby the rise of hospital midwifery practice is interpreted as a device used by men-midwives to gain ascendancy over their female colleagues, thereby instituting the convention of doctor control versus client control in reproductive care. She shows how male medical practice in obstetric cases in the eighteenth century contravened the prevailing convention of minimal body contact between doctor and patient and was facilitated in a class-divided institutional setting. Working-class women formed the bulk of hospital maternity patients in Britain through the eighteenth and nineteenth centuries, and the hierarchical control medical men were able to exercise over their bodies mapped out the female reproductive organs as male territory. Such a strategy was intrinsic to the beginnings, and thus to the success, of male reproductive medicine.

Exposing the values of one's own culture is perhaps easier for a historical than a contemporary investigator, since distance from these values brings them more sharply into focus. The same could be said of anthropological accounts of reproduction. These have provided a very fertile field indeed for expositions of women as maternity cases: 'Some societies define childbearing as ultimately dangerous, and the Aztecs saw the heavens red with the blood of men who died in battle and that of women who died in childbirth', said Margaret Mead in one of the earliest accounts of the differential cultural phasing of childbirth.

> Whether childbed is seen as a situation in which one risks death, or one out of which one acquires a baby, or social status, or a right to heaven, is not a matter of the actual statistics of maternal mortality, but of the view that a society takes of childbearing. Any argument about women's instinctive maternal behaviour which insists that in this one respect a biological substratum is stronger than every other learning experience that a female child faces, from birth on, must reckon with this great variety in the handling of childbirth. [Mead, 1962, p. 222]

Several stimulating accounts of cross-cultural variation in the management of reproduction now exist.[13] It is interesting to note that the prototype in this field was not in fact a sociological treatise, but a volume written in 1883 by Engelmann, an enlightened and inquiring obstetrician, entitled *Labor Among Primitive Peoples* and subtitled 'showing the development of the obstetric science of today from the natural and instinctive customs of all races, civilised and savage, past and present'. Engelmann contended that nineteenth-century obstetricians had a lot to learn from the customs of non-medicalized childbirth, most importantly the efficacy of the vertical delivery position – standing, squatting, kneeling – in ensuring 'natural' labour:

> I deem it a great mistake that we in this age of culture, should follow custom and fashion so completely to the exclusion of reason and instinct, in a mechanical act which so nearly concerns our animal nature as the delivery of the pregnant female. If we wish to obtain any idea of the natural position, we must look to the woman who is governed by instinct, not by prudery. . . . [Engelmann, 1883, p. 55]

Engelmann was, of course, quite right in this assessment of 'prudery' as representing a cultural constraint on unfettered reproduction; to the Victorian doctor it must have seemed a nuisance in more ways than one. The idea that women giving birth are closer to (animal) nature is a familiar one, and was, indeed, propagated by the founders of the modern 'natural childbirth' movement.[14]

Citing Engelmann, a British paediatrician in the pages of the *Lancet* in 1976 was unable to attract any serious medical attention to the view that cross-cultural data can be a helpful corrective to the limitations of some current obstetric practices (Dunn, 1976). Critics of the maternity services recognize the usefulness of the anthropological perspective in demonstrating the 'irrationality' of current obstetric techniques. 'The Cultural Warping of Childbirth', a report published in 1972 by Doris Haire, Co-President of the International Childbirth Education Association, and often cited by critics of contemporary maternity care, draws on international data and includes mention of birth practices in some non-industrialized cultures. Various recent medical volumes on reproductive care do include chapters on cross-cultural reproductive care systems, though how much these are read by doctors is an unanswered question. One instance of sustained cross-cultural analysis is Niles and Michael Newton's 'Childbirth in Cross-Cultural Perspective' in a volume entitled *Modern Perspectives in Psycho-Obstetrics*. The Newtons' piece treats American obstetric customs as of equal status with those of non-industrialized cultures, and argues that 'In learning how others have done it, it is possible to get new insight into current patterns, their possible origins and interactions' (Newton and Newton, 1972, p. 169). The Newtons are critical of American birth practices, pointing out that they allow women little achievement satisfaction. While the Ila of Northern Rhodesia, and many other peoples, praise, congratulate and thank the woman who has given birth for her success, in America 'The obstetrician says, "I delivered Mrs Jones" using the active voice. . . . The husband and family are more likely to thank the obstetrician for the delivery of the baby than to thank the wife for giving birth' (p. 155).

Periodically, the cross-cultural literature gives rise to the suggestion that a male-supremacist ideology has motivated modern patterns of reproductive care and modern medical paradigms of women as mothers. Mead (1962) makes this suggestion, as does the psychoanalyst Peter Lomas in a consideration of 'Ritualistic Elements in the Management of Childbirth' (1966), and Niles Newton has made various pointed comments about the distortion of female achievement in childbirth. Addressing the Third International Congress of Psychosomatic Medicine in Obstetrics and Gynaecology in London in 1971, she said (to a predominantly male audience):

> If you wish to understand the psychologic impact of pubic hair shaving during labour, may I suggest that next time you face some special extra hurdle in your life – like giving a speech at a medical society meeting – you take time off to have your pubic hair shaved off. You will learn that it is distracting and irritating and may bring a feeling of humiliation. Furthermore, it itches when the hair grows... [Newton, 1972, p. 17]

But it is in the third and fourth of Macintyre's categories – patient-oriented studies and patient–services interaction – that there has been the greatest growth of work. Although apparently informed by a less paradigmatic approach to the question of what reproduction means to women, studies in these categories range from the clearly programmatic to the straightforwardly descriptive. Accounts of patient–services interaction are less likely than others to be programmatic, because of their declared concern with both sides of the picture. Nevertheless, medical typifications of women as maternity cases may be pervasive in the investigator's account,[15] perhaps reflecting a tendency for sociological researchers to be drawn into an identification with the medical enterprise. Nancy Stoller Shaw's *Forced Labor* (1974), a study of maternity care in five institutional settings in the United States, is, as far as I know, the only published account, based on systematic participant observation, of staff–patient interaction in maternity care that does not resort to typifications. Shaw charts the powerlessness of maternity patients within the hospital system, showing how the bureaucratization of medical care and enforced deference to medical authority serve to interpose a dehumanizing dependence as a condition for the 'giving' of birth.

Macintyre's research on gynaecological work is not concerned with maternity care specifically, but has made a valuable contribution in articulating the various presumptions about women and reproduction that lie behind gynaecological decisions (1976a, b). She has drawn attention to the coexistence of two potentially contradictory tasks within gynaecology – the promotion and the prevention of childbirth – and to the techniques that minimize conflict between these in clinical decision-making. These techniques include the spatial/organizational separation of gynaecology and maternity work. There is also appeal to various typifications of women in which the term 'normal' is prescriptive rather than statistical. The effect of these is to justify marital rather than extra-marital reproduction, and to propose the notion that proper femininity equals a desire for children but precludes much interest in the means of acquiring them, i.e. sexuality. Sexuality itself – in the doctor–patient encounter – has contributed another, more esoteric, theme in the sociology of reproduction. Joan Emerson (1970), devoting herself to the task of describing constructions of reality in gynaecological examinations, provides an account of how medical definitions of a man's intrusion into a woman's vagina are sustained in the face of counter-themes. Modes of desexualizing the vaginal examination are also discussed by James Henslin and Mae Biggs (1971), who state the doctor's dilemma as the need to convert the sacred to the profane – to render the vagina violable, not inviolate.

There are also individual accounts, legitimated by the blossoming status of ethnomethodological inquiry within sociology, in which female sociologists spell out the nature of their own encounters with reproductive medicine (Hart, 1977; Comaroff, 1977). These offer important insights into the experience of reproductive management and the effect of paradigmatic conflicts between doctor and patient, because they portray the subjective experiences of the reproducer as valid data. Yet such accounts have to be based on the ultimately fragile equation between sociologist and social actor roles. A personal predicament can lead to valuable sociological insight, but it does not necessarily justify sociological generalization; it is no substitute for the collective predicament, the recounting of those experiences that groups of women hold in common.[16]

Patient-oriented studies vary in the extent to which they may propose or support special notions of womanhood. Studies of antenatal care include some, such as those by McKinlay (1970), Collver (1967) and Donabedian (1961), that are concerned to elucidate the reason for late antenatal booking. The assumption is that late take-up of medical care is medically bad and therefore a morally irresponsible act on the part of women, who must be re-motivated to behave more in accordance with the medical model.[17] (That this is not far from the equation in psychological studies between such behaviour and rejection of the feminine role is clearly evident.) On the other hand, there are surveys of patient attitudes that exhibit no such moral stand, taking as their brief the simple elucidation and measurement of responses to medical maternity care.[18] (The design of such studies may, of course, make it more or less difficult for patients' views to be represented. A yes/no choice does not allow for the inclusion of complex and/or radical responses to the whole cultural phasing of maternity care.) A few studies have focused in a broader way on the meaning of maternity to women – for example Jane Hubert's study of thirty-four working-class women in South London (1974). Hubert's data demonstrate the clash between the medical paradigm and women's own attitudes to reproduction, and show how the cultural presentation of childbearing and childrearing acts against a realistic anticipation of these.

It is clear from this that what the sociology of reproduction has lacked to date is a repertoire of first-hand accounts. Until very recently, the reproducers themselves have been represented merely as statistics and/or they have been manipulated to fit the contours of a largely ungrounded theory. This has also been the case in medicine and psychology, where preformed paradigms of women as maternity cases have been all-pervasive in the selection, methodology and analysis of research studies, and where, in obstetric medicine especially, a paradigmatic 'feminine' representation of women has been crucial to the whole evolution of the specialism.

In sociology the feminine paradigm is given yet another twist, and the reproductive activity of women is yoked to the axis of marriage and family relations. In all three fields, it seems that the general cultural idealization of femininity and maternity has been projected wholesale into the scientific representation of reproduction. (This point is returned to in chapter 11.) Science has not been 'scientific', and it seems that we have not yet found a way to reconcile the nature of childbirth and the representation of women in culture. It is perhaps for this reason that the medical paradigm – the medical management of reproduction – has only lately come to be conceptualized as a potential influence on the meaning of reproduction and maternity to women themselves. For this is to study culture in its effects on nature; and it is the concealed equation of women's perspectives on reproduction with the lowest common denominator of nature that has constituted the weakness of much scientific work. Not coincidentally, all the areas I have discussed – obstetrics and gynaecology, the psychology of women and sex differences, medical sociology and the sociology of the family and marriage – have had to contend with the stigma of low status. Within their disciplines, these specialisms are not highly evaluated. Women's inferiority contaminates, and is not diminished by the covert replication of cultural stereotypes in the name and guise of 'science'.

PART II

The Subjective Logic of Reproduction

Beyond the presumptions of knowledge and value-neutrality that medical and social science project, lies unveiled a repertoire of patronizing moral precepts about women's nature; but the nature of women must also be described by women themselves. First-hand accounts substitute a subjective logic for the pretentious dicta of 'science'. A presentation of this alternative perspective occupies the next six chapters, which describe a study of a group of women having their first babies in 1975–6. Beginning with the logistics of the research process, and ending with some speculations on the psychology of subordinate groups, this section proposes a new way of understanding women's reactions to childbirth. Having a baby is essentially a kind of social transition, one source and cause of life change. The key that unlocks the mystery of women's feelings after childbirth is to be found in human beings' responses to such life change. Tracing the connections between women's reactions to birth and their social circumstances in this way suggests a new interpretation of the manner in which women become either victors over or victims of their childbirth experiences.

CHAPTER 4

Researching the Transition to Motherhood

Women's maternal role has profound effects on women's lives, on ideology about women, on the reproduction of masculinity and sexual inequality, and on the reproduction of particular forms of labor power. . . . Most sociological theorists have either ignored or taken as unproblematic this sphere of social reproduction. . . . [Chodorow, 1978, pp. 11–12]

How 'normal' women experience childbearing has, as we saw in the previous section, rarely been identified as a legitimate research area in either medical or social science fields. *A priori* judgements of this experience have been imposed through adoption of a particular paradigm of women's 'nature'. This has served to confirm researchers' opinions instead of allowing those of the reproducers themselves to be heard. The research that is reported in the next seven chapters was designed as a corrective to this approach. It takes the eliciting of women's own accounts of reproduction as the chief research goal, and attempts to allow the viewpoints expressed in these accounts to shape any interpretative theories generated as a research 'product'. The accounts themselves are published separately – as the ethnography of *Becoming A Mother* (Oakley, 1979b). Taking the words of the reproducers themselves as the best descriptions available, this book charts the passage to motherhood from conception to five months postpartum, identifying the key characteristics of each phase. *Women Confined* is geared to the 'factorial' analysis of this process: in this chapter I shall briefly describe the research plan and methods; in the next six I present and discuss the main findings.

BASIC IDEAS

Out of a previous research project on housewives' attitudes to housework (Oakley, 1974b), I derived the idea that the social construction of adult femininity has certain crucial stages, among which becoming a mother is probably the most important. While women's identification with, and commitment to, the housewife role can be explored and their attitudes to, and satisfaction with, housework assessed, the core of the female tie to the home is not housework but children. Through the 'love' women feel for their children, the contingent necessity of domesticity becomes absolute, and rejection of the label 'housewife' is emotionally difficult. ('Love' is of course a problematic but nonetheless – or therefore – appropriate designation of the relationship's character.) The welding of women to the home through their children must begin with the birth of the first child, so it is logical that this should be the starting-point for any investigation of the hidden charter of motherhood.

In contemporary industrial society, parenthood is experienced by most people. Official statistics provide no figure for the proportion of the population who become parents at least once, but Busfield and Paddon in 1977 placed the figure at around 80 per cent (1977, p. 133). Given the tendency towards smaller families, proportionately more experiences of parenthood will be first-time ones: in 1976 in Britain 42 per cent of all legitimate births in first marriages were first babies (OPCS, 1978); the total figure, which would include all marriages and illegitimate maternities, is probably nearer 50 per cent. This, then, is the statistical base for the argument that the transition to motherhood is a key phase in most women's lives.

There were various other important reasons for taking first-time parenthood as a problematic area for women today (and also, in different ways, for men, though this was not a main research focus). In the first place, the *decline in family size* and increase in geographical mobility that have marked family life in the last hundred years have resulted in the restriction of most close adult–child contact to the nuclear family. Women, when they become mothers now, have rarely experienced the intimacy with small children and babies that counted as an apprenticeship for motherhood in past female generations. Looking after one's own child is therefore much more of an unknown quantity than it used to be, and first-time motherhood has become a major career transition for many women. And because motherhood is based in the nuclear family, it tends to be a relatively isolated experience – both emotionally and practically. This is a common source of personal difficulty.

Second, the structural relationship between *domesticity and work* is increasingly felt as a strain by many people in the modern industrialized world. Women's lives exemplify this competition of interests in a chronically disjunctive way. Who should look after the children is the generic issue; other conflicts stem from this. The alternatives are not only male versus female childrearing, but isolation versus cooperation, intrafamily or inter-family childcare, social versus individual responsibility. These issues are very problematic in all so-called developed cultures, as are those to do with the depth and nature of people's commitment to employment work. Women are 'carriers' of this cultural crisis since in becoming biological mothers and in retaining their social value as workers they perpetually manifest and experience the conflict of interest between production and reproduction.

The third reason for regarding the transition to motherhood as especially problematic lies in the *social management of reproduction* itself. Chapter 1 charted the way in which, in the twentieth century, reproduction has been transformed by its definition as a medical phenomenon. The process of medicalization has accelerated particularly in the last ten to fifteen years, as pharmacological and technological innovation has been introduced into obstetric work on the untested assumption that more means better. Quite apart from the impact such methods have on accepted medical indices of mortality and physical morbidity, there is the question of how medicalized reproduction affects the reproducers themselves. The contribution of medical practice to stress is one suggestion

(Grimm, 1967, p. 4). But the possibility is that the medicalization of reproduction has changed the subjective experience of reproduction altogether, making dependence on others instead of dependence on self a condition of the achievement of motherhood. What impact this may have on women's experiences of motherhood, on children's experiences of being mothered and on family and social life in general is an urgent question. Such a question cannot be answered in a historical framework because comparable historical data do not exist: we do not know how random samples of women felt about reproduction and its management in 1900 or 1600. But this does not rule out the validity of more specific inquiries. To ask what the experience of first reproduction is like in the early 1970s is one such inquiry. It is based on the supposition that although the experience of reproduction and its management must be cumulative, the first such experience may well be the most memorable and influential of all.

These are the particular reasons why I have singled out first childbirth. But they do not mean that what follows is applicable only to women having their first babies. The element of 'shock' and the social transition experience may be enhanced with first childbirth as opposed to others, but much of what is said about the impact of medical management and social factors on mothers' feelings applies equally to all maternities.

METHODS

SELECTING A SAMPLE

A sample of women booked for hospital delivery was interviewed twice in pregnancy and twice in the early postnatal months about social and medical aspects of the transition to motherhood. The women's names were chosen from first bookings at a London hospital antenatal clinic between May and July 1975 according to the following criteria: age between eighteen and thirty-one; married or cohabiting with the child's father; no previous fullterm pregnancies or second/third trimester spontaneous abortions or terminations; not booking in after 25 weeks pregnant; Irish-born, British-born or North American-born; living in certain postal districts within a restricted radius of the hospital. The object of using these criteria was to obtain a group of women without pronounced medical problems (such as might be expected for example in very young mothers or in those in their late 30s/early 40s, or in women booking in for antenatal care during the last trimester of pregnancy); to look at first-time motherhood in a sample of women having their first babies at a nationally typical age (the average age of the sample women at first interview was just under twenty-six years and the average age for first birth in Britain in 1975 was 24.6 years[1] – OPCS, 1975); to ensure a degree of cultural homogeneity in reproductive attitudes (which would be disturbed by the inclusion of ethnic minorities, for instance – see Kitzinger, 1978); to exclude those women who had already experienced the 'birth' of a child (thus late miscarriage but not early miscarriage was excluded on the assumption that, although reactions to early miscarriage may be profound, they will probably not include the feeling of having given birth to a child); to reduce the over-representation of the middle classes in the population of the sample hospital by restricting the sample to its socially mixed catchment area; and to be able to focus on the impact of motherhood on the female–male couple relationship.

This last point needs some explanation, in view of my earlier criticisms of sociologists' preoccupations with married women as research subjects. One of the areas I wanted to look at was how the birth of a baby affects the relationship between its parents. For the majority of women having babies this is an important consideration, though it does not necessarily involve marriage per se. Moreover, such a research focus does not have to entail the assumption that childbirth represents the maturity or normalcy of a marriage, nor does it have to involve the assumption that marital 'adjustment' is the most important way of measuring women's satisfaction with parenthood. The collection and analysis of data on 'domestic politics' (see Oakley, 1979b, ch. 9) in the present study reject these traditional notions. But one constraint the goal of looking at parental relationships did impose was that all the women should be living with the fathers of their children during the research project; only in this way could the day-to-day effect of parenthood be examined.

Eighty-six names were collected from the antenatal clinic records and eighty-two of these individuals were contacted; the other four could not be traced. Sixty-six women were interviewed initially; the reasons why sixteen of the contacts were not interviewed are shown in Table 4.1. The sample size fell

TABLE 4.1 *Selection of the initial sample*

	No.
Completed first interviews	66
Definite refusal	2
Other refusal*	4
Not traced	3
Agreed, but aborted before interview	7
Agreed, but appointment not kept†	4
Total	86

* These women agreed to the interview in principle, but had social problems that complicated their inclusion.
† On four occasions.

from sixty-six at interview 1 to fifty-six at interviews 2 and 3 and fifty-five at interview 4. This attrition had been allowed for in the design, a final sample of around fifty being the goal. Two interviewees miscarried shortly after the first interview, two had intrauterine deaths at about twenty-six weeks; one had a premature birth at another hospital; two went to live abroad; two moved out of London and booked beds in hospitals elsewhere and one was reluctant to be re-interviewed due to marital problems. Because the focus of the research was on becoming a mother those women who miscarried or experienced intrauterine deaths were not re-interviewed – although they were contacted and encouraged to talk about their experiences if they wanted to. Those women who delivered at other hospitals were also excluded from re-interview since the object of the research was not to compare medical experiences in different hospitals but to look at the possible connection between these experiences and outcome in a group encountering similar types of medicalization. The drop from fifty-six at interview 3 to fifty-five at interview 4 is accounted for by the return of one Irish woman to live in Ireland.

The marital and reproductive status and country of origin of the final sample of fifty-five is shown in Table 4.2, and their social class distribution in terms of the Registrar-General's occupational categories in Table 4.3. According to partner's[2] occupation, 66 per cent of the sample were middle class; according to the interviewee's own, 93 per cent were. This

TABLE 4.2 *Some sample characteristics*

Characteristic	*No.*	(%)
Marital status:		
At interview 1: married	48	(87)
cohabiting	7	(13)
At interview 4: married	51	(93)
cohabiting	4	(7)
Reproductive status:		
No previous pregnancy	49	(89)
Previous early miscarriage	2	(4)
Previous termination	4	(7)
Country of origin:		
Britain	46	(84)
Ireland	5	(9)
North America	4	(7)

$N = 55$.

TABLE 4.3 *Social class*

*Social class**		*Interviewee*		*Partner*	
		No.	(%)	*No.*	(%)
I	Professional and	2	(4)	13	(24)
II	managerial	15	(27)	13	(24)
III	Skilled non-manual	34	(62)	10	(18)
III	Skilled manual	0	(0)	15	(27)
IV	Semi-skilled	4	(7)	3	(6)
V	Unskilled	0	(0)	1	(2)
Total		55	(100)	55	(100)

* Based on previous occupation in the case of unemployed people.

'middle-classness' in the case of women's occupational classification is accounted for largely by the concentration of their work in social class III non-manual occupations: this is a pronounced feature of occupational gender differentiation in the industrial world generally. Examples of class III non-manual occupations are shop assistant, typist/secretary, clerk, telephonist and receptionist: 25 (46 per cent) of the present sample of women held jobs in these five particular categories. Social class (in the Registrar-General's sense) was not used as a criterion for selecting the sample because of the difficulty that as a sociological variable it is almost certainly an epiphenomenon of other more basic modes of social and economic differentiation. It is a 'blunderbuss' rather than a 'carefully calibrated instrument' (Stacey, 1976, p. 3). Selecting a sample according to social class presupposes that in the analysis of data this relatively crude index will turn out to be an (often the most) important factor. This may pre-empt the central question, which is not what factors are associated with social class differences, but what does the term itself 'measure' with respect to the quality of people's lives? The relevance of this alternative formulation is especially clear in the case of women, between whom occupational social class differentiates much less than it does in the case of men, and for whom the tradition of categorization by husband rather than by self can be seen as participation in the cultural typification of women that relegates them to a second-hand status (Hutton, 1974).

THE INTERVIEWING

The women whose names were selected from the hospital antenatal records were contacted (in most cases personally, in a few by telephone), told about the research and invited to participate. It was made clear that although the names had been drawn from the hospital medical record, the research itself had no connection with the hospital. All the interviews except one were done in the women's own homes; the exception was the last interview with a woman whose partner was unemployed and who was having quite severe difficulties in her relationship with him. Out of the total of 233 interviews, I did 178 and a research assistant did 55 – a division of labour accounted for by the sheer arithmetic of the overall interviewing load. The first interview was carried out as soon after hospital booking as possible – at what turned out to be an average time of twenty-six weeks before delivery (range thirty-two weeks to fifteen weeks); the second was planned to take place a few weeks before the birth and the average time was in fact six weeks before (range nine weeks to one week). The two postnatal interviews were spaced at five weeks (range nine weeks to four weeks) and twenty weeks (range twenty-seven weeks to seventeen weeks). Ending the research at five months postpartum was in one sense arbitrary (limitation of funds, etc.), but was also selected deliberately to represent the end of the transition to motherhood proper: a time when the early 'settling down' period with the baby was over and the sameness of the daily routines of motherhood had established itself. At the opposite end of the process, the idea of interviewing women as soon as possible after the confirmation of pregnancy was to elicit pre-pregnancy and early pregnancy attitudes, given that attitudes during pregnancy to many factors, for example the baby and the labour itself, are liable to change quite considerably. In the event, interviewing after hospital booking was the earliest date that was technically feasible. The time of interview 2 was chosen to occur during a period when most women would have given up employment and would be actively preparing in a number of ways for the baby; that of interview 3 at five weeks postpartum was planned as a time when interviewees would remember the birth and early postnatal days with clarity, yet would not be too exhausted to tolerate the intrusion of an interview.

All the interviews were tape-recorded and generated a round total of 546 hours of material. The average length of the first and fourth interviews was 2.4 hours each, that of interview 2, 2.1 hours and of interview 3, 2.5 hours. The interviews themselves were a mixture of structured, loosely structured and unstructured 'guides' to conversation. At certain points what was asked for was an account by the interviewee of a particular experience – for instance, her first attendance at the antenatal clinic, the labour and delivery, or daily life as a mother five months after the birth; at other points a question about, for example, her partner's reactions to pregnancy or encounters at antenatal classes could be phrased in various unspecified ways;

sometimes the interviewee was required to answer a set question, for instance 'would you say that becoming a mother has been an easy experience for you or a difficult one?', or 'do you feel you have enough time to yourself these days?' The purpose of these set questions might be to elicit either information or attitudes but they were also used as a way of getting the interviewee to sum up her own experience.

Aside from the use of such direct questions, each interview was standardized in the sense that specific areas to be covered were listed in the schedule as proper topics of conversation between interviewer and interviewee. These were:

Interview 1

A Background data
B The pregnancy
C First medical consultations
D Understanding of medical terms/procedures
E Present physical and emotional state
F The marital relationship
G Significant others
H Gender role socialization
I Sources of knowledge about motherhood
J Expectations of pregnancy and labour
K Future employment plans/feminine role ideology

Interview 2

A Present physical and emotional state
B Medical consultations since interview 1
C Parentcraft/childbirth preparation classes
D Giving up employment
E Feelings about pregnancy/expectations of baby
F Expectations/mental rehearsal of labour
G Expectations post-delivery and homecoming
H The marital relationship

Interview 3

A The baby
B Account of labour and delivery and prior medical consultations
C Labour and delivery: general
D Rest of hospital stay
E Feeding

F Homecoming
G Daily routine, attitudes to babycare and motherhood
H Present physical and emotional state
I The marital relationship

Interview 4

A Introductory
B Daily routine
C Attitudes to babycare/relationship with baby
D General feelings about present life situation
E The marital relationship
E Present physical and emotional state
G Medical consultations since last interview/ understanding of medical terms
H Expectations and reality

OTHER DATA SOURCES

In addition to the material gathered by interviewing women experiencing the transition to motherhood, three other sources were used to build up a picture of the medical side of motherhood:

(1) the interviewees' hospital medical notes, which were read in full at the end of their patient careers;
(2) observation of a small sub-sample (6) of the births;
(3) extensive observation of obstetric work in the 'research' hospital.

There were two reasons for the first exercise: to obtain more detailed information about medical procedures than interviewees were able to give (for example about the type of instrumental delivery carried out), and to look at possible discrepancies between the medical care givers' and receivers' perspectives. Sometimes this involved factual discrepancy (concerning, for example, the length of labour) and sometimes the typification of the latter by the former ('pleasant caucasian', 'unsuitable for breastfeeding', 'rather emotional', and so forth). Attending the births was seen as important because the delivery of the child is the moment of becoming a mother. Moreover, events and behaviour in the delivery room are known to be important in terms of the mother's later 'adaptation' to motherhood (Macfarlane, 1977, Chapters 5–7).

The third supplementary source of data produced a very much larger body of data than the first two, and amounted to a research project on its own. For a period of about nine months, I carried out regular observations of obstetric work in the research hospital. The result was tape-recordings of well- and ill-baby clinics, recordings and notes on parentcraft classes run by the hospital, systematic notes on interaction between staff and patients on the labour ward and notes on 'ward rounds'. Most time was spent in the outpatients' antenatal clinic where I attended ninety clinic sessions covering 906 separate doctor–patient consultations: these were written up in note form. The original reason for observing staff and patients in this way was to produce some basic information about the character of medical maternity work, which could be used to design those parts of the interview schedules concerning perceptions of medical treatment. Once this was accomplished, the place I had earned in the hospital as 'resident' sociologist seemed to justify the expenditure of further time there, since, as anyone who has researched the medical field will know, the effort of gaining medical trust tends to be rewarded in the long, but rarely the short, run by the opening of further doors and the offering of unexpected confidences. Given the then (1974) paucity of material on communication between medical staff and patients, this seemed too good an opportunity to miss.

None of this observational work covered the same population of patients as did the interviewing; it was done before the interviewing started so as to avoid a possible confusion in interviewees' perceptions of the interviewer as a person (a) carrying out a university research project and (b) seen to be working in the hospital. In this way and in its general contribution to a picture of medical maternity work in the 1970s the observational data act as a background for the interview data, placing it within a broader context of a much larger patient population.

MODES OF ANALYSIS

Listening to the tapes, transcribing them or having them transcribed, and developing and applying rating and other summary scales to the mass of material this produced, were the main techniques used to 'make sense' of the data – in the sense of establishing connections between them and the basic ideas and hypotheses that generated the research project in the first place. A profile of each respondent was written onto a series of index cards divided by topic: social class, antenatal preparation, employment, fertility and contraception and so forth. These cards included simple data (number of childbirth preparation classes attended, whether the husband was present at the birth, and so on) as well as rating scales (of, for example, satisfaction with delivery care, attitudes to experts, the marital role relationship). Analysis of the possible association between variables was done directly from these cards using a pocket calculator and (mainly) the chi square test of statistical significance.

There is nothing particularly sophisticated about such a methodology; indeed it could be said to reek of an outdated empiricism and/or an anachronistic cottage industry approach. With small-scale research, the problem – and the opportunity – as I see it is two-fold: to allow the totality of the situation as described by those studied to emerge, and to examine the components of what is said for their possible interconnections. Unless the first goal is achieved, the people become merely statistics and the centrality of their own positions is jeopardized. But without the second goal, without the attempt to unravel the interconnectedness of human experience, the research does not really move beyond a descriptive level. Of course it is interesting to know how frequently in people's experiences certain events or feelings occur, and such intra-sample frequencies can be generalized to a wider population provided the sample is a representative one. General information about these 'real' frequencies is important to combat received wisdom, to establish a base for more accurate predictions and so on. But the extent of a happening is a relatively uninteresting fact apart from the 'why' of its genesis. People want to know why things happen because of a basic curiosity, and because they hold values that give them a vested interest in the possibility of curative change in those conditions that are seen as disordered:

> Social research is political because the researcher has interests which may coincide with or contradict the interests of the

> researched. All social research has an end: the formulation of policy; the conservation, reform or radical transformation of the social situation being studied... [Cass *et al.*, 1978, p. 143]

In other words, the rationale for studying what happens to women when they have babies is to suggest why they react to childbirth in the way they do and (the more overtly political question) how their experiences of reproduction might be improved. Both these goals require a confrontation with the idea of causality, since they demand a disentangling of the factors that influence maternal outcome from those that do not and they assert the need for a theory about why independent and dependent variables are related in the way they are. As Denzin says, 'A theory is nothing ... if it is not explanation. Explanation, in turn, is nothing if it is not causally based' (1970, p. 213). The complexity of the notion of causality accounts for its absence in much social analysis today. It is pointed out, quite correctly, that no non-experimental research design allows causal relationships to be identified with perfect certainty. This leads on to the argument that causal language is impractical in the analysis of social data because it calls for infinite testing of relationships (Galtung, 1967, pp. 474–5). Moreover, the process of attempting to establish a causal relationship can bring about the appearance of 'methodolatry'[3] – the ritualistic pursuit of method for its own sake.

Causal analysis demands that three properties be demonstrated: (i) the fact that the 'causal' variables are associated with variations in dependent variables (evidence of concomitant variation); (ii) the temporal occurrence of the causal variable before the dependent variable; and (iii) proof that the relationship between causal and dependent variables is not spurious, i.e. contingent on other, unexamined, variables. I am aware of the problems associated with the idea of causality, but believe, nevertheless, that what is discussed in chapters 6–9 is basically a causal model of how women's feelings after birth are affected by certain medical and social factors. Post-birth feelings are the dependent variable, against which a variety of social and medical factors are tabulated for their capacity 'independently' to influence this. The strengths of my research design are three. First, by interviewing women during pregnancy, their attitudes, satisfaction and mental health *before* the birth could be established. (It would, of course, have been even better to have interviewed them before they became pregnant, but it is not easy to see how a sample of about-to-become-pregnant women could be obtained.) Second, by selecting a relatively socially and medically homogeneous sample of women, comparison of the different effects of various social and medical factors on maternal outcome is less likely to be confused by the influence of other, extraneous variables. Third, by distinguishing a number of different components of outcome, the possibly causal effect of independent variables can be more finely discriminated than is usual in research dealing with women's 'adjustment' to motherhood.

Having said that, I would also acknowledge that I have not *indisputably* established any causal relationships in the data analysis. One example would be the central idea that emerges in chapters 6 and 7 that postnatal depression is explained in part by the degree of technology used in labour and delivery. The depression cannot explain the technology, since it followed rather than preceded birth. But there are various competing explanations along the lines of there being some underlying predisposition in the women who had high technology births and became depressed that is responsible for both these occurrences. I discuss this more fully later (pp. 148–50) but note here that, while I can show such hypotheses to be unlikely, I do not claim to be able absolutely to rule them out.

The value of small-scale research is that it can unite the two chief strategies of social data analysis: describing the processes that are going on and identifying the factors that bring them about (see Brown, 1973). I would argue that these processual and factorial inquiries are more likely to be linked in small-scale than in large-scale research, particularly where use is made of the unstructured interview. Since the researcher is in constant contact with the data at every stage of its collection and processing, he or she can be more sensitive not only to the experience but also to the explanations that are cited by the interviewee, and is more likely to be able to integrate such explanations into the data analysis. The advantage usually cited for factorial research is that it may yield insights that are not provided by the explanations given by those who are interviewed. Yet I would contend that such insights can much more often be derived (though not, of course, 'proved') from the interpretations of events and processes provided by the people whose lives are being studied than is usually regarded as being the case. In the research project described in this book, all the theories presented as to why the sample women reacted to childbirth the way they did were suggested to me by one or more of the women who were interviewed. The fact that I have published two books based on the research, one presenting processual and the other factorial analysis, is because I want to present both more fully than is possible within the scope of one book – not because their union within the research exercise proved difficult.[4]

This type of small-scale research has been labelled 'feminine'.[5] Preoccupation with individuals rather than with large groups, masses or institutions, sensitivity to individual biography rather than statistical summation, personal involvement rather than hierarchical direction of the research process, are all aspects of women's engagement in social science research that connect with the feminine cultural stereotype. (They may also, of course, reflect the fact that more 'female' than 'male' research projects are done on a monetary shoestring because of discrimination against women in research funding itself – see Platt, 1976, pp. 108–9, 123–6.[6]) Such labelling is implicitly derogatory: the standard to which all researchers should aspire is 'masculine' and the only research that is worth doing involves a detachment from concern with individual case-history in the interests of the manipulation of large numbers. The discomfort that is often voiced about the use of tests of statistical significance in small samples may be something to do with this juxtaposition of 'masculine' and 'feminine' research methods. Although such tests, by their nature, allow for the constraints of sample size, their application to small samples appears to confuse the two modes of doing research, importing a masculine preoccupation into an essentially feminine exercise. I am, of course, only speculating here about the reasons why critics dismiss this type of research. I would add that it seems to be particularly the combination of processual and factorial analysis as applied to small samples that generates this dismissiveness. Much social analysis, especially that of the Chicago school in America, has been rooted in the ('feminine') biographical approach, and has been widely regarded as a valuable contribution.

The use of rating scales – placing individuals in categories in which they do not necessarily place themselves – is another aspect of small-scale research that can be criticized for a confusion of 'masculine' and 'feminine' methods. While the small numbers involved suggest an emphasis on empathy and description, the use of rating scales implies a positivist bias towards measurement. Where the research has a 'feminist' orientation, the status of such a 'masculine' methodology is further in doubt. Cicourel (1964) has termed researchers not mere collectors of discrete facts but active interpreters of events. Although the logic of rating scales may be spelt out by the researcher, it may still be difficult for those judging the research to understand how the scales relate to the interview data: the intervening variable is the researcher's own imposition of meaning. His or her integrity, and capacity to reproduce the meaning of events and experiences as others see them, is a quality that has to remain open to question.

One essential consideration is that the capacity of sociological research to uncover an interconnectedness in social experience is an empirically verifiable characteristic. The proof of the pudding is in the eating; what is crucial is whether such explanations explain and, even more important, whether they can act as bases for predicting action (Goldthorpe, 1973). If they can do this, then it is unlikely that the researcher has distorted the data by imposing an irrelevant meaning upon them. While the language of rating scales (the word 'assess' for example) may convey the impression that it is the researcher who sits in judgement on the researched, he or she *is* better equipped through contact with the data to judge the grouping of individuals than are those individuals themselves.

In using rating scales to analyse women's feelings before and after childbirth, I have had one particular problem in mind, and that is the need for grounded theory (Glaser and Strauss, 1968) to be grounded in two kinds of data: the old and the new. Previous research and theory formulation provide a resource from which are gained ideas for new research and theory development; dialectically, the new data that are collected establish a base for theory revision and reformulation. The same is true of research methods, which must be grounded in the logistics of each particular research exercise, but in relation both to previously used methods and to their eventual re-evaluation. Both these features of research are especially marked in the area of women's experiences of reproduction, where the large body of existing research outlined in chapters 1–3 calls both for a radical reassessment of its paradigmatic base and for a new approach that is capable of connection with the old. I have tried to accomplish both these goals, not without difficulty but with, I hope, the degree of success that will stimulate at least some new thinking about what it is that happens to women when they have babies.

CHAPTER 5

Assessing Outcome

I am nothing, a no thing, an avant garde experiment in God's spacious laboratory, a chain of sensations, a thinker of fringe thoughts. My body is a map of feelings and my mind like a convoluted cauliflower; or like a record library . . . What am I? Who am I? is the riddle. [Jessup, 1973, p. 9]

As Part I of this book observed, women's experiences of reproduction have usually been seen within both medical and social science in terms of some kind of 'adjustment'. This adjustment may be to the 'reality' of birth and the demands of newborn babies, or it may be to the requirements of the social role of mother as located in a specific cultural context – marriage, and the socially isolated and gender-divided nuclear family. A second important focus has been on the outcome of clinical postnatal depression: axiomatically the occurrence of postnatal depression counts as 'bad' adjustment and its absence as 'good'. And, as we saw in chapters 1 and 2, both the syndrome of depression and the syndrome of maladjustment have overwhelmingly been sited within a paradigm of femininity; not as examples of human reactions to human events but as unique catastrophes of womanhood. In this chapter and those that follow I want to propose a different way of analysing the outcome of the transition to motherhood. In turn this proposal will suggest a new approach to the study of the transition itself: one that stresses variables of *human* responses that are unconnected with traditional reductionist models of femininity. In order to achieve this end, it is necessary to 'assess outcome'. This is the subject of the present chapter, which is a preliminary spelling-out of some key concepts central to the data analysis and theoretical model presented in chapters 6–10.

OUTCOME VARIABLES

By 'outcome' I mean how mothers feel after the birth. To assess it I have retained an emphasis on the two traditional outcome labels of adjustment and depression, adding to them several others that seem to make the necessary distinctions between the different component parts of what is, in fact, a very complex process. There are three reasons why I look at how mothers adjust and whether they become depressed: in the first place it makes sense to ask whether women have adjusted to the level of cultural expectations concerning their role as mothers (this being a reinterpretation of older notions of adjustment); in the second place there is no doubt that one of the things women suffer from after childbirth is 'depression' – in both common-sense and clinical meanings of the word. And third, as noted in chapter 4, the point of any new model is in part its capacity to be legitimated by the old – a characteristic that can only emerge if both models share some common universe of understandings.

It is, however, necessary to break down some different meanings of the term 'postnatal depression': in the Transition to Motherhood study, out of six outcome measures used, I distinguish four 'mental health' variables. The fifth way of measuring outcome is 'satisfaction' with motherhood – 'adjustment' renamed to avoid the connotations described earlier (pp. 57–66). The sixth way refers to the feelings mothers have for their babies. I use the term 'mental health' to describe the four postnatal depression variables in order to distinguish them from the other two measures, though I do not thereby mean to imply that how a woman feels about her baby and how satisfied she is with motherhood are not equally reflections of her 'mental health'.

MENTAL HEALTH OUTCOME

The four 'postnatal depression' categories are:

Postnatal 'blues': a condition of emotional lability characterized by crying and occurring during hospitalization (the average length of hospital stay among the sample women was nine days).

Anxiety: a condition of anxiety about the baby/the responsibilities of motherhood characterized by extreme sensitivity to the baby's behaviour, feelings of being 'on edge', inability to sleep soundly or to concentrate on other tasks; reported on homecoming and lasting up to two weeks.

Depressed mood: feelings of depression that come and go after the first three postpartum weeks but without symptoms.

Depression: a depressed state occurring at any time from hospital discharge to five months postpartum, characterized by two or more symptoms and lasting (without remitting) at least two weeks.

These distinctions were made on the basis of what women said in the interviews. They described four differing conditions, each with its own characteristic time of onset and symptomatology, but all of which were branded 'postnatal depression' – either by the women themselves, by their husbands, relatives or friends or by the medical staff involved. Each of the four outcomes was assessed on the basis of self-report.[1] Women who said 'yes' to questions about feeling depressed or suffering from 'nerves' were also asked a series of questions derived from the Present State Examination Schedule, a standardized clinical-type interview developed for the detection of psychiatric morbidity at the Institute of Psychiatry in London.[2] In the following quotations from four interviews, the differences between the four mental health outcomes are demonstrated.

Postnatal blues

One day I wept and wept, I just couldn't stop, I just prayed that nobody would come and visit me, because I don't know how I would have coped. But they do say that nearly everybody has one day. I was just surprised at how weepy I was, because I'm not the kind of person that gets depressed. Mind you, I wasn't really actually depressed. It was funny, I just felt terribly, terribly worried about the baby and I just couldn't stop crying, you know, for a whole day. And so that night, that was about the fifth day, and that night they took him off to the nursery and they bottlefed him for that night, and they gave me some sleeping tablets because they said I was so tired, and I was so tensed up I wouldn't have been able to sleep, I was just getting terribly tense. And the next day I was as right as rain again. (Rosalind Kimber)

Anxiety

I was ever so nervous, especially the first night. I kept waking up to make sure he was still there, you know, he hadn't stopped breathing or anything. I felt nervous for the first couple of days and then it was allright. [Felicity Chambers]

Depressed mood

INTERVIEWER: *Are you depressed at the moment?*

SHARON WARRINGTON: *Not today. Not very often, really. Sometimes, especially when Alan goes out and the baby's gone to bed, about nine o'clock or something I might sit down and have a good old bawl. I'm crying over nothing, really. Really, I've got nothing to be depressed about, I've got a roof over my head, I've got food in the cupboard, I've got things that other people haven't got, so I can never find a reason that I am depressed. I mean, like Alan going out, that winds me up. . . .*

Depression

If you knew how long it was going to go on, you'd feel alright. But it was just the fact that day after day after day I felt the same. That was the worst thing. Every morning that sort of dread – another day. And then I used to say, now today I'm really going to make the effort. I can't today, but tomorrow will be better. And I did make myself go out just to stop crying really – I mean I used to walk around the streets pushing her, just so I wouldn't cry. . . . It wasn't as if I knew why *I felt like that . . . it was just a sort of* nothingness. *I just felt that nothing would have made any difference. If someone said to me, you can go on a lovely holiday and we'll look after the baby, it wouldn't have been any help . . . I can see how people do get completely desperate. I just wanted to sit down and do nothing. I just didn't think about* anything. *And I couldn't read a book or a newspaper – I used to switch the telly on. . . .* (José Bryce)

While the 'blues' and anxiety on first coming home with the baby were usually no more than temporary impediments to normal behaviour, both depressed mood and depression had a more pernicious influence on the satisfactions of motherhood.

On the whole the literature on postpartum mental illness does not, as we saw in chapter 2, deal with these distinctions. The main division is seen as being between psychotic and neurotic (depressive) states, with the statistically much less frequent postpartum psychosis receiving more attention than the far more common depressive syndromes. (Psychosis occurs in perhaps 0.2 per cent of women following delivery; depression, depending on its definition, in 10–80 per cent – Kaij and Nilsson, 1972.) Within the category 'postpartum depression', many investigators do not distinguish the blues from temporary anxiety states or from either brief or more enduring periods of depression.[3] However, others recognize that the emotional lability of the early puerperium is such a distinct and frequent phenomenon as to be regarded as 'normal' (Yalom *et al.*, 1968). It is, as Pitt (1972) has pointed out, in the grey area between the two extremes of the blues and postpartum psychosis that understanding of the symptoms, aetiology and prognosis of postnatal depressive states is notably deficient.

There is widespread agreement in the literature on the character of the 'blues', which concords with the definition adopted in the present study, as does its incidence – 84 per cent here, 76–80 per cent elsewhere. At the other end of the spectrum, psychotic illness would not be expected to appear in a sample of fifty-five (given its incidence of around 0.2 per cent) – as indeed it did not. It is more difficult to connect the definition of depression used with that adopted in the literature, much of which is concerned with depressive disorders serious enough to warrant hospital treatment. As Brown and Harris (1978, p. 23) observe, the separation of clinical depression and depressed mood has received little attention: there is no agreement among psychiatrists as to whether it is 'a question of different degrees of the same type of phenomena or of different types of phenomena that separate clinical depression from a disturbance of mood'. The women who experienced what I have called depressed mood in the present study were not so handicapped as those who were depressed, all of whom felt disabled by their depression: it interrupted normal behaviour, routines and social life, and was characterized, in psychiatric terms, by the presence of two or more symptoms (e.g. insomnia, appetite disturbance). In three instances it was associated with drug treatment, but no case led to hospital admission (although in two this was discussed as a possibility). It is my impression that, in terms of what psychiatrists would consider 'clinical' depression, about 15 per cent of the Transition to Motherhood sample would be defined as depressed.[4] The fact that a larger proportion (24 per cent) appears as depressed in the current analysis would seem (if replicated in further research) to indicate some discrepancy between psychiatrists and depressed people in their assessments of what depression 'is', at least in the particular instance of depression following childbirth.[5]

So far as the fourth mental health outcome – anxiety – is concerned, it is in some ways an artificial distinction to categorize this separately from depression. The two are closely linked in many disorders, and it is often only the overall preponderance of type of symptom within a disorder that enables the separation to be made. In the present study, the definition of anxiety is restricted to the period immediately following coming home from the hospital with the baby since it seemed that the emotional, physical and behavioural disorders the women reported during this phase in the transition to motherhood were related to an underlying, and usually articulated, feeling of anxiety about the responsibilities of their new state. Pitt has noted something of this order in his study of 'Neurotic (or Atypical) Depression Following Childbirth'. His patients, on going home with the baby, suffered from

> despondency, tearfulness, feelings of inadequacy and inability to cope (especially with the baby), hypochondriasis and fears of the baby's health, tension, irritability and undue fatigue, diminished appetite, difficulty in getting to sleep and decline in sexual interest. [1972, p. 348]

As a characteristic phase in the assumption of the mothering role, the anxiety syndrome identified in the current study appeared to be distinct from a depression that might or might not have anxiety symptoms attached. It was distinguished from the occurrence of depressed mood (which again might be mixed with anxiety) by being confined to the first two weeks following hospital discharge, whereas depressed mood was a syndrome occurring after this period.

All the mental health states were classed as either present or absent – a woman either experienced postnatal blues, anxiety, depressed mood or depression, or she did not. Women could, of course, experience various combinations, or all, of these syndromes over the five postpartum months of the study.

SATISFACTION WITH MOTHERHOOD

Again based on self-report, this measure relates to feelings about the role of mother, about the work of childrearing and about coping behaviour. It refers simply to the extent to which the sample women felt they were or were not coping with the baby and with motherhood.[6] There are three categories: 'high', 'medium' and 'low' satisfaction, these designations referring to normative definitions of motherhood, i.e. contentment with the maternal role and with childcare work, and feelings of being able to cope with the baby's requirements.

FEELINGS FOR THE BABY

This concerns the quality and strength of positive and negative feelings towards the baby and anxiety about/towards her/him, as expressed either spontaneously or in answer to certain questions.[7] Positive feeling, negative feeling and anxiety were all rated separately and a composite index arrived at that reflected these. The designations were of 'good', 'medium' and 'poor' feelings, taking the referent of normative views of the mother–baby bond as characterized by high positive and low negative emotions and by a certain, but not disabling, input of anxiety about the baby's health and behaviour. Although the words 'good' and 'poor' are evaluative, they are so in terms of the women's own descriptions. For example, mothers who experienced strongly negative feelings about their children were often worried because they believed they should not have such feelings, which they saw as constituting a 'poor' relationship with the baby.

All these definitions of outcome are based on postpartum state – on what the women said during the two interviews carried out at five weeks and five months after the birth. Every possible step was taken to ensure no 'contamination' between the different ratings.[8] The distribution of the various outcomes among the sample women is shown in Table 5.1. Another way of presenting the figures in Table 5.1 is to say that only two women out of the fifty-five experienced no negative mental health outcome *and* had high satisfaction with motherhood *and* 'good' feelings for their babies. This finding, together with the prevalence of

TABLE 5.1 *Different outcomes to the transition to motherhood*

Outcome	*% of women having*
Mental Health:	
postnatal blues	84
anxiety	71
depressed mood	33
depression	24
Other:	
satisfaction with motherhood:	
'high'	69
'medium'	20
'low'	11
feelings for the baby:	
'good'	42
'medium'	46
'poor'	13

$N = 55$.

negative mental health outcome found in other studies, should perhaps lead to a reformulation of the question 'why do some mothers get depressed or "adjust" badly?' as 'why do some mothers "adjust" "well" and avoid any kind of postpartum depression?' I believe that this is, in fact, the correct perspective to adopt, given the characteristic features of the transition to motherhood and motherhood as an institution in modern industrialized societies today. But to argue the legitimacy of this approach, it is necessary first to show just how negative outcome and particular aspects of the social and medical passage to motherhood may be connected.

This of course requires a process of selection. Since not *all* aspects of the transition to motherhood can be included in the analysis, *some* must be chosen as the most likely to show a relationship with the indicators of outcome. Among these, a smaller proportion will turn out to link in a statistically or theoretically meaningful way with the indicators of outcome used. In fact, six groups of factors emerged as particularly significant: those relating to *birth, antecedent socialization, baby condition, work conditions, marriage* and *general background.* According to the dual criteria of statistical and theoretical significance, these all proved to be related to outcome. The next section discusses the rationale for selecting these, the dimensions of each chosen and their operationalization in terms of the interview data.

OTHER VARIABLES

BIRTH FACTORS

The idea that the manner in which a birth is accomplished affects maternal outcome (mental health and satisfaction and feelings for the baby) is an idea that has gained currency in recent years. Behind it is the notion, foreign only to 'civilized' cultures, that birth is an event with great psychological, emotional and social meaning for the mother. Most of the protest about current methods of handling childbirth that has come from consumer and other pressure groups over the last ten to fifteen years centres on this idea.[9] Although not necessarily at odds with what Stoller Shaw (1974) calls 'the medical monopoly of childbirth care' it does in fact seem to be easily forgotten within a medical system – the very medicalness of the system calling for the primacy of narrowly medical, i.e. physiological, goals. The 'medicalization' of childbirth was gradually achieved in the first decades of the twentieth century and seems to have been characterized by a similarly slow process of intensification. An official commitment to a 100 per cent hospital confinement rate was, for instance, a gradual process, rising from 15 per cent in 1927 to 66 per cent in 1958 and 96 per cent in 1974.[10] Recently, medical developments in controlling childbirth have accelerated:

> Development and innovation in the management of childbirth over the last 10 years has taken place at an unparalleled rate. Care during pregnancy has been extended and elaborated to include assessment of foetal well-being by placental function tests and serial ultrasound cephalometry. Early recognition of chromosomal, biochemical and neural tube abnormalities in the foetus has become possible. Efficient pharmacological control of labour with oxytocin and prostaglandins has increased the scope for induction and aug-

> mentation of labour, and this in turn has prompted the development of techniques to assess the gestational age and functional maturity of the foetus more accurately than previously. Because labour itself poses a particular threat to the safety of both mother and baby, policies of universal hospital confinement have been promoted, and, in many maternity units, the use of partography, cardiotocography, foetal scalp blood sampling, and lumbar epidural blocks has become routine. [Chalmers, 1978, p. 44]

As Chalmers notes, the diversity of obstetric practice in Britain suggests some intra-professional conflict about the benefits of such a high technology system. But in the main, opposition to this system has come from clinical psychology, from medical sociology, from the consumer movement and from the media – fields in which detachment from medical involvement promotes an easier critique of what all these machines might be doing to the women who actually have babies.

In the last four years criticism has reverberated to the point where it gets written up in medical journals.[11] For the most part it is anecdotal (a word I do not use in a derogatory sense) or statistical – based on the statistics of precoded satisfaction with medical maternity care. Some research has shown identifiable links between birth management and maternal outcome (for example in the case of premature delivery, caesarean section and post-birth separation of mother and child), though mothers are seen in the bulk of this research as important only to their children (as shapers of the mother–baby relationship); their own feelings and satisfactions are a secondary concern (see Macfarlane, 1977).

To look at how birth styles might be related to maternal outcome in a broader sense, the following dimensions of birth and its management were selected:

(a) the amount of technology used during labour and delivery;
(b) the degree of control experienced during labour;
(c) satisfaction/dissatisfaction with the management of the birth;
(d) instrumental delivery;
(e) satisfaction/dissatisfaction with the second stage;
(f) epidural analgesia.

The assessment of (d) and (f) is self-explanatory – either a woman had an instrumental delivery/epidural or she did not. Technology was 'scored' as high, medium or low on the basis of the use of different medical interventions.[12] For (b), (c) and (e) the assessment of satisfaction and control followed the general principle of self-report used throughout the research analysis.[13]

TABLE 5.2 *Different experiences of birth*

Experience	*% of women having*
Technology:	
high	29
medium	46
low	25
instrumental delivery	48
epidural	79
Control:	
good	31
medium	31
poor	38
Satisfaction with birth management:	
high	59
medium	24
low	16
Satisfaction with second stage labour:	
high	38
medium	28
low	34

N = 55 for technology and satisfaction with birth management.
N = 50 for control and second stage satisfaction.

Table 5.2 summarizes the values exhibited by the sample women on these factors. Considering that they were 'normal' primigravidae, the level of intervention in birth seems high. This is not an accident of the sample chosen. As Table 5.3 shows, the pattern in the total patient population of the sample hospital during the same time period was similar. The sample hospital is a large maternity unit with (in 1975–6) around 3000 deliveries a year. Comparison with *national* practice is difficult, since some of the figures (for example of the incidence of epidural analgesia) are not available. But induction preceded 39 per cent of all births in England and Wales in 1974 (Chalmers

TABLE 5.3 *Some types of birth technology: Transition to Motherhood sample and sample hospital compared*

Sample	*Induction of labour*	*Instrumental delivery*	*Epidural block*
Transition to Motherhood sample, 1975–6*	21%	52%	79%
Primiparae, sample hospital (a) 1975†	22%	48%	76%
(b) 1976‡	24%	46%	73%

* *N* = 55.
† *N* = 1088.
‡ *N* = 1086.

and Richards, 1977, p. 22) and 26 per cent in the sample hospital. On the other hand, the instrumental delivery rate in the sample hospital was 28 per cent in 1975, which was probably about twice the national figure (Chalmers and Richards, 1977, p. 39), and accompanied an epidural rate that was substantially in advance of the national trend. In all these respects – lower induction, higher instrumental delivery and epidural rate – practice in the sample hospital foreshadowed general developments in obstetrics from the mid-1970s on.

ANTECEDENT SOCIALIZATION FACTORS

Chapters 1 and 2 showed how the guiding theme of much medical and psychological research on reproduction has been that women's 'adjustment' to motherhood is somehow determined by their pre-motherhood experiences – especially those of female biology and feminine socialization. From this viewpoint motherhood is achieving femininity, not in the sociological sense of meeting cultural expectation and facing the classic 'women's role' dilemmas, but in the internal psychological sense of completing a feminine personality agenda.

While it seems both difficult and misleading to operationalize in research any such fixed notion of what constitutes femininity, it is undoubtedly true on a *human* level that previous experiences help to shape reactions to major life events. So far as the advent of motherhood is concerned there is, for example, evidence that a woman's identification and relationship with her own mother may result in the perpetuation of certain themes when the daughter herself becomes a mother: a rejection or espousal of domesticity, the ability or inability to feel and act 'maternally' towards a child, particular patterns of childbearing and childrearing (see Hoffman and Nye, 1974; Chodorow, 1978; Illsley, 1967). The whole interface between self-image as a person, as a woman and as a mother is probably profoundly influenced by early family relationships.

In the current study, three variables were picked out as indicators of such effects: ***feminine role orientation, self-image as a mother*** and ***previous contact with babies.*** The object of using these indices was not to replicate any Freudian map of feminine personality development and 'adjustment' to motherhood, but to indicate where the sample women lay as regards the culturally normative typification of women as feminine and maternal people.

Feminine role orientation

Questions were asked about childhood gender role socialization, about the women's mothers' attitudes to employment work and housework, about adolescent ambitions for marriage and/or careers and educational and job decisions, about feelings concerning the role of housewife and housework, about the importance of motherhood to women, about sex discrimination and the women's liberation movement, and about masculine domesticity. The feminine role orientation of respondents was labelled 'traditional', 'instrumental' or 'radical' on the basis of answers to these questions. A traditional orientation accepts the definition of women as primarily devoted to the housewife–wife–mother role triad as a definition applied to oneself. An instrumental orientation means that a woman accepts as important other activities and goals in her life (such as work outside the home) but retains some view of men and women as differently suited for domesticity. A radical orientation implies a feminist rejection of female domesticity and of biologically based arguments for gender role differentiation.[14]

Self-image as a mother
Here one specific component of attitudes to femininity is identified: the extent to which women see themselves as mothers. A set of questions was asked in each interview about this.[15] The women were categorized as having a 'high', 'medium' or 'low' maternal self-image.

Previous contact with babies
Aside from doll play, having experienced childcare in the past is the only job qualification of relevance to the new occupation of mother. It may have been undertaken as a paid job or career, but it is more likely to have consisted of informal contact with siblings and/or other babies in the extended family. Some women have also done babysitting on a casual neighbourhood basis as adolescents. All these areas were asked about, and from the women's answers the amount of such experience was categorized as a lot, a medium amount or little/no contact.

TABLE 5.4 *Antecedent socialization factors*

Factor	*% of women having*
Feminine role orientation:	
traditional	54
instrumental	41
radical	5
Self-image as mother:	
high	52
medium	22
low	27
Previous contact with babies:	
a lot	30
a medium amount	20
little/none	50

N = 55.

Table 5.4 gives the range among the sample women of values on the three antecedent socialization variables. Between a third and half the sample women had a high value on these factors – the kind of value that in the psychological research would be taken as predictive of a 'good adjustment' to motherhood.

BABY CONDITION FACTORS

But even if socialized 'correctly', a new mother's work cannot be shaped by her alone. In this sense the kind of baby she gives birth to must be seen as an independent variable: a separate influence on her interpretation of motherhood. Such a view is relatively new to research on maternal behaviour. For a long time the idea persisted that maternal attitudes and behaviour determined the child's personality – that what happened in childhood was irrevocable and one-sided, with the child as innocent, vulnerable tabula rasa and the mother (not, of course, the father) as some kind of omnipotent purveyor of personality and imposer of culture. The *failure* of research to demonstrate a direct relationship between maternal influence and personality outcome was taken as a failure of research methods, not as a sign of deficiency in the model itself. In the last five to ten years awareness has grown of the need for a new 'transactional' approach:

> Both parents and child operate within a system of mutuality where the behaviour of one produces effects on the other that in turn modify the behaviour of the first ... from the beginning the baby is active, not passive; his (*sic*) behaviour is organised, not 'absent'; and even to the earliest social interactions he brings certain characteristics which will affect the behaviour of other people towards him. [Schaffer, 1977, pp. 30–1][16]

In terms of research the contribution the infant makes to his social interactions is very hard to measure. No way has yet been found of categorizing infant 'personality' at birth.[17] Moreover, *by* birth the differential impact of culture on nature has already been established – male babies, by virtue of the special chemistry that exists between them and their mothers[18] and by their greater size and weight,[19] are more likely to meet with medical intervention, which can have a behavioural effect. The behaviour of parents to boy and girl babies has been shown to be different from birth,[20] and these gender impositions may veil infants' different personality contributions to the pattern of parent–neonate interaction. In any case, the search for biologically derived gender differences in babies has mitigated any inquiry about personality individuation per se. What research has been done suggests that babies' behaviour cannot be computed from the parents' own. Richards and Bernal (1974), for instance, have shown that sleeping and crying patterns cannot be satisfactorily explained as outcomes of parental behaviour. Certainly poor sleeping and persistent crying are two features of infant behaviour parents find it hardest to tolerate.

Night sleeping

Night sleeping and crying time were asked about in the present study and cross-tabulated with outcome. Only night sleeping at five months proved to have any capacity to differentiate between types of outcome, probably because maternal report of crying time is so affected by comforting techniques used (whether the baby is picked up when it starts to cry, whether it is given a bottle or the breast or a dummy when it cries) that the result reflects the different use and impact of these techniques rather than the infant's disposition to cry.[21]

The women were divided into two groups on the basis of how long they said their babies slept at night five months after the birth: those (11 per cent) whose babies slept six hours or less and those (89 per cent) whose babies slept more than six hours.

The baby's sex

In a society where biological sex signals a complex cultural system of gender differentiation, the femaleness or maleness of a baby is liable to be endowed with more than a narrowly biological meaning. There is evidence that at birth medical, midwifery and nursing staff attach more importance to this than mothers do,[22] but certainly in the days, weeks, months and years following birth a mother's feelings about having a daughter or a son will be part of the feeling she has towards and about that child. Sex preference studies show that pre-birth ideas about the appropriate sex for a baby are clear in parental minds. The preferred sex ratio is 110–165 male to 100 female (as compared with the natural sex ratio, which is about 105:100) (Williamson, 1976). Fathers are more likely than mothers to prefer boys; boys are particularly likely to be desired more than girls as first-born or only children; and a family of two girls is more likely to be added to than one of two boys (Williamson, 1976). Of the Transition to Motherhood sample, 54 per cent of the mothers-to-be wanted boys and 22 per cent wanted girls (25 per cent said they didn't mind). Of those who had boys, 93 per cent were pleased, compared with 56 per cent of those who had girls.

A mother's reactions to her new son or daughter thus reflect imagined and desired as well as actual sex. Previously accepted concepts of femininity and masculinity ('boys are greedier than girls', 'girls are easier to bring up') are attached as diagnoses or predictors of the baby's actual (or parentally perceived) behaviour. These are reinforced, refined or disputed by the sex-typing messages sent by others – and verbal sex typing is an overt aspect of our cultural ideology of childhood and our methodology of developing gender differences. During pregnancy, 54 per cent of the Transition to Motherhood sample said that they believed boy and girl babies behaved differently; afterwards 38 per cent said they felt their relationship with the baby was affected by its sex. Thus, although biological sex is more or less equally distributed by nature – 29 women had boys and 27 had girls – the social impact of the chromosomal difference is asymmetrical.

WORK CONDITION FACTORS

Both housework and paid employment work are affected by motherhood. Feelings of domestic 'overload', social isolation in and restriction to the home, a sense of boredom or monotony and the repetitive 'sameness' of life – these have been documented as especially characteristic of mothers as a group in our society (Gavron, 1966; Oakley, 1974b; Ginsberg, 1976). Giving birth to a child that one expects (or is expected) to bring up impinges on the whole of life by engineering membership of the social category of 'mother'. A 'good' mother stays at home for the first three, preferably five and ideally eleven or twelve, years of her child's life: she provides her child with a comfortable physical and emotional environment for growth. To do this, she has to be tied, in some measure, to the home.

Certain aspects of mothers' working conditions were associated with their feelings after birth. These were: whether or not they were employed, to what extent those who were not employed missed work, whether they found babycare monotonous and whether they felt tied down by the baby.

TABLE 5.5 *Mothers' work conditions*

Condition	*% of women*
Employment:	
employed	33
not employed:	67
miss work	61
don't miss work	39
Babycare:	
monotonous*	43
not monotonous	57
feel tied down	80
don't feel tied down	20

N = 55.

* This relates to the five week interview only.

Table 5.5 gives the answers to these questions five months after the birth. 'Employment' here means *any* employment: only one woman went back to full-time work; the rest (29 per cent of the sample) worked occasionally and/or on a part-time basis. This reflects practice in the country as a whole, where, in 1974, 26 per cent of mothers of pre-school children were employed, but only 5–6 per cent on a full-time basis (Moss, 1976). The large proportion who missed work and felt tied down by the baby confirms the widespread character of such discontent.

MARITAL FACTORS

The paradigm of reproduction as a marital event was discussed in chapter 3. In the present study the aim was not to interpret childbirth in terms of its effect on marital satisfaction, but to examine parental relationships from the mother's point of view as one of the areas affected by childbirth. This is one of the subjectively important dimensions of becoming a mother according to the women's own accounts.

Parenthood and marriage are interdependent: they affect each other. Hence not only is it important to look at the possibility that parenthood affects marriage, but it is also crucial to consider the way in which the experience of parenthood is shaped by the marital context. We know that the advent of motherhood disturbs pre-existing patterns of division of labour in the household, as also does the retirement of pregnant women from employment work (Oakley, 1979b; Hoffman and Nye, 1974). Conversely, Minturn, Lambert *et al.* (1964) have shown that release from too much domestic work may very well be a condition of nurturant maternal behaviour. In this way, what husbands do in the home has a capacity to shape the parameters of maternal satisfaction.

The two-way relationship of parenthood and marriage was a theme running through all the interviews, and many dimensions of this were assessed: emotional closeness, separation versus identity of interests, the domestic division of labour in housework and childcare. Among these, the segregation – jointness dimension of the marital role relationship and the amount of help given by partners with childcare proved to have a relationship with maternal outcome.

Segregation – jointness of the marital role relationship
Following the practice set out in *The Sociology of Housework* (which in turn is based on Elizabeth Bott's original discussion of segregation and jointness in marriage – 1971), the women were grouped into two categories of segregated or joint marital role relationships. Those who had a 'joint' role relationship with their partners shared leisure activities and decision-making; those with a 'segregated' role relationship on the whole did not. 'Jointness' is associated with middle-classness[23] and probably also with different patterns of communicative behaviour. The type of role relationship was measured at the first pregnancy interview and therefore represents these dimensions of couples' relationships in the pre-parenthood phase: 34 per cent of the couples had segregated, and 66 per cent joint, role relationships.

Masculine participation in housework
Since the domestic division of labour has a certain ideological and practical autonomy, it was assessed separately from general segregation/jointness of marital role. It was based on what the women said their partners had done in the previous week in the way of cleaning, shopping, cooking, washing up, washing and ironing. (The methodological problems associated with this

type of inquiry are discussed in *The Sociology of Housework*, 1974b, Chapter 8.)

Masculine participation in housework was inquired about at each interview; Table 5.6 shows the developmental pattern – though only the five month postpartum index is statistically related to outcome. The trend is downwards, with 23 per cent of partners contributing 'a lot' of help in early pregnancy but only 6 per cent doing so five months after the birth. The same pattern, incidentally, characterizes post-birth childcare help. Table 5.7 evidences a decline in the proportion of fathers giving 'a lot' of help with their babies, from 20 per cent at five weeks to 11 per cent five months after the birth.

TABLE 5.6 *Masculine participation in housework*

Level	*Early pregnancy*	*Late pregnancy*	*Five weeks postpartum*	*Five months postpartum*
A lot	23%	22%	14%	6%
Some	27%	30%	38%	33%
A little/none	50%	48%	48%	61%

N = 55.

TABLE 5.7 *Fathers' participation in childcare*

Level	*Five weeks postpartum*	*Five months postpartum*
A lot	20%	11%
Some	29%	26%
A little/none	52%	64%

N = 55.

BACKGROUND FACTORS

Both social class and housing could be seen as flowing from the context of couples' relationships. Housing situation is closely tied to family income, which means, for many couples having children, principally father's income. And a woman's social class is usually derived directly from the occupational status of the man with whom she lives, irrespective of her own current or past occupation or any other personal index – for instance educational background.

The rationale of this tradition has been undermined by a critique of its ideological charter: the second-hand status of women is primarily the way women are *supposed* to be. But the problem is – and this is the problem of how to *revise* the social class categorization of women – that the ideal and the actual are linked. Official statisticians argue that assigning a married woman to her husband's occupational status category merely reflects social definitions of her status, definitions that parallel her own status perceptions. At the same time, the gap between men's and women's occupational statuses is recognized; in 1971 it appeared as a separate tabulation in British official statistics (see Oakley and Oakley, 1979).

This incongruity has not been resolved – either by those who work in government offices or by sociological theoreticians. From a sociological point of view, the enduring character of social class as a differentiator of life chances and life-styles indicates a continuing need for some such classification. The problem is a substantial one that cannot be dealt with here (a fact that should not preclude, but rather necessitates, its being mentioned).

Housing problems

Any report of housing problems at any point in the pregnancy was counted as evidence. In this sense, 25 per cent of the women had housing problems.

Social class

The overall social class breakdown of the sample by female and male occupation was shown in Table 4.3. Of the sample, 66 per cent were middle class according to partner's occupation, 93 per cent according to the woman's own occupation, with most of these (62 per cent) concentrated in the social class III non-manual group. This clustering of feminine occupations in the service industries is one of the difficulties about a female-based definition of class. It suggests that some other basis for differentiating between groups of women must be found, since occupation, in its conventional male classifications, does not differentiate enough.

In this chapter I have outlined how maternal outcome to first birth was measured and defined in the Transition to Motherhood study. I have also picked out six groups of factors – birth, antecedent socialization, baby condition, work conditions, marriage and background – that turn out to be related to outcome, and discussed their operationalization in terms of the analysis of the research data. In the next chapter I present a model of some relationships between these variables that, I hope, begins to offer an understanding of why childbirth provokes different kinds of outcome.

CHAPTER 6

Only Connect

Why, after more than 150 years of systematic research does the area of postpartum disorders remain clouded in ambiguity?
[Brown, 1972, p. 351]

To recapitulate, mothers' reactions to birth in the Transition to Motherhood study were measured in six ways: by the presence or absence of postnatal blues during hospital stay, and of depressed mood and depression in the first five postpartum months; by the extent of a mother's anxiety when she first came home with her baby, and by her overall satisfaction with motherhood and feelings for her baby at five months postpartum. These outcome measures yielded the conclusion that unproblematic adaptation to first-time motherhood is unusual. Only two of the fifty-five women experienced no negative mental health outcome, had high satisfaction with motherhood and 'good' feelings for their babies. The proportions suffering from poor mental health ranged from 24 per cent (depression) to 84 per cent (postnatal blues).

The challenge of these figures can be seen in two ways: the task is either to explain why poor outcome occurs, or to understand how some women achieve parenthood without apparent emotional difficulty. The two goals are interdependent: what explains one will presumably explain the other. Yet the different phrasing has important *political* implications. To ask why some mothers adjust badly is to imply that they 'ought' to adjust well and, vice versa, inquiring why some do not have such difficulties validates these as 'normal'. For most of this chapter I use the phraseology that implies that 'adaptation' is normal for the important reason that this enables comparisons with other studies to be made.

In chapters 10 and 11 I discuss some of the connections between the social expectation of women's suitability for motherhood and their oppression as a minority group. Two areas of connectedness are the concern of this chapter: between the outcome variables themselves; and between outcome and the six groups of factors described in chapter 5, pertaining to birth, antecedent socialization, baby condition, work conditions, marriage and general background.

RELATIONSHIPS BETWEEN OUTCOME VARIABLES

Figure 6.1 shows how the six outcome variables are related (and not related). Adhering to the usual criterion of statistical significance, only three associations deserve comment: those between satisfaction with motherhood and depression, between anxiety and depressed mood and between depressed mood and postnatal blues. The most striking feature of this diagram is in fact the lack of connectedness between depression and other mental health outcomes. Moreover, the association between depression and satisfaction with motherhood suggests that whatever explains the occurrence of depression may also have a capacity to distinguish between those women who do, and those who do not, 'adjust' to their situation as mothers.

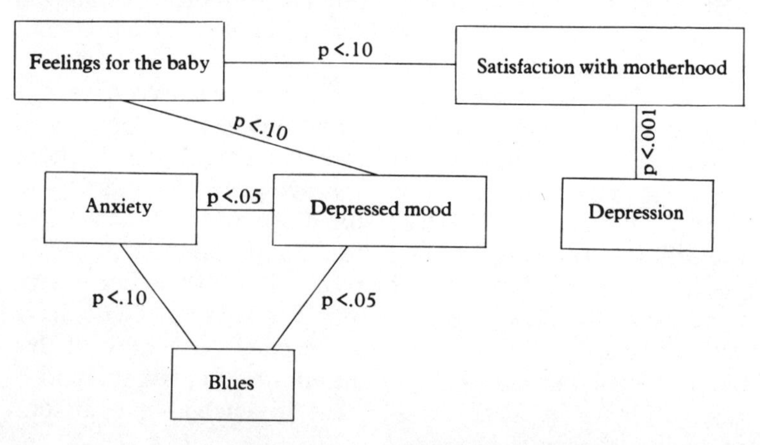

FIGURE 6.1 *Relationships between outcome variables*

Previous research has treated postnatal depression holistically and, in addition, has frequently overlapped its definition with general criteria of women's satisfaction with the social role of mother and with the kind of feelings they develop for their babies. Such research consequently offers little in the way of guidelines about the interrelatedness of different indices of women's feelings after birth. One example of this inadequacy is noted by Kaij and Nilsson, who point out that whether a woman experiences postnatal blues does not predict whether she will become depressed at a later stage:

> To the 'blues' is also ascribed a prognostic value for later neurotic reactions ... however ... this percentage [70–80%] is hardly compatible with any prognostic value ... firstly tearfulness is not a very characteristic sign of depression, and, secondly, the crying of the puerperium is not accompanied by a depressive mood. [1972, p. 371]

Depression is often taken to indicate a rejection of the baby and/or the social role of mother (as we saw in chapter 2); no such connection is evident in the Transition to Motherhood data. One other manifestation of the feminine paradigm is that poor satisfaction with motherhood and depression evidence a generally depressive ('neurotic' feminine) character. In the present study, of the four mental health outcomes, only depressed mood was associated with poor mental health in pregnancy ($p<.05$ with depressed mood in pregnancy) and there was actually an *inverse* relationship between depression in the pre- and post-birth periods. This may have to do with the shock feature of first birth and early motherhood, which is often greatest where expectations have been most idealistic and where the experience of pregnancy has been particularly smooth. The general failure of pregnancy mental health state to predict postpartum mental health state is a conclusion other researchers have reached (for example, Zajicek, n.d.; Nilsson, 1972).

Figure 6.1 shows that postpartum depressed mood and anxiety were related, as were the blues and anxiety, though less so. So far as this second connection is concerned, since both anxiety and postnatal blues were common (71 per cent and 84 per cent of the sample), some women were likely to get both – and both can in this sense be regarded as normal concomitants of first-time motherhood. (The 'normality' refers of course to a specific cultural context: institutionalized childbirth and socially isolated motherhood.) The same kind of argument applies to the association between anxiety and depressed mood. In mothers' accounts of how they felt when they first came home with their babies, being on their own and lacking social supports in their newly responsible maternal role were common themes. Social isolation, in particular, figured also in accounts of depressed mood, and it would seem that both anxiety and depressed mood were, in part, responses to the same set of circumstances.[1] This is shown in the interviews with Dawn O'Hara, a twenty-year-old Irish girl who lived in one room with her husband of one year and her five-week-old son:

Anxiety

When I came home with the baby I thought I'd crack up, I did. It was so strange, I can scarcely explain it now. I felt very anxious, I did you know. I felt it was difficult kind of getting used to the baby. I could feel myself – like when I got into bed – I could feel my head going around and I would feel as if I was going to get dizzy: I felt that, as if I was on a bus. And, you know, it can get to your tummy – sick. I felt tensed up, sort of, in case he was going to start. It's only natural. I think it was just getting used to the baby really. You can get easily upset, I think.

Depressed mood

Sometimes I feel I'm doing good – sometimes. But then when I hear him crying, I can't face it. And you start thinking of everything . . . have you enough money? And is your baby going to be alright? Are you going to make him happy? Even last night I was so fed up. I think I'm doing everything to please him, and when you feed him and change him and then he's still crying . . . then he gets me crying as well, when I can't please him. I feel that I'm not pleasing Kevin and I'm not pleasing the baby. I just go out and I slam the door and I go into the kitchen and have a good old cry. Stupid. But I feel like that sometimes. I feel sometimes that he doesn't understand.

When he cries all day it gets to me . . . I think I've smoked more cigarettes now than in my life. About twenty a day. I do get depressed. I get depressed with this room. You know what I mean? No matter how many times you clean it – every day – you get fed up with being here. Say you were going out to work, it'd be different.

Another factor underlying the relationship between postnatal blues and depressed mood may be the tendency to *express* the negative feelings that are felt. A woman who articulates her complaints of mood disturbance in the early puerperium may be more likely to do so later on in her experience of motherhood. Since the two outcomes referred to different phases of the transition to motherhood, there was not likely to be a 'contamination effect' here. Such an effect was, however, probably in part responsible for the associations between depressed mood and feelings for the baby and between feelings for the baby and satisfaction with motherhood. Here there was likely to be interaction between groups of attitudes and feelings. A mother who is prone to feel depressed may feel resentful towards her baby for placing her in her current predicament, or difficulties in the mother–baby relationship may make her feel depressed. Similarly, such difficulties are liable to overflow into her assessment of whether she is satisfied with motherhood, and feeling dissatisfied may influence feelings about the mother–baby relationship. Much the same kind of link could characterize the association between depression and adjustment.

Different outcomes are connected in terms of what is 'really' going on in the emotional lives of new mothers. Some aspects of this logic are revealed by Lily Mitchell, who is here talking about her life with five-month-old William. Lily was depressed, had a low satisfaction with motherhood and 'poor' feelings for her baby.

INTERVIEWER: *Do you like looking after the baby?*

LILY: *I do. I do and I don't. I'm having to adjust really, and there's times I miss a little of my own independence. I really do miss it now, I think. You know, I've never really put it into words for anybody before, but there's times when I feel if you went out for an afternoon, twice a week, just you, you'd be much better the other times. I find you're tied hand and foot every minute of the day . . . I mean other people can get on and do things, but if he's crying I stop doing what I'm doing. People say you just carry on doing what you're doing until you've finished and then you pick him up. You see I can't do that. So now I don't start to do things. I find I do less now than what I used to do when I was working. You know, generally about everything. I don't sort of cook the same. I don't, you know; I just think there's no point in starting this, because it won't get finished.*

Sometimes all you want is for somebody to just take that baby for a hour off you. You do. One of the neighbours took him just when I was getting a bit of depression, she came up and she'd never had him before, you know. And she said, what on earth is the matter? She could see something was wrong. And I said, everything's got on top of me. I said I just feel like throwing everything out in the street. Because I couldn't tidy it up, do you know what I mean?... She said, for goodness' sake, come on, we'll do it. And I said, actually I'd prefer it if you took William, because if you took him for an hour, I could do such a lot. And I just started and worked my way through. I felt so much better when I couldn't see dust.

INTERVIEWER: *How about feeding?*

LILY: *No, I don't mind it. It's part of the day: in fact it's a ritual of the day. The day really hasn't anything in it, unless you put something into it, really, has it? So I think, well, feed times are milestones through the day: just things to be done.*

INTERVIEWER: *Is there anything you especially dislike?*

LILY: *No. The only thing I find is that it's a very long day. Sometimes you get a bit tense at the end of a long day, so to speak. If he's particularly cranky, you know, it's your personality comes out, I think. He can be bad-tempered. I mean the doctor told me, when he tried to examine him, he said he's going to be a very strong-willed fellow when he grows up. And I said, he already is one. He wouldn't let him examine him, you know, he was screaming and kicking and fighting. He is bad-tempered and if he is, it's from me. And I do get bad-tempered with him.*

I don't feel I do anything. I feel I've done nothing, yet I still feel tired at night. I've become very apathetic. I'm just not interested in anything, really.

INTERVIEWER: *Do you feel you've done what you always wanted to do in having a baby to look after?*

LILY: *I never always wanted to have a baby. I didn't.*

INTERVIEWER: *Do you feel that there are parts of yourself you're not using at the moment?*

LILY: *I do. I just think that every day's going to go on like it is now. To me, there's nothing: I don't see anything back from it. Not back from William, I don't mean that way; every day just seems much the same as another... There's nothing I want to do and nowhere that I want to go and there's nobody I want to see. It's not a nice way to think; it's not a nice way to feel in fact.*

Everybody says it's too late for postnatal depression . . . I can only put it down to adjusting generally . . . I'm not trying to blame hormones or anything else. I feel it is just me finding it hard to adjust to being at home, I really do. I mean, when I was at home before, it was before I had him and things were different, do you know what I mean? But I think now, I've been home six months, and I think the next six months are going to be the same, and the next six months after that . . . I think depression is something which people can't understand, it is in a way self-indulgent, self-pity, feeling sorry for yourself, really it is: you know what I mean? You only have to see somebody worse than yourself. I mean I might be complaining, but the thing is, you do feel fed up sometimes, no matter who you are or what you are.

We can see how for women like Lily Mitchell depression and dissatisfaction may be two sides of the same coin: how the fragmentation and isolation of daily life as a mother prevents satisfaction and promotes depression. It is also clear how failing to derive satisfaction from performance of the social role of mother may rebound on feelings towards the baby, who comes to represent, even if it is not seen to cause, its mother's situation.

EXPLAINING OUTCOME

Since the data given in Figure 6.1 cannot tell us how these different patterns of outcome are created, it is necessary to move on to Figure 6.2. Figure 6.2 is the key ('mistress') diagram of the whole book. It summarizes the role of the groups of factors outlined in chapter 5, and the lines between the boxes are the contours of the argument presented in the rest of the book. Across the middle are the outcome variables. On the left-hand side are birth factors and on the right are factors related to work and baby conditions. At the top are marital and background factors; across the bottom those to do with socialization.

The following propositions can be argued from the relationships shown in Figure 6.2. They suggest that the four mental health outcomes – different components of the holistically

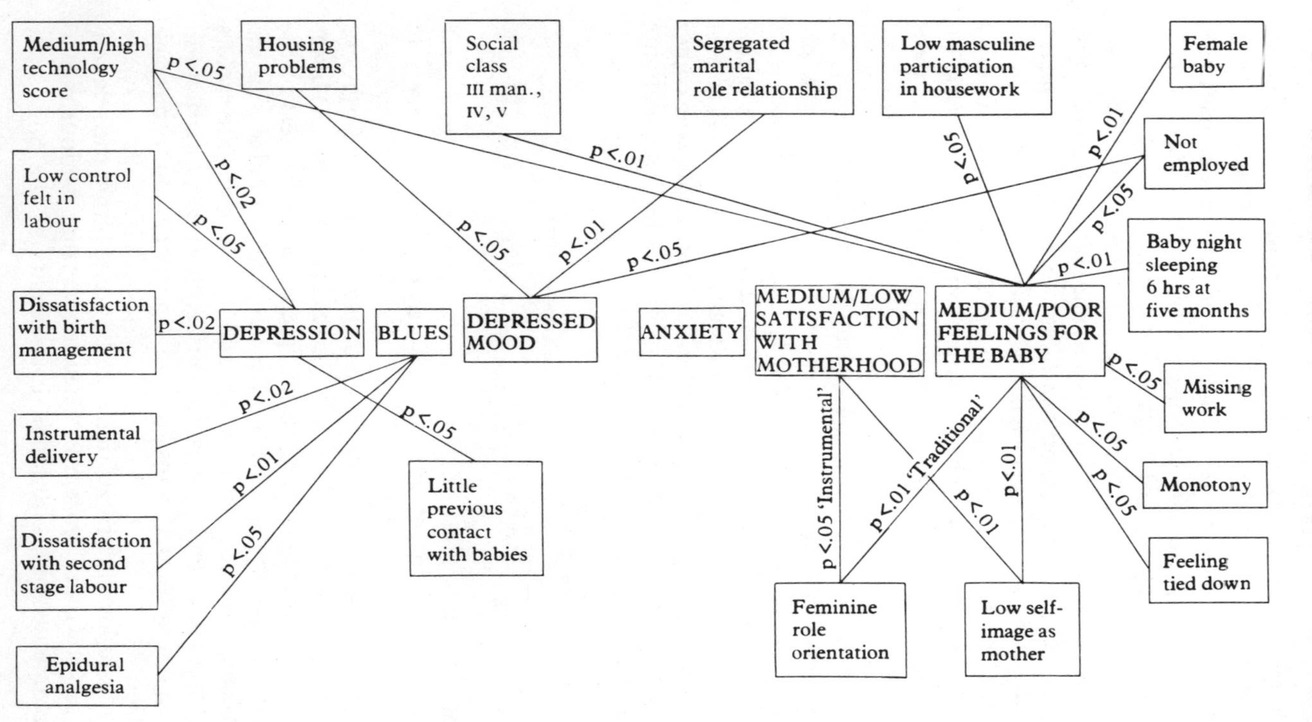

FIGURE 6.2 *Connections between outcome and other variables*

termed 'postnatal depression' syndrome – have differing aetiologies, and that satisfaction with motherhood and the type of relationship established between mothers and babies is influenced by past experience and present situation in ways that are not adequately represented by the feminine paradigm.

(1) *Postnatal blues* are related to aspects of birth management: instrumental delivery, epidural analgesia and dissatisfaction with second stage labour.
(2) *Depression* is associated with facets of the birth experience: a medium/high level of technology, a low degree of maternal control, and dissatisfaction with birth management; it is also more likely when previous job experience (contact with babies) is small or non-existent.
(3) *Depressed mood* is related to current life situation: bad housing, a segregated marital role relationship, lack of employment outside the home.
(4) *Anxiety* is not related to the experience of birth as such – only to birth as a provoking factor for first-time motherhood.
(5) *Satisfaction with motherhood* is linked with previous socialization – with the strength of the maternal self-image and with the kind of orientation towards the feminine role a woman displays.
(6) *Feelings for the baby* are also linked with feminine role orientation; but the baby itself – its sex and sleeping habits – is influential, as is current life situation – not being employed, missing work, experiencing monotony and feeling tied down, not having much help from fathers with housework, social class categorization in general.

POSTNATAL BLUES

Figure 6.2 shows that, in the Transition to Motherhood study, having the blues during postpartum hospital stay was associated with epidural block, dissatisfaction with the second stage of labour and instrumental delivery. These factors are themselves connected: epidurals cause a loss of reflex stimulation from the perineum and possibly also a general loss of muscle power, so that the incidence of instrumental delivery is increased two- or three-fold (Rosen, 1977). The risk is even higher in primigravidae who have not previously experienced the expulsion of a baby: in the sample hospital, 57 per cent of primigravidae given epidurals had forceps compared with 30 per cent of multigravidae who received epidurals (1975 figures). Dissatisfaction with second stage labour is liable to be greater when the achievement of pushing the baby out on one's own cannot be claimed. In some hospitals, babies delivered with forceps are routinely admitted to special care baby units for a short period, thus adding mother–baby separation to the list of epidural hazards; this, however, was not the practice in the sample hospital.

No pharmacological mechanism for the association between epidural block or/and instrumental delivery and postpartum blues is known. Although the drugs used in epidural analgesia and in other types of analgesia employed in instrumental delivery (and in any preceding induction or acceleration of labour) all pass into the maternal circulation (Moir, 1974), no specific tendency to provoke emotional lability in the immediate puerperium has been established. It may be that a pharmacological effect is mediated by the baby's behaviour. Sensitive neonatal neurological and behavioural tests show consistent changes in babies born after epidural block: they tend to be 'floppy', their muscle strength and tone are decreased, they are more irritable and prone to cry, and their sucking responses and food intake are also abnormal (Scanlon, 1976; 'Obstetric analgesia', 1974). A baby that is difficult and unresponsive in this way may make its mother more likely to suffer from the 'blues'.

Postnatal blues in this sense can be a response to a 'bad' birth – one that is characterized by unwelcome intervention and by the feeling that the mother was not her own baby's deliverer. Janet Streeter had a difficult forceps delivery:

I was in floods of tears the whole time [in hospital] . . . I hadn't been through it naturally, it was just that I'd been through that pain and this was just something that may have come from next door, you know? . . . I said the other day to Mike that I felt that had it been natural . . . I may have felt differently.

There is some evidence that postnatal blues is particularly related to the experience of a hospital birth. Over a third of the women explicitly attributed the blues to features of hospitalization: being separated from husband and home, problems in getting enough rest and in adapting to hospital routine, and conflict with staff over topics like feeding and baby care. For example:

I think actually all this business about postnatal depression is a load of rubbish. You only get upset when they upset you and you just tend to get a bit more *upset. I had no sort of real depression – no sort of sitting in bed feeling depressed for no reason at all. I don't think that exists. I don't think that people do get depressed for no reason. I think they get depressed because the baby won't feed properly – stuff like this.* (Cary Wimborne)

I think it was wanting to come home – I think probably I would have been like it if I'd had my appendix out. At home you wouldn't have to say goodbye to people and see them *come home. It's all circumstances.* (June Hatchard)

I didn't actually feel depressed. I was just exhausted: you don't get enough rest in there, do you? That's why I was crying. (Deidre James)

No systematic comparison of the incidence of postnatal depression syndromes in home- and institution-delivered mothers has been carried out. This is, as I contended in chapter 2, a consequence of the widespread idea that postnatal depression stems from some defect either in the mother's personality or in her hormone balance. The influence of social factors has simply been discounted. Cone (1972), reporting on a study of 193 Cardiff patients gives a 64 per cent depression (defined as weepiness during the first nine postpartum days) rate among hospital-delivered mothers compared with 19 per cent among those who had their babies at home. Conversely, Tod (1972), who studied 700 pregnancies over a five year period, 1958–63, says there is no difference in the incidence of 'puerperal depression' (not defined) between the two groups. A more recent study than either of these is O'Brien's (1978) survey of home versus hospital experiences in a sample of 2179 women delivered in mid-1975: she reports that there was no difference in the proportion of mothers who described themselves as 'weepy' some time after the birth according to place of confinement –

though she does state that in many ways the social and psychological experience of childbirth is described by mothers as more satisfactory when it takes place at home.

DEPRESSION

Becoming depressed at some point in the five months following birth was also preceded by obstetric intervention and feelings of dissatisfaction about the birth per se. In Figure 6.2, the relevant associations are with high/medium technology score, with low control in labour and with feeling dissatisfied in general with the way the birth was managed. Unlike the association between birth and the blues, these links were not usually made by the mother herself. Though the explanation might be put, the core of the depressed feeling was a sense of personal inadequacy that might not easily, at the time, be channelled into accusations of blame:

I kept thinking that I'd never be able to cope with him and do anything else at all. When the doctor came round, he told me exactly what I was going to tell him. He said, you're useless, he said, and, he said, you'll never be able to manage. But he said, probably what it is, he said, you had a bad time, and it's just taking it out of you like that. It's just a shock to your system. I don't really know. I had been so well when I was expecting, and it was just the shock, because I had a bit of a rough time. But I don't really know.

Maureen Paterson had earlier described her son's birth, which was marked by medical intervention and by a personal feeling of inability to control outcome:

They said being as how the water had broken, they couldn't sort of hang about. They fitted me up to one of them things [a syntocinon drip to accelerate her labour], *and then I had an epidural and I was having strong contractions sort of most of the time. . . . But the epidural didn't take very well, you know, and I kept getting terrible pain and he kept coming and topping it up, and in the end he said, I can't give you any more . . . I think it was because of the shape of my pelvis, it was the pressure of his head. I think he said there was just nothing they could do to stop* that *pain. Anyway, that went on . . . and the doctor kept coming round. And he said try for an hour to push the baby's head out: he said, there isn't much room. Otherwise, he said, we'll have to make a decision as to what to do. But, you know, I was too small, so at twelve o'clock he said, we'll take you upstairs, he said, and I'll try with forceps, he said, or else you'll have to have a caesarean, you know. They delivered him with forceps. And I was right out. . . . All I could remember was they took me up there and the anaesthetist put a thing over me face and he just said keep breathing deeply. And that was the last thing I remember until I woke up.*

Maureen Paterson did not directly blame the hospital for her dissatisfying birth experience, but was inclined to associate this with her later depression. Ellen George was also depressed, underwent a high technology birth (an epidural and a manual removal of the placenta under general anaesthetic) and felt little control during labour, but she articulated a hostility towards the medical managers of her birth:

It was such a nightmare. . . . I had an epidural and the first one didn't work – the woman who did it was a right South African bastard. . . . She strode into that delivery room and said I'm supposed to be at St Mark's in ten minutes: in other words, I don't want to have to come in here and do another bloody epidural. She stuck it in me and she left and it didn't work at all. . . . The other thing about the labour, looking back on it, was that I was supposed to be induced on the Monday. I went to the antenatal clinic with my suitcase, all keyed up, and was told I was ready to pop – I'd been ready to pop for ages. And was told that they were so busy on the labour ward not to come in – we can't face you. So come in on Wednesday and we'll do you on Thursday. Of course I started in labour that night and I knew *they were very busy. And I was received very cursorily by some nurse who did me and left me alone for ages and ages. . . .*

And I think that doctor who did the removal of the placenta disagreed with the sister. You see, I think I stopped having contractions after the birth and that was why they couldn't get it out, but at the same time the baby went slightly blue and they were working very hard on her. And I think he thought they should have done something to me but they couldn't – the baby was obviously more important. . . . I think they slipped up – no, not slipped up – but they attended to Emma to the detriment of me.

I think it was the whole childbirth . . . I do blame the hospital. I felt that if they'd given me the blood [a transfusion for a postpartum haemorrhage] *I wouldn't have felt the way I did. It was based so much on feeling so unfit and so exhausted. . . . I really* did *blame the hospital quite violently at one stage. . . . It was such a nightmare.*

Like the relationship between the blues and epidural analgesia, it is possible that the depression following high/medium technology birth could be mediated by the baby's state and behaviour. Although the babies born to mothers in the high/medium technology depression group were not statistically differentiated from the others on measures such as Apgar score and post-birth separation, there was a definite tendency in this direction. Had more sensitive indices of the baby's condition been available, an association between high/medium technology birth and maternal depression on the one hand, and morbidity in the baby on the other, might well have been evident.

The association between technology 'score' and depression is one of the most unequivocal findings of the study. This is because most of the measures of outcome and other variables had, necessarily, to be derived from the interview data, a procedure that, despite safeguards, always raises the possibility of overlap between one measure and another. But the technology score was arrived at independently of the interview data, being taken directly from the hospital medical notes, so that the association between depression and obstetric intervention was not likely to be an artifact of the research process.

One obvious counter-argument, that being depressed *preceded* the use of technology, is not borne out by the data. None of the women who were depressed after the birth were depressed when interviewed five weeks before it, and in twelve of the thirteen cases the onset of postpartum depression was clearly dated as occurring after the first two postpartum weeks. The only challenge to the analysis is presented by José Bryce, whose postpartum depression was mixed with mourning for her father, who died (not unexpectedly) of heart disease three weeks before her baby was born. When she described her feelings after the birth, both elements – grief for her father and the 'shock' of a technological birth – were manifested:

She [the nurse] *said why are you crying? . . . And all I could say was I want him here to see her . . . . I just wanted him to be alive just for one week or something so that I could have shown him the baby . . . But it was a postnatal thing as well; I mean I would have felt heartbroken about my father, but this was just illogical because I wasn't thinking about him. I'd just look at her and start crying . . . I did have nightmares about having her, about the forceps . . . I don't know, it was just horrible, you know. I just thought you'd be pushing away and it* [the forceps] *would just sort of lever it out and you wouldn't feel it. But it felt like a huge suction – as though everything had come out: as though I was all* empty . . .

If being depressed at the time of going into hospital to have the baby *causes* higher birth technology, the main way in which it might be expected to do so is through maternal requests for more technological aids, especially analgesia. To test this, a separate analysis of postpartum depression and birth technology was done omitting analgesia from the analysis:[2] the relationship still held ($p < .05$).

A second objection to the argument that technology is a direct cause of maternal depression might be that the degree of intervention in birth was a response to some pre-existing morbidity in the women involved. There were, in fact, more problems of high blood pressure, foetal malposition and 'post-maturity' in the high/medium technology group. But, on the other hand, there were more cases of (mostly minor) cephalo-pelvic disproportion and instances of delay between membrane rupture and the onset of contractions in the low technology group. What kinds and degrees of morbidity merit what kinds of interventions is far from generally agreed among obstetricians in the 1970s, and even among the women in this sample there were substantial variations in birth management according to the different policies of the consultants under whom the women were booked. Even if medical intervention in pregnancy, labour and delivery is in some degree a response to physical problems, it is difficult to see how these problems could themselves explain depression.

A third argument that could be put against the association between high/medium technology and depression is that there was some intervening characteristic of the women who experienced both that explains the technology–depression association as spurious rather than causal. There might, for example, be some non-medical aspect of patients that leads to doctors imposing technology, but that is also independently related to an increased incidence of depression. The most obvious possibility, social class, does not fulfil this role: neither women's own, nor their partners', social class was associated with depression or with degree of technology in the present sample. It is possible, I suppose, that some kind of personality factor could explain the association between technology and depression, but the only ones my research design enabled me to measure (feminine role orientation and maternal self-image) did not provide any support for this interpretation. In any case, even if the personalities of those women who received high/medium technology during labour and delivery and became depressed did differ in some way from those whose birth and postpartum experiences were more straightforward, this does not make redundant important questions about the medical use and psychological impact of technology. Indeed, if there are certain women who are more likely than others both to receive, and to respond adversely to, a technological birth, this is even more reason for a judicious re-evaluation of the use of such technology. (This argument is developed in chapters 8 and 10.) In this context, of explaining the technology–depression association, it is also relevant to note that whether or not the baby was initially planned or 'wanted' was not a factor that showed any association with outcome or with such crucial questions as the amount of technology employed in managing birth.

None of these counter-arguments constitute reasons for dismissing the association between technology and depression as a causal one. Even if there were other factors contributing to it, this does not mean that the relationship is destroyed – only that it is not a total explanation of why women become depressed. In chapter 7 I look at some such contributory factors.

The demonstration of a connection between depression and technology constitutes a major condemnation of the feminine paradigm. Instead of implicating women as the causes of their own postpartum mental disorder (either through personality weakness or hormone imbalance), the medical management of childbirth is characterized as a process that controls not only childbirth but women as well. Women's situation as mothers can thus be seen as partially at least located in their subjection to a system of medical monopoly.

Figure 6.2 also shows an association between depression in the early postpartum months and lack of job experience, i.e. little previous contact with babies. In general, lack of training for a new career appears to make transition to that career more difficult (Adams, Hayes and Hopson, 1976). Such an association in the case of mothers can be interpreted as a particular example of a general rule. (Chapter 8 develops this point.)

DEPRESSED MOOD

Unlike depression, depressed mood did not seem to be linked with the experience of birth, suggesting that, although some women might have described both in sequence, the association may be incidental rather than aetiological. In Figure 6.2 it is current life situation factors that appear to be associated with the tendency to feel depressed 'on and off' in early motherhood: housing problems, segregated marital roles and not being employed. Some of these connections, the way in which social situation mediates emotional satisfaction with maternal role, were described in the latter part of Dawn O'Hara's account of feeling depressed on p. 138. Dawn talked about the strain of living in one room and trying to accommodate both husband's and baby's demands in such a confined space; she pointed to the problems of divided marital interests and of maternal restriction to the home. Pat Jenkins, an ex-shop assistant and mother of Wayne, aged five months, expanded on the communication difficulty, on the strain of defining maternal childrearing as rewarding when the marital support system is virtually non-existent:

Wayne's just been getting me down, you know. I've just felt so tired, Alex doesn't really understand. When I get these silly ideas [about feeling depressed] *in my head he won't sit down and talk them out of me, he just thinks I'm silly.*

Every night he's coming in at ten o'clock, you know, or nine o'clock: eleven o'clock some nights, and he doesn't even say hallo to me, or anything. He goes and sits over there and works on papers or something. He's working too hard; he works seven days a week, he never takes a day off. He's in Saturdays and Sundays until about seven o'clock sometimes. And he doesn't really help with Wayne. He's never here. Sometimes I keep Wayne up for him at night, because I don't think he sees enough of him. You know I might as well not bother, because he never really bothers to play with him or anything. Just the mornings he'll play with him before he goes to work for ten minutes or so, if he's up early.

It's not so bad in the day, but, you know, you can't sort of go out in the evening, because Wayne has to be in bed. I just sit here and watch television.

Alex always scolds me, but he isn't with him all the time. The only time Alex sees him is when he's in a good mood. One time I really did shout at him [the baby] *. . . and he said, you know, you'll probably end up battering him. What a thing to say to me! Just because I shouted at him! And he said . . . if you feel tired, give him to me. But then he's never here, because he's always at work. When I was telling him about what the doctor said* [her doctor told her she was probably anaemic] *he went on watching the television. I said you're not listening to me, and he said no, because I'm not interested.*

In a marriage marked by such division of interests, there is no room to share not only the negative but also the positive side of childrearing. Where this is compounded with housing difficulties, the sense of being an unwilling prisoner in the home, the victim of a disabling domestic identity, is likely to be especially strong.

Anxiety

Anxiety on first coming home with the baby stands alone in the centre of Figure 6.2 and is apparently unique in having no connections with any of the six groups of factors otherwise associated with maternal outcome. It seems, as I noted earlier, that anxiety must be regarded as a usual accompaniment of first-time motherhood in a culture that assigns childrearing to women in a (normally) socially isolated nuclear family context. Since so many (71 per cent) of the sample women experienced it, and it was only temporary and only minimally disabling, anxiety on homecoming can probably be interpreted as a relatively trivial outcome measure.

SATISFACTION WITH MOTHERHOOD

Of all the propositions about outcome to the transition to motherhood suggested by Figure 6.2, this is the one that bears the closest relationship with the feminine paradigm contentions of the psychological literature – that how a woman 'adjusts' to being a mother is a function of her femininity. Figure 6.2 shows that a medium/low satisfaction with motherhood was associated with both 'instrumental' feminine role orientation and low self-image as a mother. Thus the data apparently support the idea that a 'traditional' orientation to the feminine role and a clear image of oneself as a mother predict well for a good 'adjustment' (self-reports of satisfaction with motherhood).

The women in the sample whose socialization and self-image were in this traditional direction did appear to feel more comfortable with the association between giving birth and the social role of mother: the feminine paradigm was one they were able to fit themselves into with relative ease. What is clear from the interview data is the importance of a motivation to *be* satisfied, which in turn can be traced through from childhood experiences and feelings about the mothering role:

When I was a child we had dogs and we used to play with dogs. Actually I remember dressing up puppies instead of dolls and wheeling them around in a pram, this sort of thing . . . At one point my ambition was to have a nice house in the country and have horses and dogs. A husband didn't really feature, but children did. I've always wanted to have a family. I hoped I would get married. I wanted to, because I wanted to be able to have children.

INTERVIEWER: *Can you imagine yourself as a mother?*

CATHERINE ANDREWS: *Yes, I think so. I'm looking forward to it, put it this way. My sister's only eleven. I used to change her nappies when she was two years old. I've always liked children. It doesn't seem strange at all to think of myself as a mother.*

INTERVIEWER: *Is there anything you're particularly looking forward to?*

CATHERINE: *Just having a child and doing everything for it, I've just got a maternal instinct.*

INTERVIEWER: *Do you intend to go back to work after the birth?*

CATHERINE: *I don't intend to. I think it's much nicer – it's nicer for you to be with your child. Okay, when they're at school you can be*

out when they're out, but I don't think a child should be left while you're out or left with somebody else, dumped. . .
INTERVIEWER: *Will you return to work sometime?*
CATHERINE: *No. Only if they were at school and during school hours. Unless, of course, I had to go out financially.*
INTERVIEWER: *Are there any ways in which you think women are treated unfairly at the moment?*
CATHERINE: *I suppose in some occupations there's discrimination. But then I think sometimes you do rather well out of being a woman . . . you get a seat on the bus, it has its perks. You don't earn as much, but then the chances are that you're going to do like me – get married and go off and have a baby – so you shouldn't get paid as much if you're going to do that.*
INTERVIEWER: *What would you think of a marriage in which the husband stayed at home to look after the children while the wife went out to work?*
CATHERINE: *It's not the way I would do it.*
INTERVIEWER: *Why not?*
CATHERINE: *I don't really fancy working for the rest of my life in an office. Particularly in my sort of job* [she is a receptionist]. *It's not the sort of job that leads to anything. It's roughly the same thing year after year. It wouldn't get me anywhere. Anyway, I'd like to look after my children – it's as simple as that.*

After the birth of her daughter:

INTERVIEWER: *Do you feel you have a maternal instinct?*
CATHERINE: *Oh, I think so, yes. It's so difficult to analyse what you feel. Occasionally I sit there and say what can I do? Why won't she go to sleep? And Justin says, this is what you've always wanted, shut up and enjoy it. And he's quite right.*
INTERVIEWER: *Are you going to have any more children?*
CATHERINE: *Oh yes. In a way I'd like three. If you have them all too quickly it's all over. Ideally what I'd like to do is have two reasonably close, then have a gap, then have two more.*
INTERVIEWER: *If you had to describe to someone who didn't have children, what it's like to be a mother, what would you say?*
CATHERINE: *Oh dear! I've always loved children, so I think it's a nice feeling being the person who matters* most *to the child. I mean I've always liked playing with babies and children and it's nice to play with other people's babies, but when it's your own, you're the*

person who means most *to them, which is what's so nice about it . . . And it is very* rewarding *watching her grow up and thriving and learning things.*
INTERVIEWER: *Do you miss work at all?*
CATHERINE: *Well, I miss the money! No, I don't think I do miss the work, not a bit of it. I think sometimes I miss the sort of – it was a jolly place where I worked, it was good fun. I think if I'd been on my own all the time since Fleur was born I might have felt a bit cut off. But once we get out of London, the village we're moving to is a very friendly place, it's not the sort of place where you go a whole day without talking to anybody.*
INTERVIEWER: *Do you feel you're doing what you always wanted to do in having a baby to look after?*
CATHERINE: *I think there are probably bits of me that are lying fallow as it were. I don't exactly use much of my brain at the moment. But I don't feel as though I'm wasting away or anything, I mean I always* wanted *to have a family, so I'm quite happy to drift along and be lazy. . . .*

Any minor discontents that Catherine Andrews did feel were quickly dismissed by a reminder that she was fulfilling a lifelong ambition in being a mother or by seeking to minimize the disadvantages of motherhood – a difficult baby, isolation from other social relationships. A contrasting pattern is described by Hilary Jackson, for whom motherhood was not a major life goal, and to whom a mother's working conditions were an enduring cause for complaint. She had an 'instrumental' feminine role orientation, a low maternal self-image and low satisfaction with motherhood.

INTERVIEWER: *When you were a child, what were your favourite toys and games?*
HILARY: *Nothing in particular. I was a tomboy. I could throw a ball further than any of them. My grandmother told me off. My sister was always being a lady. She stayed at home and looked after the home, and I was always up the park with the boys. . . .*
INTERVIEWER: *Do you remember whether as a child you wanted to be like your mother and get married and have children?*
HILARY: *I was always career-minded . . . I probably wanted to get married when I was about fifteen, and then when nothing happened I probably just gave up the idea and put it right out of my head.*

INTERVIEWER: *And when you got married you gave up your 'career' job?*
HILARY: *Yes. My husband does shift work; you'll find this if you talk to policemen's wives – it's not possible for the wife to really take up a career because you don't see enough of each other. And if you're so bogged down with responsibility in your job, it's just no good. . . . You have to be a very tolerant person.*
INTERVIEWER: *Do you think of yourself as a mother?*
HILARY: *No. I don't think about it. It's probably just like having a puppy – you just look after it and that's it.*
INTERVIEWER: *What are you particularly looking forward to about having a baby to look after?*
HILARY: *I think when it's about six months, just trotting round with it: that's about all. At six to seven months they become more interesting, they start looking at things and that and I think that's when I'm most patient with my friends' children. . . .*
INTERVIEWER: *Are you going to go back to work after the birth?*
HILARY: *I hope to go back. If everything goes according to plan, my mother will look after the baby.*
INTERVIEWER: *Do you think babies need their mothers?*
HILARY: *Oh no. I don't think it matters when you're very young . . . I've got friends whose children don't see many other adults and they're clinging . . . they hide behind chairs and they've got all sorts of phobias.*
INTERVIEWER: *Are there any ways in which you think women are treated unfairly at the moment?*
HILARY: *I think you're just as liberated as you want to be. Some women just love being looked after and being at home and I think they get very vegetable-like and enjoy it.*

After her daughter's birth:

INTERVIEWER: *Do you think you have a maternal instinct?*
HILARY: *No. I always say to her* [the baby] *Hilary'll do this, Hilary'll do that – you know, I'm chatting away to her and I say Hilary'll change you, I never think to myself your Mum'll change you . . . I just can't visualize myself as a Mum coping with all the Mum problems.*
INTERVIEWER: *Are you going to have any more children?*
HILARY: *No, my husband's going to have a vasectomy. We only ever wanted one child.*

INTERVIEWER: *If you had to describe to someone who didn't have children what it's like to be a mother, what would you say?*
HILARY: *Well, I suppose that really you've just got to live from day to day. . . . I mean you don't get the free time like you had, you just can't come and go as you please. And you just can't leave them and let them get on with it. You've got to be there and you've got to cope.*
INTERVIEWER: *Do you miss work?*
HILARY: *I'm just looking forward to going back . . . I shall have to do something, I couldn't stay home all the time. I'll need something to just get me out of the house. It's the same old routine, isn't it? Washing and cleaning and feeding and washing and cleaning and feeding: then you go to bed.*
INTERVIEWER: *Do you feel you're doing what you always wanted to do in having a baby to look after?*
HILARY: *No way. Good God, no. I don't think I was born into it, no.*
INTERVIEWER: *Is anybody?*
HILARY: *I think they are, yes. I've got a friend who – that's* exactly *what she was put on this earth for. And this is what she really believes. She does believe it. She's* convinced *of it. And she says she knows this is what she was best at since she was about twelve, oh she's convinced. She's got two girls and she's five months pregnant with another one. And she's convinced this is what she was put on this earth for.*
INTERVIEWER: *So do you feel that there are parts of yourself that you're not using at the moment?*
HILARY: *Oh yes.*
INTERVIEWER: *But they're used in your job?*
HILARY: *I hope so. I hope my brain's going to be used a bit more than it is now. I mean, I think if you're an organized person, it just becomes so* routine *doesn't it? Everything's done. I just do it automatically. It's like changing gear – it's done so automatically you don't – I mean sometimes I sit down and I think to myself oh my God, what have I done? I've done everything before about nine o'clock. And there she is, out there asleep and the room's tidy and everything.*

A charitable sociological reformulation of the widespread idea that only 'feminine' women adjust to motherhood would be that people are socialized for particular social roles and, where this socialization is effective, people on the whole do not complain about the roles they are called upon to perform as adults. Where, on the other hand, this socialization has been lacking in some way, difficulties will be experienced. So far as motherhood is concerned, women who deviate from cultural norms of femininity (by having more education, greater career ambitions and a greater propensity to combine 'work' with motherhood) are those who are least likely to be happy with the conventional domestic role.[3] At least, they may be more ready to *articulate* rejection of such a role, in contrast to other more 'feminine' women who may feel dissatisfied but who express a continuing commitment to traditional domestic identities.[4] This disjunction between feeling dissatisfaction and expressing it may contribute to the current finding – that the most stereotypically 'feminine' women adjusted best to motherhood. Motivated to identify with the role of mother as culturally defined, they might have been less prepared to acknowledge difficulties – or to say that their difficulties added up to not enjoying being a mother. At the same time, the closer fit between their socialization for adult womanhood and the social requirements of maternity might, of course, actually have engendered more personal satisfaction.

FEELINGS FOR THE BABY

Women's feelings for their babies are also related in Figure 6.2 to previous socialization factors. The two relevant ones are a low maternal self-image and a *traditional* feminine role orientation. This is a contrary relationship to that described above between medium/low satisfaction with motherhood and an *instrumental* orientation.

How can this contradiction be explained? Is it possible that the same personality matrix should prognosticate well in the case of feelings for the baby but poorly for satisfaction with motherhood? One possibility that suggests itself is that the experience of self as passive and submissive ('feminine') was more conducive to negative appreciation of the baby as 'dictator'.[5] Or, since the weakness of all such research findings is their necessary dependency on verbal reports, the kind of feeling/identity – language disjunction noted above may also be influential here. Adjusting the explanation somewhat to this different case of traditional femininity being associated with negative outcome, one possible interpretation hinges on the value attached to maternal satisfaction in the cultural paradigm of motherhood. Perhaps the mother's reward in the mother–baby relationship is so much a taken-for-granted construct that it receives little overt expression. Or perhaps, even more sinister, the mother's happiness has a low priority in a hierarchy of child-centred needs.

The label 'feelings for the baby' combines positive and negative affect with expressed anxiety. Thus, it is the balance between these three that is reflected in the overall rating. Bearing this in mind, another possibility is that readiness to articulate both negative affect and feelings of anxiety is in part a function of maternal age and of a planned commitment to parenthood. Older women who have planned a baby for several years may express fewer negative feelings and less anxiety about their babies than young women who have moved directly into marriage and motherhood in their late teens or very early twenties, motivated by a no less intense desire to experience birth and motherhood but possessed perhaps of less realism and knowledge about the actualities of motherhood and childcare. Some of these explanations are illustrated in these extracts from the postnatal interviews with Elizabeth Farrell, who was twenty-eight, used to be a publisher's assistant, and had been married for five years, and Grace Bower, an ex-switchboard operator who was twenty-three and had been married less than a year when her baby was born.

ELIZABETH FARRELL, five weeks after the birth:

INTERVIEWER: *Do you like looking after the baby?*
ELIZABETH: *Yes I do. I find I enjoy her company tremendously.*
INTERVIEWER: *Is there anything you particularly enjoy?*
ELIZABETH: *Yes, I* particularly *like breastfeeding her . . . I tell you what I do enjoy – I can be miles away from her and you can feel it* [the milk] *sort of beginning to come. And I enjoy the feeling that she's dependent on me. I enjoy bathing her, too: she enjoys being bathed tremendously.*
INTERVIEWER: *Is there anything you dislike?*
ELIZABETH: *No, I don't think so.*
INTERVIEWER: *Do you ever get cross with her?*

ELIZABETH: *No, I don't think so. I always hand her to someone else when I feel like that.*

Five months after the birth:

INTERVIEWER: *Do you feel relaxed or tense when you're looking after the baby?*
ELIZABETH: *Very relaxed.*
INTERVIEWER: *Do you worry about the baby?*
ELIZABETH: *No.*
INTERVIEWER: *Do you ever feel angry with the baby?*
ELIZABETH: *No. I sometimes feel cross. I don't feel violent, because if I feel cross, it's always my fault, because she only ever cries really when she's hungry and I'm late feeding her, and that's my fault, so I've no right to feel cross. . . . Sometimes I feel harassed, because if she's shrieking in her chair I can't concentrate on getting the food ready; I have to keep rushing in and giving her a piece of crinkly paper to play with.*
INTERVIEWER: *Do you like looking after her?*
ELIZABETH: *Yes I do. I enjoy it, yes.*
INTERVIEWER: *Is there anything you dislike about it?*
ELIZABETH: *Well, after I've been out the night before and I have to get up and feed her the next morning – that I hate. But then I think oh, it's not her fault, it's my fault. She gives me – us – so much reward because she's so* nice. *I don't really mind anything.*
INTERVIEWER: *If you had to describe to someone who didn't have children what it's like to be a mother, what would you say?*
ELIZABETH: *Well, I'd give a glowing report of it . . . I mean obviously there are times when you get harassed, but I mean so far it's very* happy. . . .

GRACE BOWER, five weeks after the birth:

INTERVIEWER: *Do you like looking after the baby?*
GRACE: *I like this stage when he's falling asleep. . . . I didn't think – I thought he'd be* sleeping *a lot longer, I seem to be* with *him all the time. And it's always a time when food – lunchtime, dinnertime – and that means I'm always behind with my dinners. . . . If at a quarter to eight he wakes up, who do I feed, my husband or the baby? This is the thing I* don't *like. I wish he'd sort out his hours a bit better. He's usually up when my husband comes home, so I'm feeding him instead of getting dinner ready for my husband.*

INTERVIEWER: *Is there anything else you dislike?*
GRACE: *Yes, when he's screaming! I wish he'd go to sleep so I could* do *something. Especially when I've* started *something, and I want to finish it, and he wakes up in between and I can't finish it. Then I tend to be in a hurry to put him back so I can finish what I'm doing.*
INTERVIEWER: *Do you ever feel cross with him?*
GRACE: *When he's like this!* [baby crying] *You feel desperate. You think, anything to keep him quiet . . . I – my husband threatened to throw him out of the window, he never would. . . .*

Five months after the birth:

INTERVIEWER: *Do you feel relaxed or tense when you're looking after the baby?*
GRACE: *I have felt tense.*
INTERVIEWER: *Do you worry about the baby?*
GRACE: *Occasionally. Occasionally if I can't hear him breathing in the night I go over and see. And if I still can't hear I tend to touch him so he moves. My husband goes mad: You're going to wake the baby up! I'm not. Especially if I've just heard about a cot death – that's what worries me, because nobody knows why these children die.*
INTERVIEWER: *Do you ever feel angry with him?*
GRACE: *Oh yes, definitely. Usually in the evening when he won't go to sleep. Usually once a day, definitely.*
INTERVIEWER: *Have you ever felt like hitting him?*
GRACE: *I have sometimes. I put him in his cot. I think if I hit him I'd hit him too hard. Sometimes I've* shouted *at him. Then I've regretted it. But I've never hit him, because I think if I do hit him I wouldn't be able to stop.*
INTERVIEWER: *Do you enjoy looking after him?*
GRACE: *Yes.*
INTERVIEWER: *Is there anything you dislike about it?*
GRACE: *Crying. I dislike him when he's crying. Especially when I don't know* why *he's crying – that's the thing. He cries, and I think why are you crying? You've been fed and you've been changed: why?*
INTERVIEWER: *If you had to describe to someone who didn't have children what it's like to be a mother, what would you say?*
GRACE: *Well, I don't feel any different. So how can I say? You're a bit more restricted – well, you* are *restricted. . . .*

Thus the data suggest that both younger and older mothers may experience more difficulty in achieving a 'good' baby relationship than those who are aged 24–29 when their babies are born.[6]

Unlike satisfaction with motherhood as an outcome, the quality of mothers' feelings for their babies was associated with groups of factors other than those relating to previous socialization. These were: the baby's predilection for sleep at five months, missing outside work, finding babycare monotonous, feeling tied down by the baby, having little help from partners with housework, the baby's sex, birth technology and the 'umbrella' classification of social class.

The reasons why the first five of these factors should impinge on the mother–baby relationship are self-evident. Having a baby who is reluctant to sleep well at night and living with a man who is reluctant to help much with the housework are both causes of 'overload'. The amount of domestic and childcare work a woman has to do is inflated to the point where, even for the most enthusiastic mother, it can begin to colour her feelings towards her child. A feeling of loss in relation to employment outside the home may be expressed either in nostalgia for the past or as intention for the future, but both it and the experience of monotony and restriction to the mothering role are symptoms of women's 'captivity'. Such dissatisfaction with isolation in the home may be difficult to compartmentalize: it may affect and/or be expressed as related to the way a mother feels about her child. Some of the quotations used to illustrate earlier points (see Lily Mitchell, pp. 139–41) convey the pervasive character of the 'captivity' syndrome.

The last three factors associated with the mother–baby relationship in Figure 6.2 – social class, sex of the baby and birth technology – require more sophisticated explanation. Social class and mother–baby relationship were associated in the direction of 'high' social class (I and II) being linked with 'good' feelings.[7] The extracts from the interviews with Elizabeth Farrell and Grace Bower cited earlier are contrasting instances. What these two women had to say about their relationships with their babies gives some evidence of indicators known to be associated with social class: housing situation, the division of labour and interests between husband and wife. Particularly interesting is the fact that Elizabeth Farrell 'always hands the baby to someone else' when she feels cross (i.e. there is always someone else to hand it to) and her definition of the context of reward as a joint one; compare this with the tyrannical meal-demanding role of Grace Bower's husband and her responses to the conflicting demands of husband and baby in a one-room environment.

Such aggravations are almost bound to detract from maternal satisfaction. So, apparently, is the production of a female baby. Dana Breen, in her study of first birth, reports a similar finding, although in relation to postnatal depression: 61 per cent of the women in her sample who were not depressed had boys, compared with 17 per cent of those who were. She interprets this finding by choosing a position midway between that of traditional psychoanalysis and the narrowly cultural explanation that women like sons better because men are culturally evaluated as superior to women:

> Without endorsing Freud's notion that a woman compensates with her son for the lack of a penis (his basic explanation for female psychology) we can retain from him the notion that a mother's reaction to her son is 'the most free from ambivalence of all human relationships', at least initially. As is so often the case with Freud's generalizations, what may be partly reflected here is a cultural phenomenon, that of the greater value of males in our society and the widespread notion that having a boy as a first baby is preferable. [1975, p. 176]

Greater depression and irritability among mothers of girls – Breen also found more anger towards female children – would, in this argument, reflect an underlying disappointment and consequent guilt.

In the present study, depression was not more likely among mothers of female children, but there was a tendency towards mothers feeling more irritability with girls. As girls are less likely to be criers than boys (association between maleness and crying for half an hour or more a day at five months, $p<.05$), it is not easy to interpret this irritability in terms of some perceived dimension of the baby's behaviour. The impact of sex – the mother's, the baby's – on the relationship between them is probably profound, and not easily measured (see p. 128 for some 'measures' of sex preference). Many women did, in fact, indicate that the production of a male baby is culturally considered to be a superior achievement to the replication of femaleness:

Well, I suppose to be really honest, people think it's a bit more thrilling to have a boy. They feel it's a bit more clever to produce a boy. I'm sure if I have a boy and somebody next to me has a girl I'll feel oh I did a bit better than you! (Jane Tarrant)

I want a son, born in his own home ... Absolutely a romantic fantasy! I want an heir, I want a Buckingham to carry on the Buckinghams ... (Emma Buckingham)

And the association, as was noted in chapter 5, between maleness and achievement is reflected in the fact that 93 per cent of the women who gave birth to boys were pleased, compared with 56 per cent of those who had girls. The occurrence of postnatal blues may be one response to 'failure' here – there was more among the mothers of girls, though not at a statistically significant level.

Chodorow has suggested a more complex mechanism underlying maternal responses to different sexed children that has to do with the different capacities boy and girl babies have by virtue of their sex to provoke feelings of maternal identification:

> Specifically, the experience of mothering for a woman involves a double identification ... Given that she was a female child and that identification with her mother and mothering are so bound up with her being a woman, we might expect that a woman's identification with a girl child might be stronger; that a mother who is, after all, a person who is a woman and not simply the performer of a formally defined role, would tend to treat infants of different sexes in different ways. [1974, p. 46–7][8]

Conversely, separation seems to be the hallmark of a mother's relationship with a male child, 'by emphasizing his masculinity in opposition to herself'.

Shereshefsky and Yarrow's study of *Psychological Aspects of a First Pregnancy and Early Postnatal Adaptation* produced data that confirm parts of this argument. They found that 'adaptation' to pregnancy related positively to responsiveness to the baby in the case of girls, but not boys, and suggest on this basis that mothers feel they 'know' baby girls but find it necessary to respond much more directly to the personality and behaviour of boys (1973, p. 233). Perhaps, then, one dimension of the association in the present research between a female birth and medium/poor feelings for the baby is that mothers simply did not spell out the way they felt about their daughters, whereas the motive for articulating feelings about sons was the mother's sense of the male child's difference from herself. Sex differences research supports the identification bias of mothers toward daughters: Moss (1970) has shown with a sample of neonates how the tendency to *imitate* the baby's behaviour is stronger in the mothers of girls than boys, and a study by Murphy (1962) indicates how maternal behaviour towards boys may be patterned by an early respect for the child's autonomy that is absent from mothers' relationships with girls.

The tendency to identify with girls received some verbal support in the current study. For example:

It's extraordinary, when I first, in the first week, I thought she was *me; it was really strange, such a strange feeling. I could just see myself, and it was as if I was feeding myself.* (Sue Johnson)

And in this context it is also interesting to note that in the Transition to Motherhood study girls were more likely to be breastfed ($p < .01$).[9]

A final association described in Figure 6.2 was that between the degree of technology used in birth and the kind of relationship that subsequently developed between mother and baby. A high/medium technology birth was linked with medium/poor feelings for the baby. This, like the association between depression and birth technology, can be seen as an especially striking condemnation of the feminine paradigm. Although the possible relationship between technological birth and maternal depression has received little investigation in research to date, the contribution of different styles of birth to the formation of affective ties with the baby is a territory that has been somewhat better covered. (Perhaps because the direct impingement on child welfare has more closely fitted the child-centred paradigm of research on motherhood. The argument that a mother's depression matters primarily as it affects the child is also to be found.) The early hours and days of the baby's separation from its mother have been studied, in particular to discern the possible influences of disturbances in 'bonding' at this stage on later baby-battering behaviour. Klaus and Kennell (1976) have established this link and they have shown that extra contact during the first three post-delivery days is tied to differences in maternal behaviour two years later – at least among working-class mothers.

One interpretation, then, of the finding of the present study that high/medium technology birth and medium/poor feelings for the baby were associated is that it signifies some of the same links between birth and maternal outcome that the 'separation' research has already shown. However, what is, as yet, unaccounted for is the mechanism whereby cultural intervention in the birth process brings about such difficulties. *Why* should separation from the baby immediately after birth lead to relationship difficulties? What is happening at the level of a woman's feelings about herself as a person, as a mother and as a childrearer that accounts for the influence of birth technology on this relationship?

To show the existence of statistically significant associations between variables is one aim of factorial research, but in this exercise not much may be said about the personal meaning of the experience under study. *Why* maternal outcome to first childbirth should be so crucially linked to particular factors is an inquiry that can only be carried out at the level of individual personality and meaning. What is needed, then, is a model that provides such a theoretical interpretation.

CHAPTER 7

Victims and Victors

A headstrong young woman in Ealing
Threw her two weeks' old child at the ceiling;
When quizzed why she did,
She replied, 'To be rid
Of a strange, overpowering feeling'.
[Gorey, 1974]

It is clear from what has already been said that the six measures of outcome to the transition to motherhood adopted differ considerably from each other. They refer to states/processes that varied in kind, permanence and connectedness with other aspects (past or present) of a woman's life. Both postnatal blues and anxiety on homecoming were short-lived reactions – in the first case to aspects of medicalized birth; in the second, to the new responsibilities of motherhood. Depressed mood was associated in a similar way with current social environment: housing problems, lack of employment outside the home, a division of interests between the parents. Satisfaction with motherhood was marked by the opposite case of an association with *antecedent* factors: both feminine role orientation and self-image as a mother, which develop mainly in relation to pre-adult gender role socialization. The last two measures of outcome – depression and feelings for the baby – related in a more complex way to multiple influences. The categories of 'medium' or 'poor' feelings for the baby were associated with antecedent socialization (self-image as a mother) and with social–contextual factors: not being employed, missing work, feeling babycare routines were monotonous and restricting, low masculine participation in housework and general social class location. But also important were the baby itself (its sex and sleeping habits) and the circumstances of its birth (the degree of technology used). In the case of depression, most of the associations were with birth factors too: technology, degree of control experienced during labour, satisfaction with birth management; but lack of previous job training – little or no contact with babies – appeared as an additional factor associated with poor outcome here.

In this chapter I want to begin by focusing on one of these outcomes only – depression (although at times the argument will combine this with depressed mood). The rationale for singling depression out in this way is three-fold. In the first place it represents a *major* outcome: it may have a quite severely disabling effect on normal life. Second, in suffering from postnatal depression a woman becomes overtly a victim of her childbirth experience: the legitimacy of the shock of first birth is publicly acknowledged. The symptoms of depression may thus tell us something about both the emotional impact of childbirth in general and the cultural ideology pertaining to women and reproduction in particular. And, finally, the apparent association between current methods of childbirth management and later depression in the mother is both striking and in need of elaboration: *why* should some kinds of childbirth be especially liable to cause depression? What distinguishes those who become victims from those who are victors over the experience of childbirth?

'The only known specific aetiological agent in puerperal breakdown is childbirth' (Lomas, 1967, p. 131). To an extent this is a tautology: of course the only antecedent factor that women suffering from postnatal breakdown have in common is childbirth – otherwise the breakdowns from which they were suffering would be differently labelled. What kind of reaction depression represents in general is disputed, but one view is that it arises out of the meaningfulness of experience.[1] If events, relationships, activities and goals did not possess meaning for the individual, frustration and loss in relation to these would not lead to depressed feelings. Pregnancy and birth are no exception to this rule; indeed, given the either supposed (according to the feminine paradigm) or actual (according to women's own accounts) importance of reproduction in a woman's life, there are grounds for believing that childbirth is perhaps more likely to provoke depression than many other life events, since its meaningfulness is so great. (It is interesting to note that this makes childbirth within the feminine paradigm *more* and not less likely to cause depression, since meaningfulness is expected to be heightened in 'feminine' women.) To equate the meaningful role childbirth has in a woman's life with the existence of a specific form of depression peculiar to childbirth would, however, be a mistake. Psychiatry has come a long way since the supposition that maternal hysteria arose directly out of the uterus; and

> It is now generally agreed that there are no specific mental illnesses related solely to pregnancy, childbirth and the puerperium, and that the mental illnesses which occur in relation to these events are essentially the same as those occurring otherwise. [Bardon, 1972, p. 335]

The trouble, as we saw earlier, with most existing 'explanations' of depression is that they assume the contrary: postnatal depression is seen as a specifically feminine disorder that must be aetiologically linked not only to childbirth but also to the whole previous development of feminine personality structure.

Depression seems to be occasioned by feelings of hopelessness that precipitate disturbances in body functioning and social activities. It has been argued that it is the *generalization* of such hopelessness that forms the core of a depressive disorder (Brown and Harris, 1978, p. 235). Such a disorder may arise endogenously, but it is more likely to be associated with changes in a person's environment. It is a *human* condition, a symptom of the difficulties human beings have in living happily with themselves and each other. Seen in this context, the depression that may follow childbirth is a condition of hopelessness in a general human sense. An understanding of why postnatal depression occurs is not a *separate* question from the question why depression in general occurs: it is one and the same question.

There is widespread agreement among those who treat, and those who study, mental illness that certain kinds of situations and events are especially likely to precede mental disorders. This category includes natural disasters, deaths, births, occupational changes, retirement, migration, major physical illness and disablement. All these are 'life events', situations that are liable to influence what Parkes has deemed an individual's 'assumptive world':

> The assumptive world is the only world we know, and it includes everything we know and think we know. It includes our interpretation of the past and our expectations of the future, our plans and our prejudices. [1971, p. 103]

The role of life events is crucial because of their capacity to disrupt a person's assumptive world in a negative sense – to cause stress and distress. Yet while life events are by definition potentially disruptive, they may be so because they are associated either with misery or with joy. People's responses to life events cannot be gauged from some objective characteristic of the event itself.

The hallmark of a life event is change; that change may affect an activity, a role, a person or an idea. Within life event research, childbirth has usually been classed along with other life events in terms of a common capacity to bring about disruptive changes in a person's assumptive world (as in Brown and Harris, 1978). Within the literature on motherhood, however, birth has *never* been ceded an equal status with other life events. Depending on the assumptions about women that are made, it is seen instead as 'naturally' more or less traumatic than other categories of social change – job changes, bereavement, etc. The language has been that of crisis rather than of life event – crisis being defined as anything that 'interrupts the flow of habit and gives rise to changed conditions of consciousness and practices' (Macintyre, 1977a, p. 63). The inadequacy of this perspective is shown particularly well by Macintyre in her study of pregnancy in single girls – a group in whom the crisis response would be most predicted, but was, in fact, often missing.

The term 'life event' carries no connotations of a particular outcome; 'crisis', by contrast, implies a turning-point in a person's life that produces marked negative emotion and requires resolution, so that pre-crisis equilibrium can be re-established. To argue that all first births constitute a crisis for the mother (or that all pregnancies represent a 'sick role' –

another historically dominant sociological perspective) is inseparably to join the event to one kind of meaning.

In their recent study of depression in London women, Brown and Harris found that although 'patients' (women receiving psychiatric treatment for depression) had a rate of pregnancy and birth events twice that of normal women (a random sample of women in the same community as the patients), the association was entirely due to the pregnancies and births that occurred in the context of a severe ongoing problem (e.g., poor housing, a disintegrating marriage). They conclude:

> . . . in our series there is *no* evidence that childbirth and pregnancy *as such* are linked to depression . . . the result clearly suggests that it is the meaning of events that is usually crucial: pregnancy and birth, like other crises, can bring home to a woman the disappointment and hopelessness of her position – her aspirations are made more distant or she becomes even more dependent on an uncertain relationship. [1978, p. 141]

This interpretation of the role pregnancy and childbirth play in the genesis of depression begs certain questions, as we shall see later on. However, it is not part of Brown and Harris's goal to define reproductive life events according to the emotions they *actually* produce in different individuals – which would be one way to approach the question of why some mothers become depressed and some do not. Their methodology rules out this type of measurement, and focuses instead on the *likelihood* of certain events producing strong emotion – which is, as they argue, precisely its strength. So to suggest answers to the 'why' question of differential outcome requires an alternative approach: one that centres on the issue of why some people have greater *vulnerability* than others to the depression-provoking character of life events.

In terms of Brown and Harris's analysis, the argument is that *social* factors have the capacity to promote or prevent vulnerability. The four they single out are: lack of an intimate relationship; three or more children under fourteen at home; loss of mother before eleven; no employment outside the home. They found that these factors distinguished between different likelihoods of developing depression in the presence of a provoking agent (life events and ongoing difficulties). Thus, while, for example, only 11 per cent of non-employed women with an intimate relationship became depressed, depression affected 100 per cent of those lacking such a relationship and with either early loss of mother or three or more children under fourteen. Of the four vulnerability factors, intimacy and employment seem to confer the greatest protection (Brown and Harris, 1978, ch. 11 'Vulnerability').

Applied specifically to the effect of first childbirth as a life event, the notion of vulnerability has an obvious relevance. The interview material suggested that different degrees of vulnerability to stress might be an important dimension: there seemed to be crucial differences between women who had a 'victim' response to pregnancy and childbirth and those who gave the impression of being in control of, victorious over, the experience.

I shall deal with this point on a statistical level first. Table 7.1 shows the rates of depression in four 'vulnerability' groups. The criteria ('vulnerability factors') are: lack of employment, housing problems, segregated marital role relationship and little/no previous contact with babies. These particular vulnerability factors emerged in the women's own accounts as related to the experience of depression. Many of those who had

TABLE 7.1 *Depression plus depressed mood and vulnerability factors*

	Depression + depressed mood		
*Vulnerability factors**	*Depressed* % (*N*)	*Not depressed* % (*N*)	*Total* % (*N*)
Four factors	100 (4)	0 (0)	100 (4)
Three factors	70 (7)	30 (3)	100 (10)
Two factors	53 (11)	47 (10)	100 (21)
One factor	20 (4)	80 (16)	100 (20)

$N = 55$.
$p < .01$.
* Not employed, segregated marital role relationship, housing problems, little/no previous contact with babies.

no paid work mentioned the lack of a non-domestic identity, a feeling that they were not contributing their own income to the household and the loss of employment-based social relationships. Housing problems featured as a direct cause of depression in these accounts, and are a difficulty that many women encounter at this early motherhood stage of family life. A division of interests/activities/decision-making between women and their partners was also cited as a factor contributing to depressed feelings.[2] The fourth vulnerability factor chosen (little/no previous contact with babies) is the one non-birth factor that Figure 6.2 shows was statistically associated with depression. On a commonsense level it is understandable how early motherhood could more readily provoke depression in those women who had no previous idea of the responsibility and work entailed by babycare. Again, this interpretation was offered by some of the women themselves.

Table 7.1 conveys a picture of a direct association between depression incidence and increasing vulnerability. Twenty per cent of women with one vulnerability factor were depressed, rising to 53 per cent with two, 70 per cent with three and 100 per cent with four. (There were no women with no vulnerability factors.) This table combines depression and depressed mood, thus implying that while differing in severity the two syndromes are linked in the sense that some cases of depressed mood would be expected to become cases of depression with symptoms. (The association of the vulnerability factors with depression only was: four factors, 20 per cent depressed; three factors, 40 per cent depressed; two factors, 38 per cent depressed; one factor, 0 per cent depressed.)

Table 7.1 clearly points in the direction of social context being differently associated with a risk of depression following first birth. Indeed, these social factors may constitute the 'social class' meaning of vulnerability to depression; as I mentioned earlier, neither the women's own social class nor that of their partners showed a statistically significant relationship with depression. In terms of the importance Brown and Harris found attached to intimacy and employment status as particular kinds of vulnerability factor, it is interesting to note some parallels here. An association between employment status as a single vulnerability factor and the occurrence of depression plus depressed mood was evident ($p<.025$) but an even stronger association ($p<.001$) emerged with type of marital role relationship considered in isolation from the other vulnerability factors. The social context of the marriage relationship, then, seems to be an especially crucial factor in a woman's avoidance of poor mental health after childbirth.

Life events, and childbirth is no exception, vary in the degree of threat[3] to mental health they pose. Figure 6.2 (p. 142) shows diagrammatically some of the dimensions of childbirth that appear to be associated with threat – they are linked with poor mental health outcome. Three of these dimensions (dissatisfaction with birth management, low control felt in labour and dissatisfaction with second stage labour) were assessed directly from the women's accounts of birth.[4] Epidural analgesia, instrumental delivery and technology score were derived from the hospital medical notes. Technology score as a composite index, including analgesia and all types of medical intervention, can thus be seen as a direct representation of the degree to which an individual birth is determined by medical–professional activity. Technological variation in birth experiences offers one criterion for discriminating between births as life events. The hypothesis would be that childbirths that were relatively high in technology 'score' would be more potentially stressful maternal experiences and therefore more likely to be followed by depression. Whether or not depression in fact occurred would then be seen as partly a function of social context – being 'vulnerable' or 'protected' by virtue of the absence or presence of social defences and supports. Tables 7.2 and 7.3 show the figures, for both depression singly and in combination with depressed mood. Evidently the relevance of the analysis is greater in the case of depression. All thirteen of the women who became depressed fell into the high/medium technology, two or more vulnerability factor group; when depression is combined with depressed mood this figure is twenty-one out of twenty-six (81 per cent).

The idea that a birth marked by considerable medical intervention is more likely than others to depress the mother is apparent in women's own descriptions of their births.[5] In terms of the manipulation of variables in the data analysis, the association between technology and depression is evident with-

TABLE 7.2 *Depression, technology and vulnerability factors*

Technology and vulnerability factors	*Depression*		
	Depressed % (*N*)	*Not depressed* % (*N*)	*Total* % (*N*)
High/medium technology:			
2 or more vulnerability factors	43 (13)	57 (17)	100 (30)
one factor	0 (0)	100 (11)	100 (11)
Low technology:			
2 or more vulnerability factors	0 (0)	100 (5)	100 (5)
one factor	0 (0)	100 (9)	100 (9)

N = 55.
Association between vulnerability score and depression in the high/medium technology group significant at 1% level.

TABLE 7.3 *Depression plus depressed mood, technology and vulnerability factors*

Technology and vulnerability factors	*Depression + depressed mood*		
	Depressed % (*N*)	*Not depressed* % (*N*)	*Total* % (*N*)
High/medium technology:			
2 or more vulnerability factors	70 (21)	30 (9)	100 (30)
one factor	27 (3)	73 (8)	100 (11)
Low technology:			
2 or more vulnerability factors	20 (1)	80 (4)	100 (5)
one factor	11 (1)	89 (8)	100 (9)

N = 55.
Association between vulnerability score and depression in the high/medium technology group significant at 2.5% level.

out the inclusion of maternal feelings as an intervening variable. To look at the contribution of maternal feelings about birth, I have introduced two other measures into the analysis: overall attitude to labour and 'achievement' rating. The first of these is simply derived from answers to the question asked at five weeks postpartum: 'would you describe your labour overall as a pleasant, tolerable or unpleasant experience?' The second is a multiple rating that includes not only overall attitude to labour but also the dimension of the degree of control experienced during labour and satisfaction with the second stage. Overall attitude to labour was related to depression irrespective of vulnerability status ($p < .01$); achievement was not. Tables 7.4 and 7.5 indicate the relevance of these measures to vulnerability status and outcome. Table 7.4 shows that 62 per cent of the group with high vulnerability who didn't enjoy labour became depressed as against 23 per cent who tolerated or enjoyed labour. In Table 7.5, which gives the analysis by achievement rating instead, 41 per cent of the medium/low achievement + high vulnerability group were depressed, compared with 25 per cent in the high achievement + high vulnerability group.

The way a woman feels about her labour clearly influences her chances of becoming depressed. This mediates the impact of a high/medium birth technology, so that if, in this situation, she can maintain some sense of herself as the person having the baby she may be effectively immunized against later depression. Enjoying as opposed to not enjoying labour is a more powerful discriminator here than an index that reflects control and second stage satisfaction, though the two measures are obviously not unconnected.

To summarize the argument of this chapter, it seems that 'victim' and 'victor' responses to childbirth have to be interpreted in terms of three sets of factors: the mother's social context, the medicalization of the birth, and the mediation of maternal feelings about this. A high/medium technology birth carried a particular risk of maternal depression that was intensified by social vulnerability (not being employed, having had little/no previous contact with babies, experiencing a segregated role marriage and housing problems). All thirteen of the women who had major depression during their first five postpartum months were vulnerable in two or more of these ways, and were subjected to the trauma of a birth characterized by above average levels of technology and intervention. But mothers are not merely passive responders to the input of birth

TABLE 7.4 *Depression, overall attitude to labour and vulnerability factors*

Overall attitude to labour and vulnerability factors	*Depression*		
	Depressed % (*N*)	*Not depressed* % (*N*)	*Total* % (*N*)
Didn't enjoy labour:			
2 or more vulnerability factors	62 (8)	39 (5)	100 (13)
one factor	0 (0)	100 (4)	100 (4)
Tolerated/enjoyed labour:			
2 or more vulnerability factors	23 (5)	77 (17)	100 (22)
one factor	0 (0)	100 (15)	100 (15)

N = 54.

TABLE 7.5 *Depression, birth achievement and vulnerability factors*

Achievement and vulnerability factors	*Depression*		
	Depressed % (*N*)	*Not depressed* % (*N*)	*Total* % (*N*)
Medium/low achievement:			
2 or more vulnerability factors	41 (11)	59 (16)	100 (27)
one factor	0 (0)	100 (13)	100 (13)
High achievement:			
2 or more vulnerability factors	25 (2)	75 (6)	100 (8)
one factor	0 (0)	100 (6)	100 (6)

N = 54.
$p < .01$.

technology; their own enjoyment or lack of it during labour and delivery distinguished victims (who become depressed) and victors (who do not) even in the presence of high social vulnerability.

In terms of the feminine paradigm that has been the chief model used in studies of postnatal depression to date, the finding of close links between maternal depression and social context is a marked indictment of the limitations of this approach. Childbirth happens in a medical, social and economic context that has the capacity to shape the contours of a woman's reactions to it. There is a crucial dialectic between the way childbirth happens in modern industrialized cultures and the way mothers are supposed to be – married, at home, economically disadvantaged and dependent, and blessed with a maternal instinct that enables them to rear children without first learning how to. The interplay between the ideology and practice of childbearing on the one hand and motherhood on the other, catches women in the dilemma of chasing personal human satisfaction across the psychological wasteland of alienated reproduction and captive motherhood.

So far what has been proposed is a somewhat limited version of the victim versus victor model: one that operates at the level of associations between measures of birth as a life event and social context on the one hand, and mental health outcome on the other. Apart from the general supposition that life events are theoretically, and can under certain circumstances be actually, stressful (and an argument that places first childbirth within this category), how the life event of first birth is interpreted psychologically and emotionally by mothers themselves has not been spelt out. This goal requires a more detailed exposition of the social and personal meaning of first birth as an example of general transition: this is the subject of the next chapter.

CHAPTER 8

Reproduction and Change

I am dumb and brown. I am a seed about to break.
The brownness is my dead self, and it is sullen:
It does not wish to be more, or different.
Dusk hoods me in blue now, like a Mary.
O colour of distance and forgetfulness! –
When will it be, the second when Time breaks
And eternity engulfs it, and I drown utterly?
[Plath, 1971, p. 43]

So far I have argued two main points. First, I have tried to show how the feminine paradigm as a conceptual tool in the understanding of women's reactions to childbirth has severe limitations. Second, I have proposed in its place the analysis of childbirth as a life event as an exercise that is more likely to produce reliable and relevant explanations. I now move on to consider the social and personal meaning of first birth in more detail. I will argue that childbirth shares key characteristics with other less gender-differentiated classes of life event, and that the personal meaning of childbirth to mothers is revealed by describing these similarities, rather than by appealing to its character as a feminine process. This is essentially an argument about the way human beings react to change, and *my* argument is that reproduction is an archetypal example of such life change, carrying tremendous physical, emotional, psychological and social implications for those who engage in it.

Having said that childbirth is a life event akin to others, one major qualification must be added. This is that first childbirth and subsequent childbirths are different – not definitionally but usually, that is in terms of women's own accounts of their reproductive and maternal histories. The adaptations that are required during and following first childbirth arc different and on the whole greater than those that attend other births. Having her second, third or fourth child, a woman is already a mother, is familiar with the experience of giving birth and looking after a baby and has grown accustomed either to committing herself to the domestic scene or to juggling the demands of motherhood and full- or part-time employment; the particular strains of combining marriage or some other heterosexual partnership with the requirements of childrearing are not new to her either. (Which is not to say, of course, that later births do not carry special problems or benefits of their own – the focus on *becoming* a parent has, as we saw in chapter 3, limited our understanding of these other aspects of parenthood.)

The point is that *in general* it makes more sense to treat childbirth as one among many life events. But, on the other hand, it is a mistake to assume that first and subsequent childbirths are necessarily the *same kind* of life event. It is another consequence of the prevalence of the feminine paradigm in reproductive research that by definition all childbirths have been seen as the same as each other and different from other kinds of life change. The conventional perspective is illustrated in Brown and Harris's treatment of pregnancy and birth in *Social Origins of Depression* (1978); laudably viewing reproduction as a life event rather than as a feminine happening, and proposing that first births are intrinsically more threatening than others, they nevertheless categorize all reproductive experiences separately from other life events (for example job changes). Their entrance into the theoretical interpretation of depression is in terms of their particular character as female biological events.

The most dominant metaphor used by the women in the Transition to Motherhood sample in talking about the process of becoming a mother was that of 'shock'. For example, in relation to the birth:

It woke me up from a deep sleep – such a sudden, strong pain . . . The way I woke up shocked *me, I was suffering from* shock *after it.*

I was in a state of shock *. . . time had stopped.*

It is a state of shock. *I was unaware – I mean I'd like to have another one, just to be aware of what's going on.*

He was so big – nine pounds six – I was absolutely shocked *out of my mind.*

And after the birth:

I felt it was lovely, holding her and everything, but I didn't really feel anything . . . because I was shocked.

I woke up in the middle of the night and I couldn't believe that I'd actually delivered him. It was such a shock.

I felt depressed in hospital. It was partly shock *really, and being away from home.*

And coming home with the baby:

I couldn't have managed without my mother, I couldn't have coped at all. I was so shocked, *I couldn't do anything.*

I think the biggest shock *was the amount of time that it required to look after a newborn baby.*

The recurrence of this term in the women's accounts portrays first-time motherhood as a powerful disturbance to established life-styles, routines and identities. Many described themselves as 'numbed' by shock, a familiar metaphor. For this reason 'shock', rather than 'crisis' (which does not imply temporary incapacity to feel and act), would appear to be a more appropriate description of the character childbirth has as a life event. A shock is 'A sudden or violent blow, impact or collision tending to overthrow or produce internal oscillation in a body subjected to it; A sudden and violent effect tending to impair the stability or permanence of something; A sudden and disturbing impression on the mind or feelings; usually one produced by violent emotion and tending to occasion lasting depression or loss of composure' (OED). These definitions encapsulate most of what women describe as disorienting about becoming a mother, and point precisely to the importance of analysing the traumas of childbirth as characteristics of a life event.

So what is the character of first pregnancy and childbirth as a life event? The interview material reported in this book suggests that it is a composite of the following dimensions:

Entry to the full adult feminine role (in the specific context of modern industrial culture).
A status passage from the role of non-mother to that of mother.
Retirement from the employment sphere.
Occupational career change.
Change in physical (bodily) state.
Entry to medical patienthood.
The experience of surgery.
A 'disaster' event.
Institutionalization.

These are the main processes that are carried on under the rubric of 'the transition to motherhood'. The point is not that each process is entailed by the passage to motherhood (though this is, of course, largely true) but that most of them constitute life events that occur independently of childbirth. Analysing individual responses to surgery, retirement, career change and so forth, may thus be expected to throw some light on the changes women undergo as they become mothers. In the rest of this chapter I shall consider each of these dimensions in turn, drawing on the relevant literature in the context of my interview data to illustrate how, and in what ways, the transition to motherhood parallels (or diverges from) other social transitions.

ACHIEVING FEMININITY

This first dimension of becoming a mother is self-evidently a female experience and in this way differs from the others. Motherhood is culturally equated with the achievement of femininity – by which I mean women's socially constructed gender role and identity, rather than the more specific and limited psychoanalytic meaning of feminine sexuality development described in chapter 2. Moreover, there is no direct parallel with the masculine gender role here, since parenthood and maturity are not linked in the same way for men. The achievement of fatherhood establishes fertility and, in the popular stereotype, by implication virility. It *alters* a man's image, emphasizing respectability in terms of ideologies of family life, but it is not held to establish the credentials of personal fulfilment as in the case of women.[1] Since research concerns develop in response to cultural paradigms, the meaning of the transition to parenthood for men in anything other than a narrow sexual sense has not received much attention. Fein (n.d.), in a study of American middle-class fathers, has shown how responses to impending and actual fatherhood among men may be stated derivatively in terms of wives' feelings. There appears to be no sense of identity confusion to parallel many women's experiences (although some fathers did say they wished they could change the balance of work and home in favour of home).

Without a child to call her own a woman in our culture falls short of cultural expectation. She has not achieved the standard that is set for all biologically female persons in that (a) she has not given birth and (b) she has not entered the feminine domestic triad wife–husband–child. Of course the standard that equates womanhood with reproduction is differently expressed and adhered to among different social groups. But the idea that only women with children are 'proper' women is remarkably pervasive even in these days of public commitment to sex equality:

INTERVIEWER: *Do you think that being a mother is important to women?*
SHARON WARRINGTON: *Yes.*
INTERVIEWER: *How?*
SHARON: *It's their life, isn't it? It's what they're born for.*

Sue Sharpe, investigating schoolgirls' ambitions in London recently, found that:

> Girls at secondary school are already very aware of their feminine role especially where it concerns reproduction and motherhood, and this necessarily affects their future hopes and ambitions in other areas of life . . . motherhood remains one of the most positive aspects of the feminine role for many girls. [1976, p. 206]

And, working with a sample of pregnant single women in Aberdeen, Scotland, Sally Macintyre points out that for many of them explanation of their attitudes

> was inappropriate since to explain something implies that things could have been otherwise. Their definitions were rooted in a social situation and world view in which motherhood and marriage were taken for granted as a part of being female and growing up. [1977a, p. 64]

Even 'those who rejected marriage and motherhood in favour of termination invoked highly idealistic versions of marriage and motherhood in the future' (p. 182). The emphasis on 'idealistic' is important, for, as Busfield and Paddon (1977) point out in their discussion of attitudes to parenthood, it is the *idea* of being a mother that dominates – the occupation of the role rather than having children per se. Childlessness is condoned only if involuntary, when it is pitied; expensive infertility treatment is regarded as a valid drain on the meagre resources of the NHS since it redresses the distressing evil of 'unfulfilled' parenthood (Newill, 1974; Peck, 1973). (These attitudes are, of course, limited to married couples, indicating the tight interlocking of wifehood and motherhood in the feminine paradigm.)

If femininity demands motherhood, then the dilemma can be put another way: it is the case that, until they become mothers, women do not confront the full significance of the way femininity is socially constructed in our culture. It is a meaning of which women themselves are aware:

> *I feel that my life before the baby wasn't* complete *in a sense. . . .* (Lois Manson)
>
> *I suppose I am different – more fulfilled . . . . I've joined the club.* (Jane Tarrant)
>
> *It suddenly dawned on me I was a mother. I think it makes you more contented . . . I feel more like a married woman now.* (Vera Abbatt)

– though the trajectory of female gender role socialization may be such that the meaning may not be articulated. Where there is agreement throughout a culture (or within a sub-cultural group) on what femininity and masculinity are, transition to these adult statuses has a taken-for-granted character. But where the cultural standards themselves are being questioned, as they are in many industrialized societies today, the path to femininity is exposed and the processes that develop it in infancy, childhood and adolescence are at risk of becoming poorly integrated with one another, thereby allowing 'deviations' from the norm to occur with increasing frequency.

JO INGRAM: *I wasn't planned – they conceived me before they were married . . . I think they probably wanted to have a girl – I think Dad certainly did. Because in the early stages I was really, well, there was the whole daughter bit. I was closer to my father, I was classed as a tomboy – very much so. There was a series of things, like my mother threw my jeans away and told me off for wearing my hair long and loose rather than plaited and neat – and I wouldn't wear skirts – that kind of thing. So there were definitely pressures there, but my father was a psychological wreck and he made me a psychological wreck too because, although Mum had to be sort of womanly, and I did too, really, being a girl, he couldn't stand it: he doesn't like softness and emotionality, and all the rest of it. So there was pressure from him never to show my feelings and never to be soppy. It was a disgusting mixture; I'm very fucked up. . . .*

I assumed I was never going to have children and I was never going to get married. It was a very, very conscious thing that I didn't want to have that life-style – whether I didn't want to have my mother's *life-style, I don't know. . . .*

INTERVIEWER: *Did you have any ambitions for a career?*

JO: *Yes – insofar as art is a career. It's not actually a monetary career, just a starving in the garret bit. My father's ego would have been better pleased if I'd gone to university . . . but I actually chose to go to college . . .*

For women like Jo Ingram the cultural connections between being female and being expected to devote a large part of one's adult life to parenthood are a trap that society sets for women: the source and cause of their oppression.

It is easier to see this connection when the wider social and economic consequences for women of their maternity are spelled out. Since the 1950s, a great deal of research has been done into women's situation and prospects for sex equality, and the conclusions have persistently been that once women have children they find it difficult to engage fully or at all in any other activity beyond the domain of childcare and related domestic work. Paid work outside the home, the most obvious example, is carried out by a third of all mothers of children under eleven;

two thirds do not have jobs. Only one in three of these employed mothers works full time, and in general mothers are over-represented in semi-skilled and unskilled job categories – both in relation to women as a whole and in relation to their own particular occupational qualifications (Moss, 1976). Mothers earn less than other people and those with pre-school children are especially disadvantaged. In one study, based on 1969–71 data, 61 per cent of employed women with children under five earned less than £5 a week (Hemming, 1975).

This situation reflects a lack of childcare facilities outside the family, which in turn is in line with social attitudes to mothers. Bowlbyism may have waned, but the social charter of motherhood attached to the biological act of birth is still strong:

> *If you're having a baby it's your place to stay at home with it. It's a man that goes out to work and a woman that stays at home.* (Felicity Chambers)

> Mothering mediates between the child's inner subjectivity and the outside 'real' world; it recognizes and establishes his [*sic*] personal identity and individuality; and her loving care is unique in the sense that it is adapted to his very special, individual needs . . . [Pringle, 1974, p. 36]

What applies to paid work follows also in the case of other areas of a mother's life – her domestic work, her marriage, leisure, political interests and so on. Here too maternity constrains, adding work, subtracting freedom, making psychological and emotional demands (Bernard, 1975; Boulding, 1977; Chapman and Gates, 1977; Tizard *et al.*, 1976). And the problems of combining parenthood and selfhood are peculiar to women, for dogmas of paternal non-involvement in routine childcare and housework have shifted only slightly in recent years, implying that our raised consciousness about 'women's role' has achieved a comfortable coexistence with traditional precepts of behaviour.[2]

It is first childbirth that plunges women into this bog of 'role' problems and it is therefore in this sense that entry into full adult femininity is one dimension of first-time motherhood. To say this is not to reiterate the feminine paradigm but to extract the paradigm of femininity from its external cultural location and regard it as one among many influences on the experience of reproduction. To identify the transition to femininity as one basic meaning of first-time motherhood is to comment on the particular way in which motherhood and womanhood are institutionalized within Western industrialized culture. It is to claim that such a perspective exposes the meaning of the passage to motherhood to reproducers themselves – that when they have a first child women are aware that having a baby counts as feminine achievement, and they discover that the social and economic circumstances of mothers tend to be different from those of men, or of women in general. One index of this is that 49 per cent of the Transition to Motherhood sample said that motherhood had changed their attitudes to the position of women, making them perceive discrimination where they had not perceived it before. Women's attitudes and responses to social definitions of motherhood may differ, but in part feelings about becoming a mother are bound to emerge in dialectic with the unfolding of cultural expectations. In this way the passage to femininity is the *context* within which the passage to motherhood takes place.

STATUS PASSAGE

The idea of a status passage is derived from anthropological work, especially that of Arnold van Gennep who, in *Les Rites de Passage*, proposed an analysis of individual changes in social status from the perspective of society: he argued that passages between age grades and occupations involved 'actions and reactions to be regulated and guarded so that society as a whole will suffer no discomfort or injury' (1960, p. 3). Glaser and Strauss (1971) have reversed this focus to concentrate on individual responses to processes of status change, and have developed a sophisticated description of the multiple properties of status passage. They stress that to the passagee, status passages may be in varying degrees

desirable
inevitable
reversible
repeatable

lonely
conscious
communicable
voluntary
controllable
capable of legitimation
clear
disguisable
central
lengthy

The different properties also vary in importance: perhaps the most crucial are those of *desirability*, *voluntariness*, *control* and *centrality* – where the new status stands in a person's own order of priorities. It is easy to see (though barely spelt out by Glaser and Strauss) how these dimensions apply to the passage from the status of non-mother to that of mother. For example, desirability and voluntariness are a function of motives for having a baby; inevitability may be assumed once pregnancy has begun and motherhood, once achieved, is irreversible – even if the child dies the mother's physical condition and probably her identity as well are lastingly affected. Thus any analysis of these general properties of status passage is as applicable to motherhood as it is to any other kind of transition between social statuses.

Glaser and Strauss do not deal in the coinage of identity crises, personal strain, etc; their main concern is with social aspects of status passages and the passagee's movement through them. (Their discussion of stress is, in fact, limited to the example of competitive social mobility among men, a general indication of the specific masculinity of Glaser and Strauss's model.) Similarly, van Gennep's orientation is a social and not a personal one. However, his labelling of the three types of ritual that accompany status passage was developed partly through an examination of the passage to motherhood in pre-literate societies and is certainly directly applicable to this passage in the modern industrialized context.

The three types of rites are rites of separation, transition rites and rites of incorporation (which incidentally apply both to the newborn child and to the mother). Van Gennep says:

> The ceremonies of pregnancy and childbirth together generally constitute a whole. Often the first rites performed separate the pregnant woman from society, from her family group, and sometimes even from her sex. They are followed by rites pertaining to pregnancy itself, which is a transitional period. Finally come the rites of childbirth intended to reintegrate the woman into the groups to which she previously belonged, or to establish her new position in society as a mother, especially if she has given birth to her first child or to a son. [1960, p. 41]

Since Britain in the 1970s is not the same sort of society as those described by van Gennep, the rites of passage that characterize reproduction are covert rather than overt – their existence and function are not articulated. *Rites of separation* include the medical recognition of pregnant patienthood (marking the mother-to-be out as separate in this respect from other women/family members), hospital/clinic legitimation of pregnancy status (providing a separate geographical setting for the care of pregnant and parturient women), the purchase and wearing of special pregnancy clothes (which are designed and marketed as a specific category of clothes in general) and giving up work, an event that normally occurs about three months before the date of expected birth and may be an occasion that is ritually celebrated by the pregnant woman and her work colleagues. Some references to these rituals are:

Medical recognition

I'd missed two periods. And he said – he gave me an internal and said yes, it looked like I was. But he wouldn't say for definite until I'd had a urine test done. And he did that and he gave me the results three days later and he said it was positive. (Felicity Chambers)

Hospital legitimation

I didn't believe I was pregnant until I went up there, and the sister said you're eleven-and-a-half weeks pregnant, and I thought I must be, or she wouldn't have said it like that. So I came out and I was ever so pleased really when it suddenly dawned on me . . . It didn't hit me till then that I was *pregnant.* (Vera Abbatt)

Giving up work

People kept coming to say cheerio and people kept ringing me up. I didn't feel anything really. I mean I did shed a few tears . . . But . . .

I just felt it was another Friday and I was just going on holiday. I didn't feel I was actually leaving.

I've been with the firm eleven years and naturally I've made a lot of friends. In actual fact when the officer – you know you usually have an official presentation – and he gave me the cheque: this is what I was dreading, that I was going to cry and I couldn't say my thanks. And he presented me with the cheque and everyone clapped, then one of the girls rushed up with a big bouquet of flowers. And that finished me ... I was so choked ... I was so excited about everything. It hasn't dawned on me yet that I've given up work for a long time. But I have. (Christina Lynch)

Entry into the career of pregnant woman means separating from the social world of non-pregnant woman. Pregnancy itself, and labour, are transitional stages, so that the medical and social phasing of, for example, antenatal care, formal childbirth preparation classes and labour/pre-delivery routines have the status of *rites of transition*. This sense of being *between* stages was described by Rosalind Kimber when she was 39 weeks pregnant:

I feel disoriented most of the time in that I don't really feel that I'm living any kind of life at the moment, because I can't visualize the future at all. I've given up my job and I'm not sort of committed to anything else. I mean you can't be committed to a baby that's not there yet. And so I feel I'm living in a kind of limbo from day to day.

Birth itself creates a new human being, but it also signifies the social production of a mother, and in this sense marks the beginning of rites that define the last stage in the passage to motherhood:

I can remember thinking that I was a Mum *and that was quite nice ... The actual minute he was born was very emotional ...* (Mary Rosen)

When they gave me the baby I wasn't interested a bit ... They took him away and the nurse said, oh poor little thing your Mum *doesn't want you.* (Jo Ingram)

Following the delivery of the child, women pass through *rites of incorporation* into a society of mothers – the social role that female reproducers are assigned in our culture. This incorporation is gradual in a culture where most mothers give birth in hospital and are hospitalized for a number of days after birth. Although biological mothers during this period, they are not in sole charge of their children – a fact that van Gennep sees as a critical rite of separation for the *baby*. Babies are social strangers and acquire membership of human society not by virtue of their birth but through specific introduction, a process that in many cultures requires care by someone other than the biological mother in the early days and is celebrated in rituals of one kind or another – placental burial, circumcision, etc. In modern industrialized society, the churching of women still survives as a religious ceremony and the occasion of christening has highly symbolic connotations. Less obviously, the rituals of hospital discharge and homecoming celebrate new status as a mother; the first visit by a health visitor to the home, or by the mother to a baby clinic, are public recognitions of social maternity.

Mother – baby separation

It was the way they treated me in hospital – now I look back on it I know it was all for the good, but at the time it really made me feel I couldn't cope, because they were feeding him, because I couldn't feed him, and they were changing him because I couldn't change him . . . They kept telling me, you know, we'll send a nurse up to help you feed him; the nurse would stand there while I was changing him . . . and I said to my husband I think they think I'm completely incapable of being *a mother.* (Vera Abbatt)

Leaving hospital

It was a really incredible feeling when I came out of hospital. I've never felt like that before. I came out of the gates and I was really petrified – nearly in tears; it was really weird. It suddenly hits you, you've got to take it home with you – you can't leave it at the hospital. There's definitely that thing about the baby belonging to the hospital. (Jo Ingram)

Coming home

I felt a mixture of a lot of things. Very proud and of course when we got home it all seemed terribly strange to actually have him [the baby] *there. I was very nervous about whether I'd be alright. My mother came the next day, so . . . I thought I can store up all my questions. It was very consoling, though, that she was coming.* (Rosalind Kimber)

Professional advisers: The health visitor

I came home on the Tuesday and she came on the Friday. I opened the door and said, thank God you've come. The first thing she said to me was have you got a fireguard? And my Mum was here and he cried and she picked him up and was holding him and she [the health visitor] *said you must put him down* immediately *after a feed or he won't settle . . .* (Christina Lynch)

Professional advisers: The clinic

I take him every Tuesday to have him weighed . . . I just presumed it was the natural thing to go afterwards, so I went . . . They weigh them, they give you a little card and they weigh them . . . And after he'd been weighed, they said do you want to see the health visitor or the doctor? And I said, what's the usual thing? The usual procedure is to see the doctor every eight weeks, and otherwise not to see the doctor unless there's anything actually wrong. (Rosalind Kimber)

Perhaps significantly, van Gennep's account of childbirth rites focuses on the social return from childbirth rather than on the process of incorporation into the social role of mother. In the cultures he discusses, motherhood tends to be a taken-for-granted aspect of a woman's adult life: it is something most women are expected to be, just as they are expected to continue with their productive agricultural or other work. Lacking cultural recognition of the 'two role' dilemma, and given the actual compatibility of motherhood and 'work', the problem of rejecting one in favour of the other does not arise. By comparison, the incorporation or non-incorporation of women into the social role of mother in industrialized society is much more variable and dependent on sub-cultural context and individual motivation.

Throughout his analysis, van Gennep stresses the similarity between rites of passage relating to childbirth and those pertaining to other transitions between age or occupational grades. Indeed, he sees first childbirth as an occupational change of a major kind needing rituals that bridge or 'facilitate the changing of condition without violent social disruptions or an abrupt cessation of individual and collective life' (1960, p. 48).

Social status transitions are, for the individual, carriers of 'identity strain'. They demand changes in personal awareness and new behavioural responses; previous self-concept may not fit the new circumstances and unknown skills may need to be developed. It has been noted that individuals' responses to such transitions as going to work in a foreign country, getting married or being made redundant share some characteristics of bereavement reactions: numbness, pining, depression and recovery are distinct stages in both. In *Transition: Understanding and Managing Personal Change*, Adams, Hayes and Hopson (1976) construct a list of transition reactions from people's accounts of the transition experience. I reproduce it here, interspersed with comments from the Transition to Motherhood study that serve to show how a general analysis of the psychological impact of social transitions on the individual is applicable to women 'as maternity cases'.

STAGE 1

> ... a kind of *immobilization* or a sense of being overwhelmed; of being unable to make plans, unable to reason, and unable to understand. In other words, the initial phase of a transition is experienced by many people as a feeling of being frozen up. It appears that the intensity with which people experience this first phase is a function of the *unfamiliarity* of the transition state. ... [pp. 9–10]

I kept thinking there's so much to do and I don't feel like doing it – I haven't got time to do it; I couldn't get anything done. I can't think what I did do, apart from sitting and crying my eyes out ... The first few days home I couldn't eat anything; my stomach was just in a knot. I never realised – it was very stupid of me – exactly what was involved. You can read about it, but they don't tell you all *the aspects. They tell you about the feeding, changing, clothing: they don't tell you about the other side. It's not until ... you have the baby that you know what's involved.* (Christina Lynch)

STAGE 2

> ... characterized by *minimization* of the change or disruption to trivialize it. Very often, one will deny that the change even exists. [p. 11]

At times I still don't think he's mine. Lying in bed yesterday I heard him crying and I thought, what's that? I still haven't quite realised that we've got a baby and it is ours, no-one else's . . . I still can't think of myself as a mother. When Bob talks to the baby about 'your mother' I think, who's that? A lot of times when I'm downstairs, I'm not with him, I forget completely *that I've got a baby.* (Grace Bower)

STAGE 3

> . . . the realities of the change and of the resulting stresses begin to become apparent. As people become aware that they must make some changes in the way they are living, as they become aware of the realities involved, they begin to get *depressed*. . . . They become depressed because they are just beginning to face up to the fact that there has been a change. Even if they have voluntarily created this change themselves, there is likely to be this dip in feelings. They become frustrated, because it becomes difficult to know how best to cope with the new life requirements, the ways of being, the new relationships that have been established or whatever other changes may be necessary. [p. 11]

I don't feel as if I'm coping very well . . . I suppose I remember the bad times rather than the times when she feeds and goes to sleep and settles and it's okay. It's more difficult than I imagined it would be. I'm pretty depressed I think . . . I haven't taken to motherhood well, I don't think . . . I sometimes think: why did I bother?

What you have to give up – you give up every freedom, really. You can't even go to the shops without thinking whether she's going to want feeding . . . It's just the freedom in the daytime to go to places: you can't hop on a bus and this sort of thing. Every time you go out, you've got to take her with you. . . . Apart from the fact that I'm so restricted physically, mentally I'm the same person . . . Well, I must be different, let's face it – I suppose I must be different. . . . (Sandy Wright, five weeks after the birth)

STAGE 4

> . . . *accepting reality* for what it is . . . a process of unhooking from the past and of saying 'Okay, here I am now; here is what I have; here's what I want.' As this is accepted as the new reality, the person's feelings begin to rise once more and optimism becomes possible. [pp. 11–12]

I don't feel I'm a fantastic mother but I feel I've adjusted to it more . . . I can't imagine being back at work again . . . I think you're free in that you can more or less do what you want to when you're at home. Whereas before I had *to get up and I had to be in by that time. I'm my own boss now . . . I go into work and see people, and I'm glad I'm doing what I am at the moment. I think I was getting tired of work . . . I find it quite enjoyable, really.* (Sandy Wright, five months after the birth)

Stage 5

> . . . the person becomes much more active and starts *testing* himself [*sic*] vis-a-vis the new situation: trying out new behaviours, new life-styles; and new ways of coping with transition. [p. 12]

I quite like the idea of being able to cope so well and *being a mother. The other day I got into a taxi, I'd been at the office* [Kate works two days a week as her husband's secretary] *and I had to get back, Mark was minding Gillian. And this taxi driver started to chat me up and everything . . . Then he got a bit sort of fruity, and . . . I thought well I'd say about my husband and the baby – and he* visibly *got more miserable about it. And I was very very* pleased, *because I thought, oh gosh, somebody's chatting me up, and there's me a Mum and a housewife and all that!* (Kate Prince)

Stage 6

> . . . a more gradual shifting towards becoming concerned with understanding and for *seeking meanings* for how things are different and why they are different. [p. 12]

I find it amusing: it's interesting and I'm lucky, he really is such a very good *baby . . . and it's not for such a large part of your life: I suddenly feel it's an awful pity just to work, because there's so much pressure on women to work. I saw this advertisement the other day, and someone had scrawled across it: 'babies get women down', and I suddenly thought: it's such a popular thing to say, but they don't get* all *women down. I'm really very happy doing what I do.*

I would say that it [motherhood] *is most rewarding in general, but that the first couple of months are absolute murder . . . I certainly don't recommend those first few weeks! A couple of my friends have got pregnant recently, and I sort of think, look at them: they're so happy, and they think it's all so marvellous: they don't know what they're going to have to go through for a bit!* (Janet Streeter)

STAGE 7

> . . . the final phase of *internalizing* these meanings and incorporating them into new behaviour. [p. 12]

No matter how good they [babies] *are, they* are *a handful when they're young, and I'm not the type of person who can* cope. *I don't mean* mentally, *but* physically . . . *I mean one time before I got married, I wanted six children. But now having gone through it I only want two . . . I just didn't realise what was involved.* (Sasha Morris)

In this analytic framework, no historical account of depression in terms of personality structure and development is necessary. Depression is simply a human reaction to the strain of adjusting to a new situation. As Adams *et al.* stress, the chronology of the different stages is not fixed: some people may take much longer to pass through them than others; some may miss out stages (e.g. stage 2 of *minimizing* the change) altogether; and some may remain depressed and 'maladjusted' until they are able to bring about changes in the situation itself. An example of this would be a woman whose initial depression with the shock of motherhood persisted until taking a paid job enabled her to define herself in terms of a non-domestic identity.

RETIREMENT

Retirement from economically productive work and from the public domain associated with it sums up one of the most important features of the transition to motherhood. Once a person retires, he/she is not expected to work again. Mothers-to-be are in a similar situation, since the cultural dogma is that motherhood and employment are mutually exclusive. A mother is expected to put full-time employment behind her until all her children are at least out of primary school. Both mothers and retired people suffer from the moral association between human value and economic productivity expressed, in the mother's case, in the phrase 'just a housewife'. They experience the same isolation to the private domestic sphere and a similar contraction of social relationships. Most studies of responses to retirement demonstrate that the aspect of work that is missed most both in anticipation and in practice is social interaction.[3] Certainly mothers are likely to feel that their lives lack sufficient colour in this respect:

I do feel lonely. Especially in the morning when he's gone to work. Especially if he's said he's going to golf and he won't be home till late in the afternoon. It gets boring. Because I don't get any visitors in the day. I see my Mum: I took him up there the other week, for a few hours, gave him a couple of bottles up there. It's the only time I've been out and seen my Mum: I used to see a lot of her during the week. (Janette Watson)

I'm so alone: so lonely. I'm not mixing with very many people and I would accept people at any *price when I meet them now . . . I think it's meeting people – that's the biggest disadvantage.* (Sarah Moore)

In the case of the retired person, having worked for forty or fifty years may be seen as a mitigating circumstance in the event of such deprivations. Negative responses to retirement may be that much less in general, because the person feels he/she has 'earned' a rest from engagement in the public world. In the case of the mother, active life in that sense is not normally felt to be over, and the consequences of retirement may thus be experienced and resented more keenly. (In the short phase between giving up work and becoming a mother, a woman's responses may be more akin to those of the unemployed worker – Bakke, 1933. See Rosalind Kimber's comments, p. 190.)

Retirement may be seen as either the end of one life phase or the beginning of another. Here it is easy to see the comparison with motherhood, which may be alternatively conceptualized as an end to the 'honeymoon' period of marriage and a brake on job/career ambitions, or as the onset of a new life phase. Marion Crawford, in her study of retirement (1971), uses the concepts of 'disengagement' and 're-engagement' to describe different orientations to retirement. 'Disengagers' are those who value their work status and do not look forward to retirement, which is consequently construed as a loss rather than as a gain. 'Re-engagers', on the other hand, define retirement as a gain, welcoming the new status with its associated opportunities for undertaking activities that were not possible when the individual was employed. The *meaning* of retirement thus reflects people's different evaluations of work and non-work spheres. For mothers also, the contrast is clear: the possession of a strong 'work' identity is not conducive to joyful anticipation of domesticity; not enjoying work and/or seeing oneself as a mother, is:

SARAH MOORE: *I was very shocked* [when she discovered pregnancy]. *And I had a slight* anti *feeling about it – a slight resentment because having really worked hard at my job, and now having got to the point where I was doing what I want to do, and had just a little bit more authority than I did have . . . I'd got to that stage, and I was enjoying work so much more, and when I found out that I was pregnant, the first couple of weeks I was almost horrified. I mean I'd have to give all this up.*
INTERVIEWER: *Will you continue working after the baby's born?*
SARAH: *No . . . It was just an automatic thing. If I was pregnant, I was going to give up work . . . I mean I think it's most important that a mother should be at home for the first three years. Not necessarily five, but definitely the first three. So therefore that's a sacrifice I* have *to make. I have to give up work. And it* is *a sacrifice. Now, I really do feel that I should try to be there while bringing up the children. . . . But I know that if I feel I must go back to work. . . . I mean I think there's every possibility that I may become neurotic or very lonely and be unhappy at home, and I'll feel that I have to go back to work and in that case I will.*

INTERVIEWER: *Do you plan to work after the baby's born?*
DEBORAH SMYTH: *No. Not until they're all old enough – I mean not in infants' school or juniors, I mean till they're a good age – eleven or older.*
INTERVIEWER: *How do you feel about that?*
DEBORAH: *I'm looking forward to it. I don't like work. I hate getting up in the mornings. I wouldn't like to go to work. I'd rather be at home than working.*

Responses to retirement or motherhood only make sense when

these underlying identity constructs are exposed. The actualities of 'adjustment' are different in each case: while both re-engagers and disengagers may be surprised by the contrast between fantasy and reality, the latter are likely to find actual motherhood more rewarding than anticipated, the former less so:

SARAH MOORE: *Now I've given up work I can't see myself going back to that job.*
INTERVIEWER: *Any job?*
SARAH: *Not for a long time at the moment.*
INTERVIEWER: *How long?*
SARAH: *I don't know. I've just not thought about it. I don't think I could go to work now. I'd worry. . . .*

I'm never bored. There's so much to do I haven't got time to be bored. I'm enjoying him . . . Obviously there are the tedious bits, but recognition and smiling: that sort of thing is tremendously uplifting. I mean obviously you feel lousy first thing in the morning; you go in and see him and he's laughing and chuckling – it's tremendous. No, I am enjoying him . . . I mean I had no idea, *I mean I thought I'd sit at home and be just twiddling my thumbs wondering what to do next. I mean that was* why *I said I was going to be so bored and frustrated.*

DEBORAH SMYTH: *When I first gave up, I didn't miss it at all.*
INTERVIEWER: *And since then?*
DEBORAH: *Well, it's just being on your own, just getting used to being on your own. But with the radio on it's usually alright. I get lonely, especially in the afternoons. Some afternoons if there's washing and ironing to do, it's alright.*
INTERVIEWER: *Do you see other people with babies?*
DEBORAH: *Only my sister and she's miles away. I'd like one friend . . . just someone to walk down the shops with.*
INTERVIEWER: *If you had to describe motherhood to someone who didn't have children, what would you say?*
DEBORAH: *I don't really know. My friend was getting married last Saturday. And she saw him, it was the first time she'd seen him, and she said, oh I want to start a family . . . And I said to her, don't start a family yet.*
INTERVIEWER: *Why did you say that?*
DEBORAH [pause]: *I don't know. We did it quickly . . . I like him . . .*

I like having him at home, you know. I don't know why I said that.
INTERVIEWER: *How would you compare your life now with your life before you had the baby?*
DEBORAH: *Sometimes I think about before we got married and that, you know. I think about going to work every morning. I never want to do it again, you know, I just* think *about it.*
INTERVIEWER: *Do you ever feel lonely?*
DEBORAH: *Sometimes I do, yes. When he's asleep or when he's crying.*
INTERVIEWER: *How often do you feel that?*
DEBORAH: *Quite often . . . Usually Friday and Saturday especially, because Patrick works Saturday, and Friday he doesn't come home dinner time. He leaves at 7.30, he doesn't get home till a quarter past six. It's all day, you know. Usually I go and meet him from work – just to get out, you know.*

OCCUPATIONAL CAREER CHANGE

From yet another perspective, what happens to a woman when she becomes a mother is not retirement but a change of career. There are two central occupational changes involved: to housewife and to mother. For some women a change in employment occupation is also involved.

On giving up work during pregnancy, a woman becomes a full-time housewife, that is, she is so labelled by society in general and to a greater or lesser extent by husband, relatives and friends. Her own self-concept may parallel this transition to domesticity, or it may not. Upon returning home from hospital with the baby, a second new job is added to that of housewife: motherhood. In most marriages, first-time parenthood is considered by husband and wife to change the wife's occupation but not the husband's: thus the actual twenty-four-hour-a-day childrearing responsibility devolves on her. Housework and childrearing are so intertwined in the cultural stereotype of women and the social phasing of their lives that the two may seem, or become, indistinguishable (Oakley, 1979b). A first-time mother, therefore, has to 'adjust' to two job transitions and then balance the responsibilities and demands of both jobs simultaneously for the rest of her life. Sometimes this juggling act has to be accomplished in tandem with a third job: employment. Those women (33 per cent of the Transition to Motherhood sample) who take up some form of employment work as mothers are, moreover, likely to find themselves in a different kind of work from what they had done prior to childbirth. Table 8.1 shows that only one woman returned to the same full-time job as before the birth; 18 per cent took up part-time or occasional work in the same field and 13 per cent in a different one. The paid work mothers do is generally lower in status, less skilled, less remunerated and more likely to be part-time than that undertaken by women in general.

TABLE 8.1 *Employment status after birth*

Employment status	*% of sample*	*No.*
Not employed	67	37
Employed*	33	18
(1) in same full-time job as before birth	2	1
(2) part-time/occasionally in same job as before birth*	18	10
(3) part-time/occasionally in different job from before birth	13	7

N = 55.
* Includes one woman who continued as a full-time law student after the birth.

Translated into the language of masculine career changes,[4] the feminine passage from secretary or factory machinist through housewifery to housewifery plus motherhood, to housewifery plus motherhood plus part-time typist or cleaner can be located in this framework:

> There are, with most organizations, generally accepted views about the 'normal sequence' of career movements, in which individuals pursue certain routes at certain rates through the organization. These views give rise to expectations about the 'normal' transitions an individual should experience. . . . Crossing or not crossing an organizational boundary at a particular point in time could lead to changes in the way a person is viewed by others, to changes in the way he [*sic*] sees himself, and to changes in his behaviour. [Adams *et al.*, 1976, pp. 84–5]

One major consequence of job transition is identity strain, which

> ... exists when an individual feels unable to implement his self-concept at work ... After people have crossed or not crossed particular organizational boundaries, they assess their role and attempt to integrate it with the way they view themselves as workers. Where the individual is unable to implement his occupational self-concept in his perceived role, he may be motivated either to modify his self-concept, or to change in some way his perceived role, or in extreme circumstances to withdraw from the situation. [p. 95]

Passages between jobs may be desired and the experience of the new job may be quite congruent with expectations: in this case no, or very little, identity strain is predicted. But, conversely, a contradiction between image and reality may be associated with considerable strain in the adjustment of self-image to current work situation.

So far as the transition to motherhood is concerned, the gap between expectations and reality is substantial. In the Transition to Motherhood study, 96 per cent of first-time mothers said five months after the birth that becoming a mother had contradicted their expectations in various important ways. Asked about the ease or difficulty of the experience, 31 per cent said it had been difficult; asked if their images of the transition to motherhood had been romanticized, 84 per cent said they had. Of the coping strategies employed to deal with identity strain, the most common in the case of mothers were the first two noted above: modification of self-concept and changes in the perceived role. For instance, one in three of the women had stronger ideas of themselves as mothers at five months than they did at five weeks postpartum or during the pregnancy:

INTERVIEWER: *Do you think of yourself as a mother?*
BARBARA HOOD [five weeks postpartum]: *No, I don't think so. I think I'll be more aware of it as he gets older.*

Five months after the birth:

INTERVIEWER: *If you had to fill in a form and put your occupation now, what would you put?*
BARBARA: *Mummy!* [laughs]

Changes in the perceived role, the second response, may involve reorganization of the tasks entailed by housewifery and motherhood to bring about a closer fit with the mother's self-concept. This is likely to involve the imposition of routines, the development of standards of work behaviour that, given the autonomy of the housewife, can only be imposed by her – or, rather, can only be seen to be imposed by her, though they are in fact pervasively shaped by 'external' forces, e.g. media images of domestic work, feminine role-modelling in childhood:

JOSEPHINE LLOYD [35 weeks pregnant]: *I went to my friend's, left there at about a quarter to five and she was expecting her husband home, and her little girl was getting all excited and I thought how lovely that is, that she's got all her work done and she's just waiting now for her husband to come home, and I, to me that seems like an ideal situation, because I like to be organized and this is why I've been so depressed, because I haven't been organized. . . .*

INTERVIEWER: *How do you feel you're coping with the baby?*
PAT JENKINS: *I think I'm coping okay. Now I've got into my own routine and that. I mean I never get behind with my work or anything like that. At the beginning I thought I'd never get anything done. Now I manage. If he wakens up and you're not finished . . . I always put him in that little chair and . . . as long as he sees you he's alright. When I'm hoovering, he'll sit as quiet as anything.*

JANETTE WATSON: *I'm doing alright now. Now I've got my own place I'm a lot happier.* [Janette lived with her husband and baby in her father-in-law's council flat until the baby was four months old.] *It was the same old thing at his Dad's – do all my chores, you know, all my washing, and then his Dad would come home and we'd fight over the kitchen . . . I think I'm getting on alright. I do all my washing early. Get that out of the way and then I bath him every day before his breakfast. Get that done and he'll probably go off to sleep for a little while.*

JANE TARRANT: *The only trouble is when Neil came in one day he said the house smelt of polish and he said I was getting the name of a friend of mine across the road complex: her place is always like a new pin. And really you spend all your time dusting and the place wouldn't get half as dusty if you didn't dust it . . . I think you notice all these things, and you begin to make more work for yourself, I think.*

I have argued elsewhere that the function of establishing such standards and routines is to bring about a feeling of reward in achieving a set pattern of work.[5]

Two other kinds of change in 'perceived role' encompass ideological inflation of the role and a move that effectively accomplishes its opposite – taking some form of paid job, an act that can have the function of asserting the *lack* of domination housewifery – motherhood should properly have over the shaping of life-style and identity. Angela King described the first response: inflation of the role:

I look on it by thinking if I can bring up a well-adjusted child, then I'm doing something useful. I always compensate by thinking about that, because I did before think I should be doing this and I should be doing that – not sitting at home. Because before I was thinking about putting her in a nursery, or getting somebody to look after her when she was about one or two, and going back to work. But now I've forgotten about that ... I'll feel as though I've done something useful *if I can turn her into a nice person and put her into the world. I'll feel that I've really achieved something ... I think they* [the women's liberation movement] *are responsible in a way for making a lot of housewives feel guilty about staying at home and looking after a baby.*

Kate Prince took the opposite view, that mothering should be just one among many aspects of a woman's life:

I do feel tied down, but I've lost the resentment. Because it's of my own making, and I've got to organize myself out of it. [She takes a part-time secretarial job.]

I want to have both things [a baby and a career]. *I know it means a lot of organization and hard work and all that. But I would feel miserable if each year went by and I gradually got older ... Now is the time to act ... I don't really mind* what *it is. I'm not a snob about the type of job people have, I think as long as you do anything properly, that's okay, and you should do what you want to do. ... I think often this business of saying I won't go out to work because of the child, they think it's unfair – it's a way of dodging the issue, isn't it?*

... It's the role thing, isn't it? Because it just seems to me so *natural ... why does anybody* ever *make a big deal about it? I don't mean about the* physical *effort involved, because that is a big deal – but the whole thing around motherhood. It shouldn't be like that: it should be just played down: it's just something you* do *isn't it: it's like getting a sofa or going to Waitrose. I don't think it should have this great effect, it should be played down so that people don't expect too much ... don't expect their life to be* changed *and don't expect their* marriage *to change. That shouldn't be the case.*

Identity strain is also particularly likely where the move to a new occupation is generally undesired, unplanned or thwarted. One study of career transitions defines four possible outcomes of 'adaptation':

(1) *acceptance* – where the individual feels it is better to accept the status quo and makes new assumptions about herself/himself part of a reworked self-concept;
(2) *ritualism* – here the individual rejects the situation and preserves an identity detached from it, but performs the work role minimally in order to maintain appearances;
(3) *rebellion* – a response that entails direct attempts to change the situation; and
(4) *innovation* – this differs from (3) in that there is no move to alter the situation, but instead strategies are developed to draw attention to the individual's disadvantaged position (Levenson, 1961).[6]

In the career transitions of first-time motherhood, all these responses occur. Their incidence cannot be explained in terms of whether or not the babies were wanted or planned. Much more important seems to be the lack of *reality* with which motherhood is anticipated. Both those who planned/desired their babies and those who did not were victims of an inaccurately imagined career change. This point is made by Marris in his discussion of *Loss and Change*, when he says that identity crises may well follow voluntary changes 'as their unforeseen or discounted consequences and latent contradictions begin to work themselves out' (1974, pp. 148–9).

Acceptance and *ritualism* as adaptational outcomes are illustrated by comments cited earlier (pp. 195–6). Neither rebellion nor innovation as responses apply to the mother's situation in quite the same way as they do to the business executive's. Unlike employment careers, motherhood is not usually reversible. Although it is possible that in some cases going out to work and using substitute childcare might constitute rejection of motherhood, it is usually the role of full-time mother that is disputed, and not the child itself. Such moves are an attempt to restructure the maternal childcare environment, an effort to improve work conditions.

Housewifery is more reversible than motherhood, though it does carry the difficulty of detachment from norms of expected feminine behaviour. The overlap between childbearing and the childcare work component of housework interposes a maternal rationale for housewifery that may be felt as emotionally binding. Thus, *rebellion* as a response to housewifery is more likely to express itself as lowered specification of standards and routines. In practice, it seems that this second possibility – rebellion against housework per se – is less common than resentment of the way housework routines are disrupted by the child's demands. This is illustrated in the comments made by Lily Mitchell (pp. 139–41).

Innovative responses to the career changes of first-time motherhood are largely ruled out by the mother's private and isolated work situation. 'Innovative behaviour within the organizational framework' is simply ineffective so far as the housewife–mother is concerned, because it is not visible to anyone but herself and (perhaps) her partner. Strategies such as threatening to leave the family home, and refusing to meet the partner's requirements in terms of sex, meals and clean clothes, may be more effective ways of mitigating maternal loneliness and unilateral responsibility – by forging changes in husband's time at home and his contribution to the division of labour, for example (Oakley, 1979b). Florid postnatal depression could also be seen as a strategy that will draw attention to the discontent of the housewife–mother, in this case by provoking a need for medical attention. However, here the 'adaptation' is likely to be pharmacological, not social in nature.

In a wider cultural sense, both rebellion and innovation as reactions to motherhood can be discerned in the ideology of social movements aimed at changing women's role. The 'wages for housework' campaign is one innovative strategy oriented towards a public recognition of the housewife–mother's discontent, and demanding public retribution for one of its 'causes' – financial dependence (Warrior and Leghorn, 1975). The women's liberation movement in general has seen the oppression of women as centred in their restriction to a domestic, maternal, family-oriented image.[7] Changing this locus of oppression is an important part of the 'rebellion' against established typifications of womanhood the movement as a whole has come to represent.

CHANGE IN PHYSICAL STATE

Becoming a mother involves gross changes in body shape. These can be summed up quite inadequately by saying that the mother-to-be loses her waistline and gains about 28 pounds over a thirty-eight-week period, most of which will be lost during delivery and the succeeding postpartum days. In fact what pregnancy entails in terms of physical change differs between individuals, as also must the personal meaning of such change.

Although certain disease conditions may be associated with excessive weight gain and some, e.g. ovarian cysts, may be responsible for a particular pregnancy-mimicking pattern of abdominal expansion, there is no direct parallel between the physical changes of pregnancy and other such changes. Moreover, it could be argued that the change in body shape associated with pregnancy is always experienced differently from other such changes (the personal meaning is different) because it is known to be caused by a baby's growth. This is then held to be associated with the emotional significance of birth and motherhood, an interpretation that translates the embarrassing vastness of pregnancy into the emotional 'blossoming' of maternity.

Such an interpretation is, of course, hypothetical: it must be tested by reference to an empirical sample of cases. As earlier sections of this book noted, the paradigm of 'adjustment' to femininity has been the theoretical construct underlying much 'explanation' of reactions to pregnancy, birth and motherhood. The bodily changes entailed in these processes have been no exception to this general rule. A woman's feelings about body change have been taken as an index of her 'femininity' (liking it is feminine, disliking it is not). Femininity has been defined as a state of being that must parallel in predetermined ways the contours of the female biological role in reproduction. Thus in the Freudian tradition, maternal reporting of most, if not all, pregnancy symptoms (nausea, vomiting, bleeding, headache, backache, constipation, etc.) expresses a rejection of motherhood and wifehood (the incorporated object – the sperm – is said directly to represent the husband himself). A general feeling of completeness (being 'full up') evidences the equating of child with penis. During later pregnancy, when the movements of the child are felt, some degree of relationship between mother and infant develops that is likely to conform to the pattern of the woman's relationship with her own mother; feelings about body shape in this and other ways reflect the model of femininity established during childhood. In general, pregnancy is 'regressive'. It provokes ambivalence about retentive and expulsive impulses, so that much of what a woman feels about her body is interpretable only in the light of this conflict. Studies of reactions to pregnancy, birth and motherhood that use this framework operationalize the notion of femininity rejection in terms of, for example, 'gynaecological-obstetrical pathology' (e.g. threatened miscarriage, breech presentation), 'psychosomatic symptoms specific to pregnancy' (vomiting, nausea, breathlessness, debility). Chertok, from whose study of *Motherhood and Personality* (1969) these examples are taken, considers such symptomatology (which includes a general dislike of being pregnant) as part of a total negativity score that ought to be related to performance during childbirth. (He finds however that this is, by and large, not so.)[8]

In such a theoretical context maternal awareness of pregnancy symptoms is equated with poor adaptation to motherhood – with some degree of rejection of the pregnancy, the baby and the feminine role (Chertok 1969; Shereshefsky and Yarrow, 1973; Breen, 1975). The symptoms investigated are invariably 'negative', i.e. those associated, in other contexts, with illness. 'Positive' symptom formation is a residual category, indicated by the absence of illness symptoms.

Given the pre-judged paradigm of femininity that underlies these equations, certain possibilities are ruled out *a priori*. First, the theory does not allow for the fact that unpleasant pregnancy symptoms may be caused by the body and not the psyche – by the hormonal chemistry of pregnancy, for example.[9] Second, no separation is made between feelings about being pregnant, feelings about the baby and attitudes to the social role of mother. There is no reason (aside from that provided by the feminine paradigm itself) why these three should be synonymous. In the Transition to Motherhood study, pregnancy 'orientation' (the way a woman feels about being pregnant as reported in answer to direct questions) was statistically related to the two outcomes of satisfaction with motherhood ($p<.05$) and feelings for the baby ($p<.01$). However, as Figure 6.2 shows, both these outcomes were themselves related to the extent to which a woman saw herself as a mother. It is to this dimension of the self-concept that pregnancy orientation may be linked ($p<.025$) – rather than to either of the outcome measures per se. The extent to which specific symptoms were reported during pregnancy was not related to feminine role orientation or to satisfaction with motherhood (though there was an association – $p<.05$ – with feelings for the baby).

A woman who dislikes her increased contours might be expected to report more illness symptoms, and certainly a negative attitude to pregnancy size would be a component of how a woman feels about being pregnant. But none of these measures of maternal responses to pregnancy directly reflect attitudes to changing body shape. The only other medium in which this aspect of pregnancy has been investigated is that of sexuality. A large number of studies have focused on the interaction between pregnancy development and sexual orientation (in, of course, *married* women).[10] The degree to which this connection has been emphasized is not warranted by empirical evidence as to the importance of sexual desire/attractiveness in determining women's overall attitudes to body change in pregnancy. Rather, the research focus seems to be yet another by-product of masculine bias, which, combined with the feminine paradigm, decrees that the most relevant way a mother-to-be reacts to her growing size is to become less sexually desirable and available to men.

Taking this definition of sexual identity as based on attractiveness to men, J. E. Rosser (1978) has recently shown that women's responses to pregnancy size and shape often conflict with the standards of sexual attractiveness they perceive as applied to women in general. There are two reasons for this. In the first place, cultural images of sexuality and maternity contradict one another: a woman who is sexy is not a mother and mothers are not sexy people. In the current study these thoughts were often expressed:

I have to hold onto the mantelpiece when I get up: I feel like an old woman . . . And I can't do *things – I can't* run *: I bounce up and down. . . . People don't look upon you as a pregnant* woman *: they just look upon you as a clumsy oaf. You just look clumsy and turn people* off. (Pauline Diggory)

I think he looks at me in a different way from what he used to . . . I don't suppose he finds me so sexy. Well, I don't suppose I look so sexy. No, I think he thinks of me more as the mother of his child. (Jane Tarrant)

A second reason for the antithetical relationship of pregnancy and sexual attractiveness is that the apposite parallel to pregnancy is obesity, which is not a desired feminine characteristic:

The only thing I think about is what to wear. At the moment everything's tight, and I just look fat. (Janette Watson)

The fact that many primigravidae are anxious to begin wearing maternity clothes illustrates their anxiety to move out of the ambiguous early stage of pregnancy, when they just seem to be a little bit fat, into a public declaration of pregnant status.

Women's clothing is designed to emphasize body contours, and its tightness and imposed restriction of movement have historically been very important in defining feminine occupations and styles of behaviour. Henley, in a study of *Body Politics* (1977), suggests that loose clothing implies a loose woman – one whose sexuality is out of control. This association may be behind negative attitudes to maternity wear that begin to predominate in the last months of pregnancy. As Orbach (1978) has put it 'fat is a feminist issue'. The absolute value of slimness in the stereotypical image of a sexually attractive woman is thematic to the social construction of femininity in our culture. Moreover, such are Western attitudes to body shape that obesity is often seen to be a physical disability for which the victim is herself/himself responsible (Bloom and Clark, 1964). At the opposite end of the spectrum, anorexia nervosa is also a cultural – and medical – cause for concern. Though opinions differ as to its aetiology, it is undoubtedly far more common in females than in males, and identity crises to do with notions of achievement (of one kind or another) are pervasive (Crisp *et al.*, 1976; Bruch, 1974; Parker and Manger, 1974). Studies have shown that women are generally more concerned about weight and size than men (Dwyer and Mayer, 1970). For all these reasons it would be surprising if women did not display some ambivalence about the change in body size and image that becoming a mother entails. And given the negative connotations of fatness in the feminine stereotype, the disjunction between contravening the feminine standard (getting fat) and conforming to it (having a baby) would be expected to be a source of personal difficulty for some women. The majority of women in the current study did voice a dislike of pregnancy for reasons to do with the inherent unpleasantness of being 'too fat', 'out of control', 'elephantish', 'heavy', and being unable to fit into ordinary clothes.

INTERVIEWER: *Do you like being pregnant?*
LOIS MANSON: *I really don't know. It's exciting but* beginning *to feel a bit uncomfortable. . . . I suppose I feel a bit like I've been taken over, because I've got no control over my swollen body.*

JANE TARRANT: *Not really. I don't hate it or anything. I thought I would really love it. But I think in fact it irks me – the restrictions . . . Everybody tells me I have no problems and I thought if you feel a bit tired and elephantish and you have no problems, what the heck is it like if you're not feeling well?*

DEIRDRE JAMES: *I feel like a pregnant elephant. Uncomfortable . . . I feel as though I've been taken over. I can't imagine what it's like to be back to normal size. I look at my wardrobe - and I think I used to be able to get into that!*

JANET STREETER: *I'm fed up actually. I find now that – really I'm quite small compared with a lot of people I've seen, but I do begin to feel much* heavier. *I mean I really am quite heavy; I feel uncomfortable and I do feel fed up and I wish to God it would hurry up and come . . . I'm fed up with floppy clothes.*

But what about the postpartum phase – the sudden 'shock' of losing the 'bump'?

I couldn't believe it was over, it took so long to really click that he had been born. I kept feeling my tummy. I had to keep reminding myself that I had given birth. (Rosalind Kimber)

This poses an altogether different sort of problem. Some analysts have stressed the difficulty of associating feelings about the baby inside and feelings about the baby outside (e.g. Heiman, 1965). In the Transition to Motherhood study this was certainly one of the tasks new mothers felt they had to accomplish, and it was one to which differences in birth management were particularly relevant. But the birth of the baby out of the mother's body is an event for which one analogy is amputation: the surgical removal of a limb or body organ.

Studies of reactions to amputation surgery have some parallels with childbirth:

> . . . the immediate reaction to amputation is often a state of numbness in which physical and mental feeling is blunted, this is soon succeeded by a phase of distress in which episodes of severe anxiety occur . . . Depression, restlessness, tension, difficulty in concentration, insomnia, loss of appetite and loss of weight are common symptoms . . . the individual has the feeling that it [the lost object] is still present. [Parkes, 1971, p. 109]

(Compare this with the comment on p. 181.) The reason why the limb or organ has to go does not account for the depressive reaction: anticipation of, and responses to, cancer surgery, for example, may be quite out of proportion to the actual malignancy of the disease (Sutherland and Orbach, 1953). One important factor involved is a change in body image – adjustment to the new image of an 'incomplete' body (Dembo *et al.*, 1952; see also Fisher, 1960), where a limb or organ has been removed, or, in the postpartum case of mothers, readjustment of their views of their own bodies to fit the new non-pregnant shape. Although losing one's 'bump' is conventionally seen as a particularly 'feminine' adaptational task, the experience is in essence similar to being deprived of other parts of one's body.

> It [postnatal depression] is similar to the reaction that follows the loss of any part of the body and is frequently seen postoperatively in surgical patients. The fetus is considered a part of the mother and is now lost. Some degree of depression is inevitable until the mother can readjust and establish a new relationship with the child. [Asch, 1965]

All such responses are essentially responses to loss, and their quality is that of grief. As Colin Parkes argues in *Bereavement* (1972), reactions to loss among amputees are the same as other 'bereavement' reactions. The person has been bereaved; the fact that the loss comprises part of the body and not a loved person outside it does not predict a qualitatively different reaction. Each case of loss – of leg or pregnancy or spouse – is a psychosocial transition in which a reorganization of the 'assumptive' world has to take place, and new meanings have to be sought to replace old ones.

PATIENTHOOD

The symptoms of pregnancy are, in other contexts, illness symptoms; reproduction itself in Western industrialized culture is defined as a medical exercise. Thus, running parallel with a woman's pregnancy career is her career as a patient. For most women having first babies, this is probably the most extensive they have ever embarked on. While individual definitions of the passage to motherhood must influence the shaping of pregnancy, delivery and postpartum medical careers, the converse is almost certainly true: how a woman feels about being a patient impinges on the way she perceives and responds to becoming a mother.

Some of the manifestations of this relationship were outlined in chapters 6 and 7. There the spotlight was on feelings about, and satisfaction with, the medicalization of birth – the degree of medical intervention in labour and delivery, and general styles of birth management. These variables were shown to be definitely associated with maternal outcome – whether or not a woman experienced postnatal blues or depression, the kind of relationship she developed with her baby. Here I want briefly to consider less specific aspects of reproductive medical careers, drawing out the similarities between them and other patient careers, and pointing to some of the ways in which responses to patienthood might be expected to influence maternal outcomes to childbirth.

Parenthood and patienthood are directly contrasting status passages. While one is basic to the self-concept, the other (usually) is not; while the control of one is (theoretically at least) in the hands of the individual, control of the other emanates from an autonomous and hierarchical medical 'profession'.[11] Among the 'problems of patienthood' are discerning and conforming to the rules of patient behaviour that operate in medicine generally, and in each institutional setting specifically. This role acquisition imposes a certain ideal identity on the patient, for medical–professional and patient are not equal, but superordinate–subordinate statuses.

In much medical literature, the language used indicates an ideal image of patients as passive, cooperative and obedient (Stimson, 1974). But while it may be possible for doctors to project this image of patients during the medical encounter, beyond its boundaries patient compliance may be fictional, since the patient becomes her/his own decision-making authority (Stimson, 1976b). For neither patient nor doctor does medical expertise apparently constitute the rationale behind the doctor's superior status and the habit of patient deference to it. More persuasive, according to various studies, are (1) the perception of general social status differences between doctors and patients (the identification of doctors with the upper class and with the traditional authority figures of this and similar superior hierarchies); (2) the doctor's control over treatment resources – prescriptions, drugs, time off work, referrals to specialists and/or hospitals; (3) the relative inability of patients to select doctors, compared with the institutionalized provision for doctors to exercise control over the selection and continuing treatment of patients (Haug, 1976). Patients' views of medical expertise are likely to reflect these other dimensions of medical status as well as their own attitudes towards illness and authority figures in general.

On the other hand, the wider cultural abdication of responsibility for health and illness to the medical profession places everyone in a position of theoretical dependence on doctors – the only exception being perhaps doctors themselves, notably, and probably not incidentally, one of the sickest groups in society (see, for example, Murray, 1974). When people believe themselves to be ill, the chances are that they will go to a doctor, and the chances are that most doctors will treat even self-limiting and socially caused illnesses medically, i.e. with drugs, specialist referrals, recommendations for surgical treatment, etc. This bias is related to the doctor's own professional and personal reluctance to bestow upon patients themselves the moral idea that suffering is a collective and individual human disorder. The inevitability of a proportion of illness symptoms, given the physical and social conditions of the way human beings live, is certainly not a message taught in medical schools, nor is it one that can be conveyed to the patient in the few minutes of surgery time he/she is allocated.

The best-known presentation of this argument about the moral and iatrogenic evils of societal dependence on medical culture is Illich's *Medical Nemesis*. Illich's treatise does not develop the argument in relation to childbirth, although he does extend it to the meaning of death in the modern industrialized world:

> Death no longer occurs except as the self-fulfilling prophecy of the medical man. . . . Society, acting through the medical system, decides when and after what indignities and mutilations he [the patient] shall die. The medicalization of society has brought the epoch of natural death to an end. Western man has lost the right to preside at his act of dying. Health, or the autonomous power to cope, has been expropriated down to the last breath. [1975, pp. 148–50]

As we saw in chapter 1, the medicalization of birth has historically been oriented to removing the capacity for autonomous control from mother to medical expert. Thus, the contention that dying patients are iniquitously dependent on the medical system applies also to patients giving birth – and those being born:

ROSALIND KIMBER [accelerated labour, epidural, forceps delivery]: *They all kept saying well done, and I remember thinking, but I haven't done anything. It was because I was very conscious that in fact the doctor was doing all the work and I wasn't doing anything . . . the responsibility for it all was out of my hands, and in the hands of people I felt were very competent . . . They were all getting on with their job . . . I didn't have much of a chance to do all the breathing and things they'd been telling me to do . . . so really it was a bit like having a tooth out or something . . . you don't actually do it yourself: the dentist does it.*

. . . I suppose in a way it's an overwhelming experience, as everybody says, except that it feels curiously detached from me now, almost as if I hadn't been through it at all.

INTERVIEWER: *How did you feel when you first held the baby?*

ROSALIND: *I felt more detached than I thought I would, because he didn't feel like my baby actually at that stage . . . I felt, you know, that he ought to be taken off and seen to, or whatever they did, so when they came to take him away I felt that was the right thing to do.*

Lack of control over birth has become a taken-for-granted feature of the transition to motherhood in most social and medical settings today. The move towards home confinement, the demand for childbirth without analgesia or anaesthesia, protests about the need to have babies born in semi-darkness or kept in bed night and day with the mother – all these are probably the opinions of the minority of women giving birth, but they are usually dismissed within the medical frame of reference as deviant and esoteric responses. (The two statistics – of how many users of the maternity services protest, and how many medics reject the protest – are in principle independent of one another, since medical control of childbirth is endemic to the medical perspective.) At the moment, it is not possible to produce research findings that show that the majority of women are dissatisfied with medical styles of childbirth management – in the sense of wanting a radically different alternative to medicalized birth. But, on the other hand, many studies, including the present one, do demonstrate a great deal of discontent. Problems in doctor–patient communication, with hospital facilities, with the notion of patient 'choice' as an arbiter of treatment decisions are well documented (e.g. Cartwright, 1979; Fleury, 1967; Graham, 1978; Houghton, 1968). These difficulties are not specific to maternity patients, but are an exaggeration of the dissatisfactions of patients in general, mediated by the specific circumstances of women having babies. For maternity patients what is important is the difference between illness and reproduction, and the reduced propensity to appreciate the illness-curing and life-saving properties of medical treatment in what is normally neither a sick nor a life-threatening situation. In Ann Cartwright's analysis of *Human Relations and Hospital Care*, maternity patients' criticisms of the medical system were very similar to those of other young women patients: the principal differentiator was first-time motherhood, which was more likely to be associated with the complaint of inadequate information (1964, p. 178). It seems that first-time mothers want more information about the parameters of their patient careers than other mothers or patients in general.

The effects of dependent patienthood on patient/maternity patient outcome are difficult to quantify. Measured satisfaction with medical services may encompass responses to the unequal structure of doctor–patient relationships, or it may not. Even in the more equal patient–as-consumer model of health care, differences in consumer satisfaction remain an important way of assessing outcome from the patient's point of view.[12] As Stimson and Webb amongst others argue, 'satisfaction' with medical care is a fluid concept, reflecting the time-dependent quality of patient attitudes as well as their constant reordering and re-evaluation. Moreover, the underlying motivation of patients 'to succeed in the interaction game' predisposes them towards a declaration of satisfaction. To be dissatisfied may be to admit personal failure (1975, p. 78).

Aside from the question of satisfaction, there are many other labels that come to mind as descriptions of what people say they feel about medical treatment: anxiety, helplessness, ignorance, fear, irritation, anger, depression, resignation. These are the negative designations to be juxtaposed with a sense of reassurance, security, happiness and gratitude that some people feel but not many people express (the precept here being, as elsewhere, that only bad news is news).

Then they come in and said something about a cyst, and I didn't quite get it. So I sat up and said, can you explain it again? So they said you've got a cyst on your ovary. We'll just take that out for you. I was thinking, well, the doctor's told me I'm pregnant – if I've got a cyst there, is that something else? Am I still pregnant or have I got both things, or what? I wasn't quite sure. I said that to the nurse. She said, well, ask them. And I didn't ask them, because they went out. . . . (Michelle Craig)

This one [vaginal examination] *was a bit painful, I suppose because you're all tensed up. And the thing was, he said that I've got an ulcer at the neck of the womb, and he made it bleed, and when I saw that . . . It did bleed afterwards and it was quite worrying, because I'm not three months. He told me not to worry, but when I saw the blood, that made me worried – I was a bit queer that night actually.* (Janette Watson)

The fellow that came round examined him [the baby] *right at the end of the bed; this sister came with him, and he was testing all his reflexes and he was saying to her, oh he's such-and-such – mumbling – and he never said anything to me! Anything I wanted to know I had to ask. And he sort of acted like I was interfering – that it was none of my business. And I found that really annoying.* (Rachel Sharpe)

Why should one have to get used to all these things? That's what annoys me about it. Like having internals every five minutes – why should one have *to get used to it? It's not a very nice thing to have to get used to. Unless you happen to like hospitals. Why the hell should one have to grow to like hospitals and get used to them?* (Alison Mountjoy)

When I finally decided to have it [an epidural] *it wasn't just the pain. I didn't mind the contractions really. The pain of somebody doing something to you is worse. I had decided beforehand when I got so scared about being induced, I had more or less come to terms with the fact that I'd probably be asking for an epidural. . . . I was just scared of what* they *would do to me and how much* they *would hurt . . .* (Alison Mountjoy)

In the Transition to Motherhood study, the women's attitudes to medical experts were rated on the basis of answers to questions about induction of labour and question-asking in medical encounters. The dimension chosen was that of 'deference' – the extent to which the women saw doctors as purveyors of intrinsically superior medical knowledge and expertise: 45 per cent of the women were highly deferential, 5 per cent low in deference, the rest in between. Differences in deference were associated with feminine role orientation, those women with a 'traditional' orientation to the feminine role being most likely to exhibit deference ($p<.05$), and with social class, in the direction of working-class women being more deferential (by partner's occupation $p<.001$, by the woman's own, $p<.10$).[13] Attitudes to medical experts were linked both with epidurals, more deferential than non-deferential women having epidurals ($p<.025$), and with the related variable of amount of technology used during labour and delivery ($p<.001$, in the same direction). Since attitudes to experts were assessed in the pre-natal interviews, the association could not be such that the experience of epidural analgesia and a technological birth led to the formation of a deferential attitude. It seems more probable that pre-existing differences in women's readiness to accept medical decision-making affected the likelihood of succumbing to medical control. The link with social class, which, defined by partner's occupation, is part of routine medical note-taking, might also of course influence medical decisions, via the doctor's perceptions of the 'type' of patient who will benefit from more technological management.

In terms of affecting maternal outcome, attitudes to experts as thus measured did not relate to any of the four mental health outcomes (postnatal blues, homecoming anxiety, depressed mood and depression) or to the other outcomes of satisfaction with motherhood and feelings for the baby.[14] But the way a woman felt about medical expertise *was* associated with different patterns of satisfaction with medical care. Among the 'deferential' women, both satisfaction with antenatal care and satisfaction with birth management were more likely ($p<.01$ in both cases) than among women with a more critical attitude towards the medical profession. The other striking association was with levels of anxiety about labour and delivery. As measured at the two pre-natal interviews and the first postpartum one, high levels of anxiety about birth before and during the event were more common among women with deferential attitudes to doctors ($p<.01$).

Perhaps it should be argued that dissatisfaction with medical care and anxiety about one's condition are both measures of the influence patienthood has upon the experience of becoming a mother. For, insofar as aspects of medical care during pregnancy, delivery and the postpartum period are themselves linked to major measures of outcome (depression and feelings for the baby), the impact of relegating control over the shaping of the passage to motherhood to a profession of medical experts is profound.

SURGERY

As the association between parenthood and patienthood is contingent on historical–cultural circumstances, so also is that between the experience of childbirth and the experience of surgery. Where most mothers deliver at home without medical intervention, the parallels between having a baby and having a surgical operation are virtually non-existent. But in a society where 96 per cent of mothers have their babies in hospitals, a third have their labours induced, one in ten have their babies delivered by instruments, one in twenty have them removed by caesarean section, and more than half are subjected to surgical incision of the perineum and other so-called 'minor' surgical procedures, the birth of a child becomes an occasion that from the 'patient's' point of view is much more like major surgery than a 'natural' family event. The similarity is that much more pronounced in the case of first birth, where the incidence of surgery (e.g. induction of labour, forceps delivery, episiotomy) is greater than among women who have had a baby before.[15]

Among prevailing conceptual frameworks for studying childbirth, there is no recognition of the fact that mental and emotional states during pregnancy and the postpartum may be bound up with anticipation of, and response to, body surgery. Anxiety and depression in relation to motherhood are predominantly seen as reflections of a feminine psyche, and not as rational concomitants of anticipated and actual surgical experiences. For whether or not the surgery consists of limb/organ removal (see the section 'Change in physical state' above), its association with hospitalization and subjection to the physical intrusion of unfamiliar medical professionals is a human stress situation. Various studies have described the reactions of groups of surgical patients to their experiences. Lindemann, in an American survey, found 33 per cent of women surgical patients expressing 'depression' afterwards: 'A characteristic type of behavior was a mild degree of agitation, restlessness, insomnia and a preoccupation with depressive thought content' (1941, p. 135). Other symptoms were irritability and 'undue' worry about the welfare of husbands and children. Such responses occurred twice as often after pelvic than upper abdominal operations, and there was no relation to pre-operative anxiety. In Janis's study of surgical stress (1958), fear in anticipation of surgery is realistically based on the perception that surgery constitutes a 'danger' situation (akin, for example, to natural disasters such as flooding or fire). After intensive interviews with a group of such patients, Janis argues that both low and high levels of anticipatory fear predispose towards post-operative emotional disturbance – though in the latter group 'bad' adjustment only occurred if the stress of surgery was severe (a major operation, intense pain, 'an accumulation of harassing deprivations'). Moderate degrees of fear prior to surgery are predictors of unproblematic mental health outcome; such patients did not, in Janis's study, become disturbed, even when exposed to considerable post-operative pain and deprivation.

In Janis's model, the gap between expectations and reality is the key to understanding the relationship between pre-operative fear and post-operative mental health outcome; this had greater explanatory power than patients' specific personality dispositions. A sense of 'victimization' resulting from a reality that was considerably more stressful than expected promoted reactive emotional disturbance, a dysphoric mood, increasing the likelihood of depression. Conversely, when the amount of suffering, pain and loss was less than expected, the resulting euphoria protected against the negative responses of anger, depression, resentment, etc. But in both groups – those who experienced a reality worse than, and those who found it better than, their expectations – the pre-operative fear and post-operative reactions were realistically based on the risk of 'suffering pain, permanent injury, or death' and on the special threat of incisions that would or might be 'near the genital region' (1958, p. 409).

The relevance of these descriptions to women awaiting or recovering from childbirth is clear. One important component about the way childbirth was imagined before it happened was fear of surgical defacement of the body and its associated pain and disruption in intact body image: the fear was realistic, given the current medicalization of childbirth. And, following birth, a dominant theme in the postnatal reactions of mothers to the birth and its product, the baby, was how they felt about birth as surgery: the capacity of birth experiences to shatter previously cherished illusions about the 'naturalness' and painlessness of having a baby or, conversely, to mitigate images of birth as especially painful and gruesome. (The actual degree of pain and discomfort felt during labour, delivery and the early post-partum is, of course, another factor contributing to the character of mothers' emotional states that is laid aside in 'feminine' explanations of maternal mental health.)

These considerations were raised by Sandy Wright, who had an over-optimistic view of birth during pregnancy, and by Caroline Saunders, whose attitude to birth construed it as a fairly unpleasant experience; the reality turned out to be less horrific than she had imagined.

SANDY WRIGHT, in pregnancy:
INTERVIEWER: *How do you think you will feel about the birth?*
SANDY: *I expect to find it painful but I would think it would be a satisfying experience as well, especially if you're aware.*
INTERVIEWER: *Do you want to be conscious when the baby's born?*
SANDY: *This comes back to that epidural thing, doesn't it?* Now *I think so . . . I feel it's a natural thing and therefore it should be done naturally if possible . . . I don't think you should have to have something . . . I feel that if people go to the trouble of working it* [psychoprophylaxis] *all out and teaching it to you there must be something in it.*
After the birth:
I thought I felt a lot of pain . . . I think possibly I was a little

over-confident about the relaxation classes. I thought I'd be able to cope. But I couldn't even think *about what I was supposed to be doing. I think it was because they* [contractions] *came suddenly and painfully and quite close together right from the beginning. It didn't give me a chance to sort things out and go into it gradually.*

I had the epidural because I wasn't taking it too well, and I was getting pretty desperate. My husband wasn't liking watching me getting like that, and also the doctor and the midwife suggested I had one. So I thought well, alright.

INTERVIEWER: *Are you glad you did?*

SANDY: *Yes and no. I think now: why on earth couldn't I put up with it? I didn't intend to have one. I fully intended to try the breathing and everything. I was getting really het up. I suppose everybody does. Let's face it: it's quite painful, whatever anyone says.*

CAROLINE SAUNDERS, in pregnancy:

INTERVIEWER: *How do you feel about the actual birth now?*

CAROLINE: *I don't dread it. If I'm in pain, I'll have the epidural, it's as simple as that. I feel quite indifferent really.*

I mean I'm not a great one for suffering pain and I don't feel that you're a full woman if you feel a lot of pain. I think that's a load of rubbish actually. The more books you read and the more they keep telling you about the pain the more I keep persuading myself: the epidural . . . I was talking to my sister this weekend and she says, oh it's a pain you forget. I said don't be silly – I've never forgotten any of the pains I've had. I mean I had a filling done without an injection once and I've never forgotten that *pain. I'm not very brave.*

Afterwards:

I wouldn't say it was pleasant. I don't understand these people who say it's a wonderful thing. I wouldn't say it was unpleasant – tolerable.

It wasn't bad actually when the baby was born, because I didn't feel any pain, it was a nice sensation the baby coming out . . . I was quite happy with the effect of the epidural, because it was nice being able to feel something. It wasn't unbearable the sensation: like a slight ache.

INTERVIEWER: *In general, was having the baby anything like you expected it to be?*

CAROLINE: *I didn't expect it to be all that tremendous and it wasn't.*

Sandy Wright experienced great disorientation and anxiety on leaving hospital and then became quite depressed; for Caroline Saunders, postnatal recovery was much smoother.

Syndromes of postpartum emotional disorder, especially the blues and anxiety states, do in fact have much in common with the 'disturbed' reactions of surgical patients. For example, reactive elation as a response to surgery (marking the realization that one has passed through danger and survived) is characterized by 'momentary breakthroughs of weeping, agitation, or depressive mood' (Janis, 1958, p. 141). Euphoria in the immediate post-operative phase is especially likely to be followed by depression, as the second phase of post-operative physical discomfort ('prolonged deprivation') succeeds the first, acute phase. In Lindemann's study, serious depression had an onset three to four weeks after the operation, which is a typical time for postpartum depression (as opposed to the blues or a simple anxiety state) to occur (Lindemann, 1941, p. 135).

Categorizing maternity patients on the basis of their patienthood rather than their biological role, therefore introduces a perspective in which postnatal depression syndromes can be seen as a species of the larger genus – psychological responses to surgical trauma. This analogy is certainly appropriate to the connection between high technology birth and depression, for the experience of surgical intervention and control in these cases both outweighed expectations and was a conscious cause of stress and 'victimization' feelings for all the women concerned. It is not necessary, in other words, to posit the meaningfulness to *women* of *childbirth* per se in order to 'explain' depressive reactions, for these are associated with the meaningfulness to *people* of surgically intrusive medical experiences – a category in which childbirth is located, not necessarily, but for specific historical–cultural reasons.

DISASTER

The emotional aftermath of surgery has been compared with the psychological sequelae of natural or human-made disasters

– earthquakes, wars, etc. A group of studies has noted that following a major threat there is a

> secondary impact phase of prolonged deprivation ... The emotional pattern is biphasic in character. First, there is an elated reaction of emotional relief and then a gradual development of reactive depression ... [which] includes the following component symptoms: feelings of hopelessness, low self-esteem, loss of pleasure in usual social activities, resentment, constriction, and irritability in daily interpersonal relationships. [Janis, 1958, p. 160]

Such a syndrome of reactive depression has been noted following exposure to a wide variety of stress situations including peacetime disasters, wartime bombing of the civilian population, military combat and imprisonment or concentration camp confinement (see the bibliography in Janis, 1958, esp. p. 176). For example, Taketoshi Takuma (1978), studying the effects of a severe Japanese earthquake in 1964, reported large increases in the incidence of many 'ill-health' symptoms in the affected population about a week after the earthquake. These included palpitations, giddiness, insomnia, general irritability, headache and diarrhoea or constipation. A wartime study of men engaged in active air combat described a syndrome known as 'operational fatigue' ('the euphemism by which war neuroses are designated'). Men who were thus labelled suffered, among other symptoms, from restlessness, irritability, fatigue on arising and lethargy, difficulty in falling asleep, subjective anxiety, easy fatigue, startle reaction, and feelings of tension and depression (Grinker and Spiegel, 1945).

In the psychoanalytic tradition, such reactive depression is seen as '... essentially a human way of reacting to frustration and misery whenever the ego finds itself in a state of (real or imagined) helplessness against overwhelming odds' (E. Bibring cited in Janis, 1958, p. 176). One reason why responses to childbirth have not been assimilated to this viewpoint is presumably because the gratifications of becoming a mother are supposed to outweigh the deprivations of the experience. Yet (as the next chapter argues) this is very much a hypothetical view that has to be evaluated against an empirical range of cases. And childbirth does not *necessarily* differ from community disasters in being voluntary and predictable: some childbirths are involuntary (in the sense of being not chosen by the individual) and those that are not surgically induced are unpredictable in their timing; equally, some natural disasters, such as hurricanes and earthquakes, may be accurately forecast, so that a population is forewarned of their occurrence and probable effects. One difference lies in the size of the population affected: childbirth impinges on a population of one. Yet one characteristic of disaster reactions is the sense of being personally immune to damage or alone in experiencing it; community disasters are rarely a collective experience in this sense (Wolfenstein, 1957).

INSTITUTIONALIZATION

You feel really happy, and hospital is the last place you want to be, because it's really like being in jail.

The analogy is apposite, because although mothers 'choose' to be 'confined' in hospital,[16] the character of their institutionalization has much in common with that of prisoners and other inmates of what Goffman (1961) has termed 'a total institution'. He has provided a detailed description of the processes that institutional confinement entails: the 'mortification' of self; role dispossession; loss of identity equipment; violation of 'informational preserve regarding self'; forced interpersonal contact; and so forth. These processes are carried to extremes in such locations as concentration camps, where the overt rationale is abrogation of personal identity, but the loss of self-determination, individual autonomy and freedom of action are characteristic of institutionalization per se (Bettelheim, 1961).

Maternity hospitals are no exception to this general rule. Their very 'nature' as total institutions imposes a conformity with the general pattern. Much current criticism of maternity care in fact centres on the psychological effects of institutional confinement on the self (for example, Arms, 1977); and comments on the various routines and rituals of the inmate world were a notable feature of mothers' accounts published in

Becoming a Mother. Such aspects of hospital confinement as pre-birth shaving and denuding of personal possessions, the childlike status accorded to patients by staff during birth and in the postnatal wards, the rigid imposition of ward routines according to the principle that all patients must be treated alike, the refusal to disclose personal medical information, and so on, comprise a large part of the response to hospital delivery and early postpartum care. The parallels with concentration camp confinement are suggested by Bettelheim in his discussion of its psychological effects:

> Sudden personality changes are often the result of traumatic experiences ... the initial shock of being torn away from one's family, friends and occupation and then deprived of one's civil rights and locked into a prison, may be separated from the trauma of subjection to extraordinary abuse ... What happened in the concentration camp suggests that under conditions of extreme deprivation, the influence of the environment over the individual can become total. Whether it does or not seems to depend a great deal on impact and timing: on how sudden the impact, and how little (or how much) the individual is prepared for it (because it is also destructive if someone has always expected something terrible to happen to him [*sic*] and it does). It depends even more on how long the condition prevails, how well integrated the person is whom it hits, and finally whether it remains unmitigated. Or to put the last point differently: whether the conviction is given that no matter what one does, no positive response can be drawn from the environment through efforts of one's own. [1961, p. 147]

The fact that women having babies are not ill, nor have they been judged to offend against a dictatorial ideology, in no way alters the effect of institutionalization: it is placement in an institution that entails the personal degradation, and not any prior status (such as being ill or criminal) per se.

It was observed some years ago by Coser (1960) in her study of fifty-one surgical and medical patients in the USA that adaptation to the patient role is dysfunctional in terms of patients' preparation for life outside the hospital. Induced passivity that makes for a 'good patient' is contra-indicated in everyday life when some ability to direct the course of one's own life is necessary. The relationship between 'adjustment' to inpatient life and mental health has not been directly examined, but many studies show the high levels of anxiety that assumption of the institutionalized patient role engenders. Again, to cite an extreme instance of institutionalization, psychiatric findings on repatriated prisoners-of-war show that on release many 'appeared "suspended in time", confused by their newly acquired status, and incapable of forming decisions regarding their future course of action' (Segal, 1954; see also Bondy, 1943).

One further finding, of particular relevance to maternity patients, is the association between sleep deprivation and the onset of illness symptoms. Reduction in deep sleep occurs in the last trimester of pregnancy and is only slowly restored in the puerperium. Maternity ward routines are noted for their sleep-disturbing tendencies (79 per cent of the Transition to Motherhood sample said they had insufficient rest in hospital). Disturbances of sleep patterns that reduce the proportion of time spent in deep sleep have been reported in psychiatric patients, and cognitive dysfunction has followed experimental deprivation of sleep in normal non-pregnant subjects (Karacan and Williams, 1970). Insofar as hospitalization intensifies this problem of sleep deprivation, it may contribute directly to the possibility of postpartum emotional disturbance. In that case, it is one among various ways in which so-called 'postpartum' reactions are actually human responses to the stresses of institutionalization with its imposed denudation of personal identity and autonomy.

Childbirth is a life event, a transition among other social transitions. First childbirth stands out among all childbirths as an emblem of change, the mark of an era. By dissecting the various levels of meaning personally and socially attached to becoming a mother, the process can be interpreted in a human rather than in a specifically feminine fashion. In giving birth to her first child, a woman is involved in a status passage from non-mother to mother, the social rituals and personal consequences of which can be compared with other such status changes. Through processes of retirement and relocation, which other groups of workers encounter, her relationship to the world of paid work is permanently altered. She takes on two new jobs, in relation to which she is likely to have held unrealistic expectations and for which she may lack training. Transition to these new occupations, like all such transitions, may be personally stressful and entail the need for developing new skills and new ideas of self. During pregnancy a woman has to confront the different physical reality and image of herself as her body expands and loses its former shape: this may be perceived by her as an unpleasant physical and sexual experience, and as analogous with obesity. After the baby's birth, loss of the 'bump' produces reactions similar to those following amputation surgery: there is a feeling of loss and a need to readjust self-image to accommodate the change in body shape. New mothers are also medical patients, and their passage to motherhood has to be negotiated through the difficult territory of dependence on doctors. Birth is an experience akin to major surgery, which is known to precipitate acute emotional reactions: both are forms of 'disaster' paralleling such events as earthquakes in their emotional impact and consequences for individuals. Finally, the experience of becoming a mother entails institutionalization in hospital, with all the implications in terms of stress reactions and loss of self that this has been shown to have for other institutionalized people.

Looking at the process of becoming a mother in this way places the interpretation of childbirth as a human life event at the centre of the stage. It translates the measurement of outcome into a question about the relative balance of loss and gain in the individual psychological domains of people who have babies.

CHAPTER 9

Losses and Gains

> *... regarded from the standpoint of the social struggle, motherhood* may *be a handicap. It is certainly so at the present time ... But from the biological point of view woman has in motherhood ... a quite indisputable ... superiority.*
>
> [Horney, 1974, p. 10]

In the last chapter childbirth was compared with other social transitions in terms of its personal and social meaning. In this chapter I continue this theme by examining in more detail the character of emotional reactions to change in general.

When the familiar routines of life are disrupted, an element of potential unmanageability is introduced. The extent of this change may be major (rehousing, a change of career, a death) or minor (a cold, one postal delivery a day instead of two). The way people interpret change is similarly variable, but the probability is that every kind of change represents both some kind of loss and some degree of gain. It is the balance between these two, an equation that must be empirically negotiated by each individual, that decides the pattern of reaction to change: 'adjustment' or depression. Essentially what the change of life events imposes is the necessity to restructure meaning. As change challenges the individual's assumptive world, old meanings collapse and new ones have to be sought and believed in. If this cognitive task is not accomplished, the 'meaning of life' itself stands in jeopardy.

The classic exposition of this perspective is Peter Marris's *Loss and Change* (1974), a powerfully argued exercise in the cross-cultural logistics of social and personal change. Drawing on studies of bereavement, urban slum clearance and African tribal associations, Marris puts forward the view that where change precipitates a dominant feeling of loss, the repertoire of personal responses is akin to mourning, and can be analysed in the same terms as any 'grief' reaction. Whatever it is that the individual has lost – a loved companion, a familiar territory, an important identity – the sense of bereavement provokes a struggle between 'attempts to retain the past, and to escape altogether from its consequences' (1974, p. 41). Those who 'adapt' successfully will eventually establish a new pattern of meaning through the gradual resolution of this conflict – and it is in such a resolution (rather than in some automatic and abrupt alteration in personal habits and identity) that the meaning of adaptation inheres.

Even if change in a person's life is eagerly sought and planned, it is still a life event – the possibilities of disruption and trauma are entailed by the fact of change (though they may be heightened or lessened by individual circumstances). Marris makes this point at the end of his chapter on grief among a sample of London widows:

> This analysis of grief and mourning has been concerned with situations of loss which we recognise as painful. But by the same argument, a similar pattern of adjustment should work itself out whenever the familiar pattern of life has been disrupted. . . . Even changes which we scarcely think to involve loss may be analysable in similar terms. [p. 41]

Marris then goes on to comment that marriage, for example, involves the loss or abandonment of previous self, relationships and commitments, though it is usually also interpreted to mean the gain of a new self, a valued relationship and deeply held personal and normative commitments to one's spouse and his or her family, interests and life-style within the context of marriage as a respected and respectable institution. Yet, throughout what is at times a moving and forceful analysis of human needs and values in the face of change, Marris never once considers that in childbirth women confront perhaps the greatest paradox of all such change. In the 'mixed blessing' of childbirth's potential for enormously meaningful gain and tremendously disturbing loss, women encounter a formula that is individually variable, but also structurally dependent on the cultural articulation of reproduction and femininity and on the cultural management and control of childbirth itself.

This is a complicated way of saying that because childbirth has the associations it does for women today – because it means medical and surgical experiences, loss of autonomy as a patient, the attainment of 'feminine' fulfilment, changes in self-concept and an altered life-style – it is particularly likely to represent both sides of the equation: the negative and the positive. The changes associated with reproduction in the specific case of first childbirth, which were outlined in the last chapter, cover four main areas: (1) becoming a patient, (2) retiring from paid work, (3) becoming a full-time housewife and (4) being pregnant and becoming a mother. Each of these areas involves losses and gains in the domains of identity, role, life-style and relationships. For instance, in becoming a patient a woman is obliged to undergo frequent, time-consuming medical check-ups, she becomes a drug-user, experiences surgical trauma, has her intact body-image disrupted and is institutionalized; she may however derive some satisfaction from her career as a patient, and during it she is 'delivered of' a baby. As a worker, the loss of income, status, occupational identity and social interaction that are frequently entailed by impending motherhood may be counterbalanced by freedom from the ties of paid work routines. Being a full-time housewife is likely to carry the consequence of financial dependence, a limiting domestic identity as 'just a housewife' and the corollary of less masculine participation in domestic work; on the other hand, women who are housewives have autonomy as their 'own bosses', and the status of housewife may be regarded as an advance. The changes of motherhood include getting fat, having physical 'illness' symptoms, experiencing the 'natural disaster' of birth, feeling isolated and restricted by the role of childrearer, and meeting conflict between this role and that of wife; conversely, motherhood may be felt to fulfil women, bestow status, create a family and entail a new and interesting career.

Many losses can be restated as gains – the loss of a wage or salary and the consequential gain of freedom from the tyranny of externally imposed work structures is a case in point. For other losses, a positive interpretation may be more difficult. Many of the losses involved in becoming a patient fall under this heading: surgical trauma creates (or adds to) the resource of story-telling about medical experiences, and may confirm a previously held sick role identity, but it can hardly be construed as a benefit in any other sense.

The balance between loss and gain, the interpretation of events and processes as personally advantageous or disadvantageous, cannot be derived from the character of the events and processes themselves. It is only as events are filtered through the medium of personal biography that the balance of meaning attached to the components of the transition to motherhood can be computed.

Feeling a failure or a success manifests the impact of events on women's *self-esteem.* It seems that the differential effect of childbirth and its management, or any other element of becoming a mother, is mediated through the level of a woman's conscious regard for herself – the way in which, or the extent to which, she sees herself as a valuable and valued person. Becoming a mother either adds to this or detracts from it. Signs of impaired or raised self-esteem are thematic to many interviews and accounts of crucial phases in the transition to motherhood (though self-esteem was not asked about directly). Below I have picked out extracts from the interviews with two women that indicate the way in which the self-esteem effect presents itself. Caroline Saunders was 28, a physiotherapist (some of her comments about the birth in anticipation and retrospect are given in chapter 8); Mandy Green was 30, a hairdresser.

'WORK'

First pregnancy interview

CAROLINE: *I feel quite indifferent about giving up work. I don't mind, actually, I enjoy work. Obviously you have to give up work, though I'll quite miss the contact with people . . . I'll do other things to occupy myself; I certainly wouldn't work before the child was at school unless it was totally necessary. I don't see any point in having a child, if you don't look after it.*

MANDY: *I've always been so independent, I've never had to rely on anybody for anything before. I'll be glad to give up* that *job – I've had enough there: I've been there for three years. So the actual job itself I'm not that bothered about, but work itself: I shall probably be bored, depressed . . . I think, you know, I can't stand over the garden chatting and this, it's just not me . . . I'd hope to go back to work anyway . . .*

Second pregnancy interview

INTERVIEWER: *How did you feel about giving up work?*
CAROLINE: *Glad, I looked forward to it. I keep going out for coffee everywhere, everyone keeps inviting me out for coffee; it's lovely. I don't miss work at all, I'm always out.*
INTERVIEWER: *Do you plan to return after the birth?*
CAROLINE: *Oh no. It's marvellous actually being at home.*

MANDY: *I find I am getting ever so particular about cleanliness* [since she gave up work]. *I used to, you know, see a bit of dust and think that's it: a bit of dust. As long as there's no actual dirt around, it didn't bother me, it could pile up there for a week. . . . But I find now that I look for it. I look to see how much dust there is around. Especially in the kitchen . . . I've always been a bit particular about hygiene, but I am terrible: this isn't normally me. I'll have to watch myself and be careful, because I know there's no two ways that I can alter things and I know it is just being changed mentally and I didn't think it would be possible, your actual mental state, you know, to change. I just didn't think that was on. . . . I feel a bit lonely sometimes . . . It's not affecting me at the moment, but I could see that if it were a long period of time it would.*

First postnatal interview

INTERVIEWER: *Do you think about returning to work at all?*
CAROLINE: *No. I quite enjoy it at home. I'm quite happy. I think Richard wants to give up work now – he keeps going off in the morning and seeing me at home lying in bed: oh I've got to go to work again!*

INTERVIEWER: *How do you feel now about going back to work?*
MANDY: *I haven't even thought about it, actually. I had anticipated going back to work, but I haven't thought about it. There's no chance at the moment: I just couldn't cope.*

Second postnatal interview

INTERVIEWER: *Do you ever compare your life now with what it was like before you had the baby?*

CAROLINE: *No. I don't like to look back on things . . . I just take life as it comes, really. I was happy in that situation and I'm happy now in my present situation. I don't think you can compare. I am working at home actually. I do paperwork – I fetch the paperwork and I do it at home for £1 an hour plus my expenses. It's quite good. I was getting bored actually. I mean I was reading, but I wasn't getting the right stimulation. So I decided to do this paperwork. It's only about six hours a week. It's just enough.*
INTERVIEWER: *Would you take a full-time job?*
CAROLINE: *No, because if I want to go out during the day with my housework, or this work, I can just leave it, and catch up. Whereas if you've* got *to go out at a certain time, it's like being at work anyway, which I don't like. I mean I enjoy the freedom I have now: it's nice.*

INTERVIEWER: *Do you ever compare your life now with what it was like before you had the baby?*
MANDY: *Yes: thinking how I could just breeze out to the shops when I wanted to, and how free I was actually. Free of consideration for anybody else except Harry who is very easy to fit in with . . . If I wanted to go for a walk, I'd go for a walk. But with her I can't go for a walk. . . . Plus the lack of money, now that I'm not working.*
INTERVIEWER: *Have you felt like going back to work?*
MANDY: *I have always thought that I would like to go back to work to sort of get outside interests. It has been so intense with her, because it has been every minute of every day thinking baby things. Which I haven't particularly liked. . . . I am not as self-confident as I used to be, I'm not as confident about this going off to work lark* [she is planning two weeks' temporary secretarial work, leaving the baby with a friend]. *I should be, but I'm wondering whether I'll be able to cope with it. I mean it's only, what, seven months, since I left there? And I've been working fourteen years: why should I be any different? But I think I feel as if I've been on a little island and, you know, I'm going to step off it and I'm not sure how the ground is, you know.*

PREGNANCY AND ATTITUDES TO THE BABY/MOTHERHOOD

INTERVIEWER: *How do you feel about being eight months pregnant?*
CAROLINE: *Uncomfortable! Indifferent really. I mean it's a funny*

old stage – I've got over the excitement of knowing that it's a baby and I'm just waiting to produce it now, really.
INTERVIEWER: *Is there anything you're particularly looking forward to about having a baby to look after?*
CAROLINE: *Well, at this stage just being back to normal, I think. Just being part of a family, I suppose: becoming a family. I mean we're a family now – but a new addition.*
INTERVIEWER: *Do you think of yourself as a mother?*
CAROLINE: *I like the idea of becoming a mother. I don't think of myself as a mother. But it doesn't strike me as a strange idea.*

INTERVIEWER: *Are you enjoying being pregnant?*
MANDY: *I think women are very different, very very different . . . to me it means absolutely nothing to be honest. I cannot imagine that in seven weeks' time or whatever there will be a baby. No way. I don't mind being as I am, in fact I am enjoying being pregnant now more than before, because this is more solid now, it's part of me, but before when I was quite large and little of it was baby it was sort of in the way and I was annoyed about it . . . It just seems to me as if I've put on an awful lot of weight.*
INTERVIEWER: *Do you think of yourself as a mother?*
MANDY: *Nope, not at all. It seems strange to me – being the mother of a baby . . . I can't think of a baby as being mine, you know. I can think of a baby quite easily, but not as being part of me.*
INTERVIEWER: *Is being a mother important to you?*
MANDY: *I think so, but I think it's important inasmuch as I'd like to go through it . . . I admit I was often curious, I wondered what it would be like to feel these things happening to you. But I can't say that the end result – a baby – is anything tied up with it. A baby is what you get, it's the feeling of the bit beforehand.*

BIRTH ANTICIPATED

INTERVIEWER: *How do you feel about the birth?*
CAROLINE: *A natural experience for a woman. It'll be fairly unpleasant. I don't think it'll be a pleasant thing. But not more so than, as some people say, having their teeth done.*

INTERVIEWER: *How do you feel about the birth now?*
MANDY: *This is where the apprehension lies. If I can carry it through the way I want to carry it through, I think I would look*

forward to it. But if I am told what I'm to do and told no you can't do this . . . I'm afraid I might panic because I would feel I can't control the situation. But if I can be left to my own devices I am sure I could control the situation . . . not easily, but quite comfortably, take it in my stride . . . Pain doesn't bother me. I wouldn't like to think, you know, that I was torn. But I am a great believer in nature, a terrific believer in nature, and I think if you are reasonably fit, well, you won't tear yourself that much, because it will hang around a bit longer until you're big enough to give birth – as long as it just takes its time, nobody's pushing you.

BIRTH EXPERIENCED

CAROLINE [induced labour, epidural, forceps delivery]: *They broke the waters, introduced the drip and I started having contractions about an hour later. And they were going quite steady – they were getting worse after about another hour. And I said to the nurse: oh I don't think much of these. And she said, well you've considered the epidural, would you like it? So I said yes, yes: so I had the epidural, it was great . . . I was exhausted. I had to have a forceps delivery in the end because I couldn't push. I did push – I pushed for an hour and a half, but there was no progress, so they decided to get the doctor. I had to wait for him coming and he delivered it. And then the placenta got stuck which I could feel. And they put the baby on me – the baby came out: they put the baby on me, and started tugging at the placenta. I said, oh take her away! – I just wasn't interested.*

The induction wasn't really bad at all. Not half as bad as I imagined. You forget about it. It wouldn't bother me to be induced again.

INTERVIEWER: *Would you say you felt in control of yourself and what was going on?*

CAROLINE: *Not really, because they're in control, aren't they? You're just there. But I didn't mind that.*

MANDY [pethidine, epidural, forceps delivery]: . . . *I can't really remember what was said except that the sister came and gave me an injection . . . so I had that, and that knocked me for six, you know I can't really remember anything . . . I was completely out, because of the pethidine, not really the pain . . . When the pains got severe I was coming round at the height of the pain and going back off again, and there was no control on my behalf whatsoever, not once I'd had the pethidine . . . I never had any control over the situation at all.*

I'd had a whole build up to the start of labour, to actually having the baby, and the whole thing was just a complete anti-climax. . . . I don't know what exactly I had expected . . . but the whole nine months' preparation had been building up to the birth and . . . there you were in the labour ward, completely nothing, just here you are, just another slab sort of thing.

If I'd been more compos mentis, yes, I would have liked to have seen the whole thing and be aware of what was happening, and, you know, ask questions . . . I would have kept my eyes a bit peeled . . . I think it would have been very interesting. I wish I had been there to be able to see it all. . . . You couldn't sort of pat yourself on the back and say haven't I done well, because you haven't really. I didn't have any particular feelings towards the baby, so there was no feeling, there was just a complete nothing really. Just something that I had to go through and I went through it, and that was it.

ATTITUDES TO THE BABY, MOTHERHOOD AND THE HOUSEWIFE ROLE

First postnatal interview

INTERVIEWER: *Are you aware of being a mother?*

CAROLINE: *Yes. You can't forget it really, because the baby's with you all the time. Sometimes when I push her in her room I quite forget and get on with my housework. But you are conscious of it, because your life just revolves around her now, so you can't be anything else.*

INTERVIEWER: *Do you feel you have enough time to yourself?*

CAROLINE: *Oh no. I just don't know where the day goes.*

INTERVIEWER: *Do you feel you have a relationship with your baby?*

CAROLINE: *I think the baby develops an attachment to you. I know it's a silly thing to say, but I don't know sometimes, I feel I shouldn't leave the baby even for a minute because I'm conscious that she might be aware I'm not there . . . I think you get to know the baby, her likes and dislikes, the cries – I find it's easy if I'm there: my mind's at rest; I know how to react to her.*

INTERVIEWER: *How much difference do you think having a baby has made to your life so far?*

CAROLINE: *A tremendous amount. It just revolves around her now. Very much so. More so than I expected.*

INTERVIEWER: *Are you aware of being a mother?*
MANDY: *No. I feel more like chief cook and bottle-washer, or chief cook and nappy changer, I should say. I think at the moment there is no sort of response, or very little, and when she shows a response to me is when I feel more attached to her: when I'm just shoving it in one end and taking it out the other I think I just feel more like a human machine.*

I'm aware of being tied, I'm often aware of that at times. There is no time to get anything done, and that's just not like me . . . I find it very hard to get anything in.

INTERVIEWER: *Do you feel you have enough time to yourself?*
MANDY: *No. No way do I have enough time to myself.*
INTERVIEWER: *How much difference do you think having a baby has made to your life so far?*
MANDY: *There seems no comparison, absolutely none. . . . It's not the same life, is it?*

Second postnatal interview

INTERVIEWER: *Do you like looking after the baby?*
CAROLINE: *I enjoy it. Probably because she's a good baby. . . . And I think it's very interesting at this age. She's a very good-humoured baby. And she gives a lot of pleasure. I mean you can look at her if you're feeling depressed – I mean I don't feel depressed – but if you're feeling low, you can look at her and she lifts you up. It's very worthwhile. . . . It's something to* love. *I mean they can't love you back, yet . . . I think everyone has a certain amount of love inside them, it's a way of expressing it, on a child . . . I mean you can release your emotions on the child which you can't on a husband.*
INTERVIEWER: *How do you feel about being a mother?*
CAROLINE: *Oh I enjoy it. It's nice. It's very rewarding – it gives you a lot of pleasure. It's very difficult actually to describe: just a very very rewarding job, actually. . . . It's just something I've always wanted. And it's lived up to expectations.*
INTERVIEWER: *Do you think people treat you as a mother?*
CAROLINE: *You don't get as many whistles from men passing by! More people talk to you if you've got a baby. It takes you far longer to do the shopping. It's quite nice, actually; it's nice, people praising your baby. I mean, you do enjoy it really.*
INTERVIEWER: *Out of being a mother, being a wife and being a housewife, which would you say is most important to you?*

CAROLINE: *I suppose being a wife comes first. Then a mother. Then a housewife's definitely last.*
INTERVIEWER: *If you had to fill in a form and put your occupation now, what would you put?*
CAROLINE: *Housewife.*
INTERVIEWER: *What do you feel about that?*
CAROLINE: *Well, there's not an awful lot you can say because what else would I call myself? . . . You do feel a bit as though you've been put into a certain category. And sometimes you feel a bit neglected in a way. That you are just a housewife. You've lost your status and you are part of your husband now – it's your husband that's the important one. I suppose that's the only difference. I only feel like that when I'm filling in forms. I don't normally. I've got my own life.*
INTERVIEWER: *Apart from the fact that you're now a mother, have your interests changed at all?*
CAROLINE: *Yes. Our old friends – I don't take as much interest in them as I used to. Even though they've got children, I tend to concentrate on the friends I've made around here, I suppose I like doing more with the people round here, so we've got more to talk about. Interests socially, no, because I'm doing badminton and things like that. No, I think we've got the same interests as we used to.*
INTERVIEWER: *Do you feel you're doing what you always wanted to do in having a baby to look after?*
CAROLINE: *I never really thought it was going to be my fulfilment to have a family. It was just one of the things that happened. I'm happy now. But it was never that I really wanted to have a child and stay at home. It wasn't anything I* planned. *I don't plan my life. It was just something that happened, and I'm very happy it's happened.*
INTERVIEWER: *Since you became a mother, have your views about the position of women changed at all?*
CAROLINE: *I tend to favour female politicians more than I did before. I tend to think of women being stronger now. Able to cope more. I'm sure if I was left in a position now where I had to cope, I probably would. And I feel that other women should as well.*

INTERVIEWER: *Do you like looking after the baby?*
MANDY: *It gets a bit monotonous. She's a bit of a baby to look after. I*

don't mind looking after her. It's just a case of I can't get anything else done while I'm looking after her, and that's why I get tired.

INTERVIEWER: *How do you feel about being a mother?*

MANDY: *No different, to be quite honest . . . I can't remember what it was like to carry her or have her. In fact sometimes when she is out of the way I still think I haven't got her . . . I object to being tied down. I suppose to the friends who know me I sort of say, she's been an absolute pain in the neck, and you think carefully before you think of having any! I don't know. I am glad we've got her now, but I don't know whether I would have been glad up to now – it has been a job. I certainly haven't experienced any of the joys of motherhood. . . . This house needs so much doing to it and I would normally be the one who would be doing the things that need doing now, like the painting and the decorating. I enjoy doing them and I can't do them, because she is such a handful. I get very frustrated.*

INTERVIEWER: *Apart from the fact that you're now a mother, have your interests changed at all?*

MANDY: *I haven't had time for my other interests. Nothing. You see, it is really baby, baby, baby twenty-four hours a day. There hasn't been time for anything . . . I am just biding my time. . . .*

INTERVIEWER: *Out of being a mother, being a wife and being a housewife which is the most important to you?*

MANDY: *Oh wife.*

INTERVIEWER: *Why is that?*

MANDY: *Well, when all is said and done eventually she's going to hop off and leave and I will be left with Harry. So, and I love him very much. There's no way I want our love to die because if it did I wouldn't be any good to anybody.*

INTERVIEWER: *If you had to fill in a form and put your occupation now what would you put?*

MANDY: *Housewife, damn it. Nasty.*

INTERVIEWER: *Why?*

MANDY: *Oh, because I'm stuck with a label, aren't I? She's one of them – with the rollers in her hair. Oh, I don't know what you're supposed to feel like when you are a housewife, I really don't . . . I don't really know how life is supposed to change. But I know that housewife doesn't sound very interesting.*

INTERVIEWER: *Do you feel you are doing what you always wanted to do in having a baby to look after?*

MANDY [laughs]: *No, not particularly.*
INTERVIEWER: *Do you feel there are parts of yourself you're not using at the moment?*
MANDY: *Um, you mean like brains, things like that? I am not really living through this period of time, I am existing through it.*
INTERVIEWER: *Since you became a mother, have your views about the position of women changed at all?*
MANDY: *I think that it doesn't matter what you feel before you have a baby, you are just going to be sort of shifted into the category of being a mother or what you presume a mother is, a housewife. I don't think you can avoid it. No matter how much you don't want to become what you dread – I dreaded it – you've got to to a certain extent.*
INTERVIEWER: *How do you feel about that?*
MANDY: *Well, I wish it didn't have to be, but it does, so that's all there is to it.*

There are many contrasts between these extracts and some similarities. Both Caroline and Mandy had epidurals in labour, for example, and both felt somewhat irked by the totality of the baby's demands in the early weeks. Yet their reactions to becoming mothers diverged critically in the contribution each felt the birth of the child had made to her self-confidence and ability to cope – not only with the child, but with her own felt needs as a person and aspects of the domestic scene – housework and its isolation; wifehood. Mandy Green felt bereft of confidence in relation to her pre-motherhood performance at work: she experienced almost total relegation of self in relation to the baby's requirements. The restrictions of motherhood were not counterbalanced by reward from the baby, nor by release from the strictures of outside work. The birth itself was endured rather than experienced, in contrast to the image she had beforehand of herself as active agent and not passive subject, delivering, instead of being delivered of, a baby. For Caroline Saunders, exposed to a similar set of deprivations (patienthood, institutionalization, epidural analgesia, etc.) the response was different. She underwent a transformation of her previous image of women to a new emphasis on female strengths. This was not corroded by her 'controlled' birth, which merely confirmed her expectation that childbirth is not a woman's most supreme achievement. (In this respect it is interesting to note that her epidural enabled her to feel the baby emerging from the vagina (p. 223). More often, in this sample, epidural block annihilated this sensation.) While the bonds of motherhood were noted by Caroline as restrictive, they were also interpreted as addictive: she was welded by the emotional rewards of motherhood into a gratifying acceptance of the role. For the social contact of work she substituted a network of neighbourhood friends, and filled her need for mental stimulation by acquiring a part-time job to do at home that in no way interfered with her new-found 'freedom'.

These differences between the two women were accompanied by different descriptions of their babies in the early weeks. Mandy's baby cried more and slept less than Caroline's, a fact that may reflect their mother's different responses to birth and motherhood, but that also points to infant temperament as an important influence on maternal satisfaction.

It is obvious that the two women balanced the account of loss and gain in the transition to motherhood in two different ways. Caroline's conclusion was that, overall, it represented gain: it raised her self-esteem and promoted a positive sense of identity and achievement. For Mandy, the effect was in the opposite direction and motherhood reduced self-esteem and gave rise to feelings of failure and loss of identity.

It is not enough, in explaining these contrasting reactions, to say that the two women differed in their resourcefulness at adapting to the new situation – or that they differed in the kind of resources (of friends, etc.) on which they were able to draw. Neither is it enough to trace the post-birth responses back to motives for having a child: these did not differ in the two cases, representing paradigms of 'family' planning. One important factor was the level of expectations about childbirth and motherhood. These appeared different for the two women, and Mandy was much less prepared than Caroline for the vicissitudes of medicalized birth and of being a mother. Experiencing a reality very different from that of one's expectations impinges on self-esteem. There is a tendency to hold oneself responsible for the self-deception of unrealistic expectations and to blame oneself for the consequences of failing to match image and reality. Alternatively, a 'conspiracy' reaction – a suspicion that other women, childbirth educators, etc., have conspired to present an inaccurate picture of childbirth and motherhood – may also result in feelings of personal worthlessness: why was one not 'worth' an accurate representation of the difficulties ahead? What kind of personal weakness elicited the fictional response? The shock of discovering things are not the way they were thought to be is a crashing blow, carrying the necessary entailment of alteration in a person's assumptive world. The closer to core values the disturbed vision lies (if it relates, for example, to the achievement of a 'natural' childbirth rather than the amount of washing a baby creates), the more central and consequential an effect on self-image it might be expected to have.

But the underlying theme of Caroline Saunders' and Mandy Green's descriptions of becoming mothers, and of all the accounts collected in the Transition to Motherhood project, was not simply that women balance the losses and gains of first-time motherhood to obtain differing positive and negative formulae. This is true; but its truth holds despite, or rather because of, the fact that through the social, economic and medical phrasing of motherhood in contemporary industrialized society, the 'achievement' of becoming a mother represents primarily and essentially a loss of identity.

Motherhood erodes the sense of *personal* identity – the feeling of being a separate person in an equal community of other persons. Once a woman has a baby she will never entirely be a person in her own right again – that is, she will never achieve a personal identity on the same terms and in the same way as before she had a baby. The effect is due not to biological reproduction per se, but to the cultural categorization of reproduction and motherhood. Becoming and being a mother affect the way a woman is seen and treated by others, and social/medical differentiation rebounds on self-perception, so that a woman enters into a parallel process of self-categorization: '. . . changes in the world's view of me are likely to be associated with changes in my view of myself. This is particularly likely when changes take place in those things I view as most intimately mine' (Parkes, 1972, p. 95). During this self-categorizing process, cultural/medical labels are imported into a woman's own dialogue with herself. Since these tend to be derogatory (a 'patient', 'just a housewife') she becomes involved in a process of self-derogation that is part and parcel of her normative commitment to the institution of motherhood and its related cultural paradigm of femininity. The institution of motherhood and its experience, theoretically separate agendas, then come to be seen and felt as indissolubly linked.

Due to the *centrality* of motherhood in the feminine self-image – of women and in society generally – these changes cannot occur without affecting self-esteem. This is one of the ways in which loss of identity with motherhood carries the rider of impaired self-esteem. The identity change and impact on self-esteem is primary: the alterations in life-style and relational identities are secondary. This explains why the character of a woman's self-esteem before the onset of motherhood is so important. In chapter 6 we saw how different maternal outcomes were associated with the three socialization variables of previous contact with babies, feminine role orientation and self-image as a mother. For a woman whose self-concept is already organized around a normative commitment to motherhood, its arrival brings a sense of reinforcement and confirmation instead of a need to reorder how the self is perceived and evaluated. And, of course, for those women who have rehearsed motherhood with other babies, the gap between expectations and reality is also likely to be narrower, thus removing one rationale for revision of self-esteem.

Having said that changes in life-style and relationships with others are secondary to the identity drama, it must also be said that reactive alterations in these have a feedback effect on self-esteem. By taking a part-time job, by developing a network of friends, by pressing for a more equal division of labour in the home, a woman may be able to restore to herself the feeling of being someone other than a mere domestic appendage. This is a response charted by Caroline Saunders, when she describes her social life as a mother and says 'I have my own life'.

Since the primary meaning of first-time motherhood is loss of identity, there is a bias towards poor maternal outcome. One sign of this is the figures for 'postnatal depression', less than 'good' feelings for the baby and medium/low satisfaction with motherhood given in chapter 5. Another is the tendency for some women to note negative aspects of their new role. Asked whether becoming a mother had affected their views of the position of women, 49 per cent of the sample said it had, making them more critical of existing social arrangements. Table 9.1 lists answers to another question about the 'disadvantages' of motherhood noted by the sample women. Two-thirds of the women felt they were treated differently as mothers, a third felt economically dependent and a quarter felt restricted by the baby. Another critical parameter of the identity changes associated with first-time motherhood is that a mother's working conditions do not simply replace her job conditions as an employed worker: they are decisively different. Thus, we must add to the total picture the facts presented in Table 9.2. The transformation of identity from woman to mother, insofar as it is seen as a drop in status, is, then, accompanied by changes in life-style that tend to be felt as restrictive in character. Over a

TABLE 9.1 *Aspects of motherhood*

Aspect	*% of women noting*
Treated less favourably as mother	69
Economic dependence	30
Practical difficulties (e.g. shopping)	20
Being tied to the baby	24

N=55.

TABLE 9.2 *Mothers' working conditions*

Condition	*% of women noting*
Social isolation*	36
Monotony*	40
Excessive pace*	66
'Tied down'	80
No time to self	67
Changed (restricted) interests	55
Baby has 'changed life completely'	67

N=55.
*These questions were asked at the five week interview only.

third of the sample women reported social isolation and monotony, four-fifths described themselves as 'tied down' in general, two-thirds said they had no time to themselves, complained of excessive pace in their work or said their lives had been 'changed completely' by the baby. (This change was described as restrictive, though it was not necessarily resented.) There are thus close connections between the sense of a lost identity and the experience of deprivation as a worker. It is important to realize that the possibility of interpreting the transition to motherhood as loss in these terrains of identity and life-style is not explicable in terms of previous work careers. Previous employment status and perception of poor postpartum working conditions (monotony, social isolation, etc.) were not associated in this sample. This reflects the conclusion other studies have come to that the attribution of 'class differences' to women's employment motivations conceals the basic competing attractiveness of almost all employment work occupations in relation to the social isolation of domestic work.[1]

The problem of loss can also be seen another way. In a study of attitudes to housework (Oakley, 1974b) I noted that affiliation to the role of housewife often contrasted with the level of housework satisfaction. Many women wanted and accepted an identification with the housewife role but at the same time felt dissatisfied with the work they found themselves doing as housewives. If this is true of housewifery, how much more true it is likely to be of motherhood, a state of being that in the feminine paradigm is coated with a glorification that mere domesticity does not have. Losing her identity as a person and as a worker, a woman acquires a new highly culturally valued feminine identity. Personal difficulty inheres in the fact that not only may the conditions of a mother's work be negatively experienced but, while the maternal character is idolized, a mother's childcare work is held in very low social regard indeed. The reality, the satisfaction, of motherhood in this sense, as experienced day by day, is bound to contrast with its image and with the commitment many women feel to the state of 'being' a mother. For women becoming mothers for the first time, this discrepancy is a further source of personal and general disillusionment – another mode in which loss is experienced.

The argument about the likelihood of 'loss' interpretations applies equally cogently to the promises of fulfilment as a woman and the achievement of family status. Maternalism is, as Alice Rossi has observed, a component of the feminine paradigm that is isolated from, and even at odds with, the others. One manifestation of this is the muting of sexuality in motherhood: the sexual satisfaction of childbirth and lactation is played down, while the pleasures of heterosexual (marital) intercourse are emphasized as the correct outlet for female sexual desire:

> We define maternity in artificially narrow ways, clearly differentiating it from sexuality, and requiring that women deny the evidence of their senses by repressing the component of sexuality in the maternal role. . . . It is to men's sexual advantage to restrict women's sexual gratification to heterosexual coitus. . . . [Rossi, 1973, p. 167]

– though, Rossi suggests, it is to the disadvantage of women and children who therefore encounter a less gratifying bond, one that stresses psychological duties instead of physical mutuality. In men's images of women, too, motherhood is a limited asset. Mothers are often perceived as less sexy than other women (although pregnancy itself may be taken as a sign of sexual abandon). The physical alterations of motherhood (thicker waistline and hips, more flaccid breasts) contravene accepted standards of feminine attractiveness: this, as chapter 8 argued, is one of the standard ambiguities of motherhood. It is as though the structure of the male psyche requires a separation between sexual partners and mothers, an identity between the two posing an obscene threat to the male's fragile rejection of the feminine element – his own childhood identification with the mother as the childrearing person (see chapter 11, pp. 286–9).

Once they achieve motherhood, these are the classic dilemmas women confront. Fulfilled as women, mothers may be denied their sexuality. The transformation of couple into family proves, on inspection, to have parallel chimera-like dimensions. The birth of a child publicly labels a couple's relationship a family, but the emotional work required to deal with the new triadic relationships can be an unforeseen drawback for the wife–mother. Moreover, families are more precise formulae of gender role differentiation (housewife and 'head of the household', father, mother and child) than couples, and women who saw themselves as marriage partners before motherhood may find themselves afterwards as members of families participating in a less egalitarian role.

TABLE 9.3 *Motherhood and parental relationships five months after birth*

Aspect of parental relationship	*Increased* % (*No.*)	*Decreased* % (*No.*)	*The same* % (*No.*)
'Emotional closeness'	20 (11)	47 (26)	33 (18)
Satisfaction with masculine participation in housework	15 (8)	42 (23)	44 (24)
Satisfaction with masculine participation in childcare	7 (4)	51 (28)	42 (23)
Jointness of couple's role relationship	0 (0)	15 (8)	85 (47)

N = 55.

Some indices of these changes appear in Table 9.3. This shows that 'emotional closeness' of the couples' relationships as described by the women deteriorated during the period from early pregnancy to five months postpartum in 47 per cent of the couples, women's satisfaction with the level of masculine help in housework decreased for 42 per cent of the sample and satisfaction with the way fathers participated in babycare over the first five months of motherhood had dropped for 51 per cent of the women between the first and second postnatal interviews. (These figures are complemented by those shown in Tables 5.6 and 5.7, p. 132, which show the actual changes in the domestic division of labour reported to have taken place.) In addition, 15 per cent of the role relationships moved towards more segregation between the first and last interviews; none increased in jointness.[2]

In this computation of the losses and gains of motherhood I have, in talking of roles and identities, omitted what many people would see as the primary gain – the child itself. Reproduction is production, not only of a worker (in the Marxist schema) but of an entire new person with whom one will be in close contact for the rest of one's life. The magic of this, the miracle of biology and uterine labour, the daily joy of rearing one's own child: surely these are sufficient to counterbalance motherhood's deprivations? I would contend that the only reason why most women do not break down irremediably after childbirth is that they *are* sufficient. I mean this not in the sense that 'aren't children wonderful!' is a cultural epithet that labels children as a specific and separate class of being (Davis and Strong, 1976), but in terms of the reward that is gained by human beings in a context where the result of their labour is the love, development and growth of another human being. The biological connection may be an added bonus, or an irrelevancy: the point is that in all philosophies of human action facilitating such growth is seen as intrinsically self-gratifying.

I just enjoy her. She's more interesting *than I thought a baby would be. I find all her little developments fascinating . . . It's like a chrysalis, like watching a butterfly coming out.* (Sophy Fisher)

I feel as though I've done something useful if I can turn her into a nice person and put her into the world. I'll feel that I've really achieved something. (Angela King)

The gain of the child itself points in the direction of an increase in self-esteem. Yet, paradoxically, and because of mothers' particular social and personal circumstances, there is no absolute guarantee of this. Earlier I argued that first childbirth has different outcomes for different women according to its effect on self-esteem. There are two prongs to this argument. In the first place, it is pre-existing levels of self-esteem that count; how a woman feels and thinks about herself as a person before she becomes a mother. Second, it is the case that different social contexts of the transition to motherhood can contribute in different ways to self-esteem; some childbirths and some motherhood transitions may be more discouraging than others. The two contentions connect: low self-esteem before motherhood increases vulnerability to the impact of particular childbirth and motherhood transition experiences; high self-esteem protects. But why should, say, technological childbirth or lack of employment lower self-esteem in the first place? What are the inner processes whereby life events and vulnerability factors act to lower a person's self-esteem? The other unanswered question concerns the psychology of women specifically. For, in the light of the data on outcomes to the transition to motherhood presented in chapters 6 and 7, two theories are possible: either first childbirth and motherhood are such inherently dissatisfying experiences in modern industrialized society that the possibility of poor maternal outcome has become a probability; or, there is something about the psychology of women in particular that renders them especially liable to disturbances in self-esteem following a life event such as childbirth. (This contention does not have to refer to the Freudian paradigm, as we shall see in the next chapter.) It is likely that both theories are relevant. But before turning to the particular issue of women's psychology and self-esteem, I want to discuss in a little more detail the self-esteem effect of particular childbirths and particular contextual definitions of becoming a mother as a social transition.

Life events constitute loss events if their major effect is to deprive a person of sources of value or reward. Faced with such deprivation, a person may struggle on and emerge without disabling emotional impairment if he/she feels in control of the parameters of his/her life space and is able to exercise this control effectively, so as to restore a sense of meaning. Otherwise the response to loss is liable to be hopelessness, and the risk of feeling this way for very long is its generalization; in such generalization of hopelessness probably lies the genesis of clinical depression (and other states thus labelled by their possessors). The key is the extent to which a person feels, and is, able to take control over her/his own life. Where the feeling is strong, personal self-regard is high; one is important to oneself through the possession of this skill to determine, at least partially, the shape of one's life. Technical difficulties may be more easily overcome, the search for alternative sources of reward may be more likely to be successful and the fight against feeling hopeless will more reliably accomplish the basic feat of warding off depression. But where the opposite case holds, and feelings of being in control are low or non-existent, the possibility of high self-regard is remote: personal efficacy belongs to other people. Practical problems such as finding a new place to live, a new job, a day nursery place for a child, become overwhelming obstacles: what they overwhelm is the fragile sense of being at the centre of one's own life. It is correspondingly more difficult to substitute new sources of reward for old (the effort is literally too much) and easier to feel that one's sense of pessimism about particular events is truly depressing in its implications.

The role of vulnerability factors in this picture is described by Brown and Harris as making feelings of control less likely. They propose that these factors (in their analysis, loss of mother before eleven, three or more children under fourteen, absence of a confiding relationship, no employment) act so as to deprive a woman of critical role identities, making a fit between aspiration and achievement in the wife and mother roles less possible (Brown and Harris, 1978, ch. 15 'Depression and loss'). One problem with this view is that in having children (particularly more than one child), in staying at home to look after them and in acting as the supportive partner in a role-segregated relationship, a woman is, in fact, precisely meeting some main requirements of womanhood in our culture. It is difficult to see how the vulnerability to depression associated with being at home, having three or more young children and lacking an intimate relationship could be manifested in the chronic low self-esteem of failure to be a 'good wife and mother'. An alternative interpretation is that the economic and social conditions under which motherhood and wifehood are practised are themselves inimical to high self-esteem, and that in certain circumstances women are protected against the mental health consequences (precipitated by life events) of low self-esteem. This is simply a reversal of the argument, for vulnerability factors are also protective when assigned the opposite value (*having* a paid job, etc.). It does seem however that, in terms of developing a theoretical understanding, it is more correct to stress their protective value as defences against the erosion of self-importance entailed by institutionalized female domesticity.

Following this argument, the four vulnerability factors analysed in relation to outcome of the present study (chapter 7) should be seen more accurately in their positive values as protective factors, rather than in their negative version as inducing vulnerability. The relevant formulation is then that a medium/high previous contact with babies, employment, joint marital role relationship and a satisfactory housing situation provide protection against the lowered self-esteem impact of first childbirth as a life event. This rewording of the relationship is of central importance to the framework of understanding that can be developed about the genesis of reactions to childbirth. It alters the emphasis from a weakness in the actor (women being 'vulnerable' to the effects of childbirth) to the problematic character of a social institution (childbirth and motherhood being so socially defined that the probability of personal damage or difficulty is high). It is essential to avoid interpretations that cast women in the role of culpable victim, for historically this has both been the dominant ideological mode of 'explaining' women's distress and provided a prescription for the treatment of personal, as opposed to social, disorder.[3] Any diagnosis that blames women individually for the collective manifestation of symptoms of oppression is theoretically naïve and politically reactionary in character.

It is clear that the four 'protective' factors must operate in different ways. Contact with children before the advent of motherhood converts the assumption of responsibility for one's own child from a sudden shock to a continuous theme. Neither are the distasteful aspects of childcare new, nor (perhaps) is the social marginalization of maternal childcare work experienced as pervasive; looking after children is simply something that has to be done, an activity separate from the status of women as mothers. The protective effect of the other three factors is accomplished differently, for they relate the experience of motherhood to its context in the present. By maximizing its advantages and minimizing its disadvantages, they encourage self-esteem to remain reasonably high. Having a 'decent' home to rear a child in, doing so in a relationship where mother and father share to some extent the same world of interests and activities, feeling confirmed as a non-domestic person by the social and financial reward of employment: these all provide a charter that stresses the values and benefits of motherhood without placing undue emphasis on its privations.

I have also said that the greatest protection against breakdown after childbirth is the child itself. 'A baby of one's own'[4] provides an alternative source of reward to counterbalance those that are, or may have been, lost: the satisfaction of a job well done, social interaction with workmates, the sense of physical and emotional intactness that is often broken or suspended by the act of birth. In the long run this seems to be evidently true. Weeks, months or, in some cases, years after childbirth there is a feeling of recovery from the trauma of becoming a mother that expresses the successful imposition of a new pattern of meaning on life. (This is one meaning of 'adjustment' as a measure of outcome, of course.) What was lost is seen as balanced by what has been gained, the 'depressing' qualities of motherhood as outweighed by the joy of loving a child. But it takes some time for this process to happen. First of all, birth is experienced in a direct physical way as loss – the loss of the baby within, which, until it is recognized as an independent person, is bound to be experienced as part of the mother's body. Also, in the short run many babies are not found rewarding: crying and refusing to sleep or to be comforted are common sources of parental anguish in the early weeks. In terms of work, and in terms of physical energy, most first babies turn out to be far more demanding than their parents anticipated they would be. To the exhaustion of childbirth is added the deprivation of broken nights; against the image of the mother as omnipotent satisfier of the baby's needs is set the depressing intransigence of the newborn's refusal to *be* satisfied.

These (usually temporary) difficulties are compounded by a further problem. To find the baby rewarding, a mother has to develop an attachment to it. Emotional attachment to the baby is not an automatic consequence of the pre-birth physical association between mother and child. The physical 'gain' of producing the baby is not a gain at the level of emotional reward until the relationship between mother and baby has been established some days, weeks or months later. In the Transition to Motherhood project, some indices of these immediate post-partum difficulties are: 70 per cent of mothers did not love their babies at first, 77 per cent said that looking after a baby was harder work than they imagined, 100 per cent found the first weeks tiring, some to the point of physical exhaustion. Table 9.4 shows some ways in which the triumph of becoming a mother may be undermined by a sense of not having gained in personal terms.

TABLE 9.4 *Loss versus gain in early maternal care*

Mothers' reactions	*% of sample*
Not interested in the baby at birth	70
Disappointed with baby's sex	25
Babycare harder work than expected	77
Felt angry/violent towards baby	70
Cannot get enough sleep	100
Feeding problems	73
Felt very anxious about baby	45

N = 55.

In most cases these difficulties were eventually resolved, though they might be neither easily nor rapidly overcome. The painful character of the process is better appreciated when it is realized that one important principle involved is that, as Marris has put it, 'loss cannot be made good merely by substitution' (Marris, 1974, p. 91). Grieving for a lost person, object, identity or relationship resolves itself not through substitution but through a reformulation of meaning. Hence the vacuity of responses that urge a bereaved person to re-invest her/his energies in new domains, to 'forget' or 'count your blessings'. Such exhortations make no sense when what is felt is the profundity of loss and an empty hopelessness that asserts disengagement from society as the correct response. They only begin to seem relevant when out of the conflict of meaning generated by loss the new attachments are already emerging and it genuinely seems to the bereaved person that all is not lost and something can be, or has been, gained: a revised identity, a new strength, a vision of alternative roles and relationships.

The argument thus moves on to the point at which depression as an outcome of first birth can be restated as grief work for the mother's lost identity. This formulation does not necessarily suppose that first childbirth will provoke a depressive response in greater measure than subsequent ones. Although the extent of the change that is capable of interpretation as loss can be seen as greater in the case of first birth, it is possible that aspects of the loss are intensified by the addition of other children to the family. A second, third or fourth child could, for instance, lead to an accelerated deterioration in parental relationships, or make a woman feel much more tied to the home than she did with only one child. Sincc postnatal depression has been attributed primarily to defects in maternal personality and has not been seen as a loss response to childbirth as a life event, existing research cannot answer even the statistical question whether depression occurs more often after first birth than others – or whether (a more qualitative question) the character of depression is different in first-time and other mothers.

That depression after bereavement is common has been shown by many studies in Britain and America. How frequently it occurs is not known, partly because research on bereavement reactions has often been limited to those who seek help, and partly because the difficulty, as Parkes has said, is that 'Grief is not a set of symptoms . . . It involves a succession of clinical pictures which blend into and replace one another' (1972, pp. 6–7). While bereavement reactions can be seen as falling into the category of 'reactive depression', the successive stages of numbness, yearning and depression that mark the bereaved person's responses can also, as Parkes argues, be interpreted as particular types of separation anxiety states: anxiety is a prominent symptom, expressing the fundamental fact of the person's irremediable separation from the loved and familiar person. Whatever the psychiatric classification, and whatever the nature of the loss that has occurred (the death of a husband for instance can have different meanings and consequences according to circumstance), the symptomatology is remarkably consistent: physical distress and health impairment; apathy, insomnia, loss of contact with reality, anger, guilt, hostility, feelings of unreality (1972, pp. 6–7), all of which are also manifested in so-called 'postnatal depression'.

Although childbirth itself has not been considered in this literature, studies of bereavement reactions have established that

(1) the sequence of responses to other types of loss, for example the amputation of a limb, are similar to those experienced by bereaved persons (this point was touched on in chapter 8);
(2) the intensity of grief is not proportional to the degree of attachment that was felt to the lost person;
(3) depression is not a symptom of pathology when it occurs following a loss; 'In fact there are some grounds for regarding

the absence of depression after bereavement as more "abnormal" than its presence' (Parkes, 1972, p. 107).

If there are grounds for supposing this in the case of those who lose a spouse, then the grounds for supposing the same in the case of first childbirth are surely clear, given what has been said earlier about the predominance of loss following this event. The second point is especially relevant, for it is sometimes contended that postnatal depression is a function of the mother's (unfeminine) commitment to an employment career: the depressive reaction expresses a non-maternal identification.

> Although it seems natural to grieve for the loss of someone or something you love, love does not explain grief ... The fundamental crisis of bereavement arises, not from the loss of others, but the loss of self. [Marris, 1974, pp. 32–3]

It is the impact of loss on self-identity that makes it so disturbing. Conceptions of self are disputed, customary habits of thought and behaviour become out of place. It is easy to see that where death is unexpected the depth of the disturbance may be greater: equally, where the realities of motherhood have been unforeseen or incorrectly anticipated, the temporary shattering of the ego may be more complete.

The implication of this argument that postnatal depression is a response to the loss meaning of childbirth is that the likelihood of depression occurring may be directly computed out of the balance between loss and gain that characterizes each experience. Moreover, the contribution of medical factors – the way the childbirth is managed and is seen to be managed – can readily be assimilated to this model. An experience of control by medical professionals, of birth by technology and surgery, with the mother as passive subject rather than active agent, simply facilitates loss interpretations: in becoming mothers, women lose their separate identity as people cumulatively, by forgoing an occupational role and by submitting to the personal degradations of patienthood. Where, for structural reasons (the practical and ideological difficulty of combining motherhood with employment work, the medicalization of childbirth), this dual loss is the probable mode of experiencing first childbirth, depression and other signs of poor 'adjustment' are to be expected as a normal reaction.

CHAPTER 10

A Psychology of Women?

> *Depression, in general, seems to relate to feeling blocked, unable to do or get what one wants. The question is: what is it that one really wants? Here we find difficult and complicated depressions that do not seem to 'make sense'. On the surface it may even seem that a person has what she wants. It often turns out, however, that, instead, she has what she has been led to believe she should want . . . How then to discover what one is really after? And why does one feel so useless and hopeless?*
> [Miller, 1977, p. 91]

The chief methodological stumbling block in the study of women's reactions to reproduction has been that only women have babies. This has encouraged an already prevailing tendency to treat women as a separate class of beings. It has seemed self-evidently true that the responses of women to childbirth must be bound up with (and therefore explained by) the character of their feminine identities.

The problem with this approach, as we have seen, is that it ignores the substratum of the *human* element. Women are 'first and foremost human beings', and they do not cease to have this status because they have babies. Human behaviour is interpreted by its human context (a dictum that in its application to men is rarely questioned). The question of how relevant gender is in any situation is hypothetical, and not a matter for *a priori* assumption. Obviously identity as a feminine or masculine person can be important as an aspect of personal identity and can act as a significant motivator of conduct. Yet the extent of its importance and the nature of its contribution to any given outcome is an issue that can only be settled empirically.

Part I of this book examined the model of maternal attitudes to reproduction in terms of traditional feminine psychology that have abounded to date in the medical and social sciences, and found it lacking in explanatory value. In Part II an alternative perspective has been proposed via an analysis of childbirth as a particular kind of life event and of becoming a mother as a type of social transition. I have argued that the character of this life event and social transition as experienced by many women is such as to involve loss, and that it is the impact of this loss on the psyche that generates the insignia of 'maladjustment' to motherhood.

The argument throughout has been anchored in the social situation of women today, since it is only in this way that the particular character of first reproduction as a life event/social transition can be exposed. But the interpretation of maternal outcome as a response to childbirth as a life event has been arrived at primarily through a consideration of how life events and transitions impinge on the psychology of human beings in general. Is this an overreaction to the constraints of the feminine paradigm? Though traditional paradigms of femininity cannot explain why women respond to reproduction the way they do, perhaps there is another sense in which the psychology of women underwrites human response – to childbirth, as well as to other critical life events?

I'm not a very confident sort of person.

I am not basically a very confident person. I always question everything I'm doing.

I don't feel confident when I'm meeting people . . . I'm not a very good judge of character . . . I always say the wrong thing at the wrong time . . . And also, you know, worrying how people look at me and what they think of me. That seems to preoccupy me quite a bit.

I'm not very confident. I've got that sort of shyness, that I'm afraid to meet people and things like that.

I've no confidence in myself at all in any way.

I just feel the same as I've always felt. I've never had any confidence.

How confident do you feel in yourself?

Oh I've no confidence at all, none at all. I never have.

Can you make decisions easily?

No I cannot, no I'm just a wreck, I'm a hopeless person, honestly . . . I'm no good.

How confident do you feel in yourself?

I've never been confident in myself, never.

Can you make decisions easily?

I've never been able to make decisions.

Why is that?

I think because I'm not a very confident person . . . so far as personal things go, for example my appearance and my personality and things like that. . . . If we go out, I never make a decision about where we're going. You know I'm always trying to please somebody else rather than please myself . . . I'd much rather somebody else made the decision for me.

These vignettes express a thread running through these and other interviews with women: the chronic self-doubt many women experience. What is doubted is inherent self-worth, and with it the capacity to control what happens to the self: if I am not worth very much, then I certainly cannot 'master' the shape of my life.

Lack of self-esteem is most commonly expressed in the form of low self-confidence. Either terminology is appropriate to the related dimension of 'mastery', a term that is intrinsically sexist through its imputation of control to the masculine gender – though not, in one sense, inappropriately so, since it seems to be women who tend, in this and other research, to feel they are passive victims and not active agents of their fate. 'Mastery', as Brown and Harris have analysed it, is of critical importance to life event reactions, underlying as they see it all four of their vulnerability factors (loss of mother before eleven, three or more children under fourteen, no employment, lack of an intimate relationship) by interposing an axis of optimism–pessimism with which personal difficulty is confronted (Brown and Harris, 1978, ch. 15 'Depression and loss'). A woman who feels 'master' of her own life is more likely to feel basically optimistic in the face of threatening change: she is able to visualize recovery from loss and the restructuring of identity and reward that this entails. Conversely, someone who does not feel 'mastery' is more likely to respond with enduring pessimism to change or difficulty: she cannot see 'the light at the end of the tunnel'; her vision of recovery is obscured by the image she has of herself as a victim.

Neither response is contingent on circumstances: both proceed from dimensions of the self-concept. The self as controller or controlled is a feature of identity that is probably formed in infancy as part and parcel of the child's developing sense of being (becoming) a person among, but different from, other people. It is a function of the *differentiation* that is learnt about, and then applied to, the separateness of the self and other selves – a mode of experiencing oneself in the world. In Brown and Harris's model it is particularly important to isolate the development of mastery in childhood because only in this way can the impact of loss of mother before eleven be linked with increased risk of depression in adulthood. They contend that in such cases individual mastery is not learnt, or is not learnt sufficiently, because until about the age of eleven control of the child's environment is exercised mainly by the mother (in the conventional family situation where the mother is the childrearing parent). This learning failure intensifies the chance of adult depression per se, but also probably helps to promote a sequence of events that itself militates against an ability to feel in control (becoming involved in a non-intimate marriage, having three or more children under fourteen, for example).

In theory, the argument about the childhood learning of mastery being a necessary precursor to adult feelings of self-esteem is applicable to both sexes. There is no reason why the *way* in which mastery is developed should be gender differentiated. But, on the other hand, since childhood and childrearing *are* gender differentiated, there is every reason to suppose that the opportunity to learn mastery is differentially provided in the socialization of female and male children. This would be a necessary contention if the argument about the relevance of mastery to self-esteem is to hold any explanatory value so far as the differential responses of men and women to the stress of life events is concerned. The sex differences literature does, in fact, show female–male differences on various dimensions related to the development of 'mastery' including aggression, dependency and spatial ability. Insofar as it is possible to connect these gender differences with different socialization pressures (the methodology of much sex differences research is often not adequate to this task) there does seem to be a general parental concern for the fragility and physical vulnerability of girls as opposed to boys. Girls are restricted more and their dependency meets with more approval than does that of boys: parents' views of how boys and girls differ emphasize the greater physical activity and environmental control of boys and their greater resistance to parental manipulation (Maccoby and Jacklin, 1974, ch. 9 'Differential socialization of boys and girls'). In later childhood and adolescence males see themselves as higher on the dimensions of personal strength and potency than females; girls are more likely to believe that their achievements are due to factors beyond their control ('luck' rather than hard work – ch. 4 'Achievement motivation and self concept'). 'The greater power of the male to control his own destiny is part of the cultural stereotype of maleness' (p. 157) – as conveyed by the media, as well as in the heads of men and women.

Having argued that first childbirth impairs self-esteem by provoking a sense of loss in people who are already low in 'mastery', the next step is to ask *why* the hopelessness that is occasioned by loss is so often generalized into frank depressed mood or full-blown clinical depression. The link with specific 'vulnerability' in the Transition to Motherhood study (little previous contact with babies, no employment, housing problems, a segregated marital role relationship) draws attention to a set of social circumstances that facilitates the impairment of self-esteem with the loss of first childbirth. But it is the mediation of a specifically female psychology that attaches a high probability to this outcome. (I use the term 'female psychology' as opposed to 'feminine psychology' to indicate the difference between what I am about to say and the psychoanalytic paradigm of women's psychology that was criticized in chapter 2.)

Thirty years ago a short article by a sociologist, Helen Hacker, entitled 'Women as a minority group' appeared in the American journal *Social Forces* (1951). Often cited, but never taken up as a research brief, the article's theme outlined the parallels between the social situation and personal character of women and 'negroes' as two minority groups within a white masculine cultural ethos. 'Minority group' is not a statistical term, it refers to 'any group of people who because of their physical or cultural characteristics, are singled out from the others in the society in which they live for differential and unequal treatment'.[1] Hacker aligns many so-called feminine characteristics with the introjection of the dominant group's attitudes of inferiority and dependence. Thus, a comparison of ideal–typical 'negro' and 'feminine' character reveals many similarities: the attribution of inferior intelligence, emotional instability, poor superego, 'natural' deference, mythical contentment, and actual social, economic, political and legal discrimination. 'Helplessness' is a key attribute of both ethnic and gender inferiority, because it is a label attached to the character of minority group members by the dominant group and because such labelling promotes the formation of parallel attitudes among minority group members themselves. The connection between labelling by others and labelling by self is an intimate and mutually reinforcing one. Moreover, it is likely to be mediated by features of the social structure (e.g. the segregation of negroes and of women in the family) that encourage intergenerational transmission of such imputed inequalities. The social/economic division of labour, the attitude of the dominant group to themselves and to subordinates and the inculcation of minority group personality, all coexist in an arrangement that seems ordained by 'nature' but is in fact part of a cultural strategy on behalf of the male white world to maintain supremacy.

More recently, Jean Baker Miller (1977) has explored this mode of analysing feminine personality in greater depth. Beginning with the basic precept that the character of women is formed dialectically with the fact of male supremacy, she argues that the opposition between femininity and masculinity is secondary and the conflict between superordinate and subordinate is primary: gender identity styles are a *particular* manifestation of the cultural hierarchy, and it is only by viewing the relations between men and women as a specific instance of the oppression of one class by another that the social differentiation of sex can be understood.

Characteristic of the modus operandi of a dominant group is the assignment of preferred values, roles, activities and personal qualities to itself. Subordinates become the repository of inferior versions; assigned and behavioural modes of inferiority become, significantly, indistinguishable. However the matter by no means ends there. The division of responsibility is most unequal (as one would expect it to be), but it is so in the sense that the subordinates (women) have become the 'carriers' of certain crucial but problematic aspects of human existence: those concerned with emotional connectedness to others rather than with the enhancement of self-autonomy; with helping others to grow rather than oneself; with serving others' needs rather than establishing and satisfying one's own. (This is one reason why much women's work is not perceived as genuine labour: it is associated with helping others' development and not one's own, a quality that runs counter to the dominant value.) Women's crucial oppression as a subordinate group is thus not being able 'to feel that their life activities are for themselves' (Miller, 1977, p. 62). And, correspondingly, male society is engaged in a permanent fight to prove its self-directedness by maintaining the subordination of women who give that self-directedness the *appearance* of truth. In reality, of course, men are only where they are because of women's constant emotional and personal/social 'housekeeping' support.

It is difficult to summarize the implications of this complex position. But it could be said, as Miller suggests, that women have been put in charge not (or not only) of humankind's lowest needs but of their highest necessities – the capacity for emotional cooperation and creativity. The result of this is often not reward, but disability. Through their intense attunement to the needs of others, women are likely to suffer from feelings of weakness, vulnerability and helplessness in far greater measure than men. These qualities are labelled disabilities by the dominant culture (of men and the male-led psychoanalytic and psychiatric professions), and indeed they *feel* like disabilities to women who have internalized the dominant values and are trying to match their inner experiences with the outer reality of conventional feminine roles. But if the constrictions of the male ideological paradigm are loosened, it becomes evident that symptoms of emotional connectedness with others (which include feelings of vulnerability and helplessness) are very far from the 'sickness' they appear to be. They are optimistic signs that an individual is embedded in relations with others and, in more general terms, that society as a whole possesses an important dimension of psychic health – is concerned with the way human beings develop their potential for living 'together'.

To see this, women have to be capable of an ideological transformation. They have to be able to recognize that the image of their characters conveyed by masculine culture is one-sided and limited in its representation not only of human potential but of female reality. As Miller points out, the problem for women has always been one of creating a basis for worthiness that differs from that bestowed by the dominant culture.

> They have effected enough of a creative internal transformation of values to allow themselves to believe that caring for people and participating in others' development is enhancing to self-esteem. [1977, p. 44]

– even though the expression of these alternative values has to be in the language of the dominant culture: 'just a housewife'. Most women have simply not had sufficient opportunity to recognize the ideological substitution of weakness for strength and the legitimacy of their own contribution to the social order.

This point can be generalized beyond the individual case-history to research on the generality of women's situation. For it seems likely that what has not been sufficiently appreciated is the chronicity of low self-esteem in the psychology of women, the fact that a low estimation of self stems not from the possession of a different genital organization or from a disturbed pattern of family relations, but from the simple impoverishment of being female in a male world and experiencing a life-long syndrome of personal and institutional subordination. Whereas particular women may be especially low in self-esteem (those who have lost their mothers before eleven, those who have no employment, and so on), the generic difficulty is not the specifically dissatisfying social context but the underlying cultural demarcation of women as inferior, which makes impaired self-esteem the probable response to all personal difficulty.

'Mastery' in women is not a highly developed quality: according to the dominant paradigm of relations between men and women, it is not supposed to be. Similarly, because affiliation with others is such a valued feminine characteristic, loss of a sense of being affiliated is likely to be experienced as especially threatening. Is this what happens when women become mothers? How can women be said to lose in emotional connectedness when they simultaneously gain the richly meaningful relationship with a child?

As we have seen in both the Transition to Motherhood and other studies, motherhood is generally experienced as a constriction of the social world. Friendships are often narrowed down to a circle of biological relations and geographical neighbours and, of course, to the nuclear family itself. Such a reduction means qualitative as well as quantitative loss, for what is given up is the chance to interact with others as a person in one's own right, that is independently of the fact of motherhood. The extent of affiliation is changed, but so is its character. Interaction on a social-role basis is not the same as self-motivated interaction.

A similar process of attrition takes place within the nuclear family. Here, the necessity of putting motherhood first is substituted for the opportunity to define the female–male relationship as one between equal partners. Compensation for this loss of companionship with her partner is not necessarily provided by the mother's relationship with her child for, as we have seen, this is the product and not the precursor of social interaction between them.

In becoming a mother a woman loses the main basis for self-worth provided by male-led society: the social and financial rewards of employment. 'Work' counts as the basis for self-estimation in a somewhat complex sense, which can be conveniently summed up as 'masculine'; it does, however, include the specific contribution of a capitalist economic organization and protestant ideologies about the benefits of 'work' to the soul. So long as 'work' is held in high regard as the economic mainstay of capitalist society; so long as it is seen to reflect (or develop) a person's moral character; and so long as it is equated with personal growth and achievement, then those who are barred from its world (women, mainly) are deprived of perceiving their value as people. It is important to realize that these consequences of motherhood appear to some extent even in women who continue to be employed. For them again, as we have seen earlier in this book, employment is never again likely to be on the same basis as it was before the onset of parenthood: it will be temporary, or part-time, or subject to interruptions caused by maternity, and even if full-time and relatively uninterrupted it will be contingent on the fact of motherhood, since the shape of a woman's employment life will be determined by the extent to which she is able to solve the problems of her life as a mother. The automatic confirmation of self in 'work' is lost through the induced primacy of the commitment to child-rearing.

Having said this, it is, however, essential to note that, so important is the status attached to 'work' in masculine society, maternal involvement in it supplies some protection against vulnerability to depression. It would seem that any opportunity to receive public reward for one's labour encourages feelings of being worthy and of being in control – at least of the work-process – that help to balance the perceived deprivations of motherhood. The only viable alternative is, as Miller notes, the development of a counterbelief that caring for a baby makes one a worthy person per se, and this is a more radical step than many women are able to take, given their socialization to masculine horizons.

There is another interpretation of postnatal depression in terms of the psychology of women as a subordinate group that is suggested in Miller's book, although it is not offered as such. She says:

> It has long been recognized that there are so-called paradoxical depressions, which are most often observed in men. They occur after a man who has been competent receives a promotion or other advance that presumably should make him happy and even more effective. Such depressions may reflect the fact that the individual is forced to admit to increased self-determination and to admit that he, himself, is responsible for what happens. He is not doing it for someone else or under the direction of someone else. Women do not get promotion depressions so commonly because they do not get many promotions. [1977, p. 92]

They do, however, get promoted from non-mother to mother, a promotion that, in terms of responsibility and autonomy, is very definitely a gain.[2] And if men, trained in habits of self-determination, are liable to experience fear when opportunities to engage in it are increased, how much greater might be the terror of women, who are not used to self-determination as a principle of action.

The promotion to motherhood is a double-edged sword in two further senses. It may bestow responsibility and the capacity for self-direction, but it also carries the rider that if these are fully taken up the basis of a woman's evaluation by the dominant group may change. The sting in the tail of the psychology of subordinate groups is that it is on the maintenance of this psychological status quo that the evaluation by the dominant group of the worth of subordinate group members rests. Once subordinate group members begin to emulate the psychological structure and social/economic statuses of the dominant group, they cannot be 'loved' (needed) by the dominant group in the same way. The dilemma for women is how to use the autonomy they are offered as mothers without seeming to – and certainly without being affected by it.

In the second place, the opportunity to direct one's own life as a mother is limited by its condition: the child. The paradoxical reason for 'becoming one's own boss' is satisfying 'the baby as dictator' (Andrewski, 1966). Babies are not malleable objects of maternal labour, but independent variables whose nature and behaviour daily shape the extent of self-determination mothers are able to exercise in their work. Moreover, it is a salient facet of masculine paradigms about women and children that although (because?) they share the same subordinate status women exist to serve children. A 'good' mother is one who is especially attuned to the needs of her child; one, that is, in whom this 'feminine' sensitivity is particularly well developed.[3] By making it a condition of motherhood that women are vulnerable to children and their needs in this way, masculine culture ensures the covertness of conflict: the strength of women's connection to their children is also their weakness.

All the evidence is that women on the one hand look forward to the promotion of first-time motherhood and, on the other hand, experience great shock when the reality of this promotion impinges on them. They find that emphasizing their new self-directedness threatens marital harmony, to which disappointment is added the discovery that babies very often demand the upper hand. These realities, in a social context where motherhood as an occupation is idolized but socially downgraded by the dominant culture, are usually sufficient to block any attempt to reform dominant values and salvage the reward of enhanced self-esteem.

The impact of disappointed expectation underlies many of the connections shown in Figure 6.2 (p. 142) between work conditions and 'background' factors on the one hand, and the outcomes of depressed mood and medium/poor feelings for the baby on the other. What is common to all these associations is the revealed reality of motherhood behind the disguise of the dominant paradigm: the discovery of the effect of motherhood as it is, rather than as it is supposed to be.

Yet if such an approach to female psychology is genuinely an aid to interpreting 'loss' reactions to motherhood, it must, in addition, be able to throw some light on the connections outlined in chapters 5–8 between maternal depression and the medical control of childbirth. Patienthood and femininity are similar stereotypes: both patients and women are thought of as dependent and passive persons. One aspect of a dominant group's stereotyping of subordinates is the attribution of child-like status, a cluster of personality characteristics organized around submissiveness, passivity, dependence and lack of initiative. This has been true of ethnic minorities and of women and is an integral part of the patient role as it has evolved within professionalized medicine. Thus, to begin with, whatever loss women experience in becoming mothers is likely to be compounded by the attrition of personality accompanying patienthood. The match between femininity and patienthood can be phrased differently, however; it could be contended that patienthood (in an ideal–typical sense) comes more easily to women than to men because their socialization as women has prepared them so well for its role demands and associated personal deprivations.

In an important sense this is true. But it is probably also correct to say that, *because* of the fit between patienthood and femininity, women's vulnerability is increased. The imposed dependence of patienthood magnifies the dependent response of subordinate group status and a double deprivation is experienced. The effect of such deprivations is cumulative. Women are victims of a situation of 'learned helplessness'.

The aetiology and consequences of a disposition to feel helpless are discussed by Seligman (1975) in a book that generalizes from the motivational consequences of uncontrollable shock in dogs to the syndrome of depression in human beings. The dangers of importing models of animal behaviour wholesale into explanation of human conduct are many (some are discussed by Seligman), but his basic argument does seem not improbable as an interpretation of one of the fundamental mechanisms involved in human responses to stress. It is particularly pertinent to female psychology, though Seligman himself does not appear to visualize this connection.[4]

The original experiment concerned the giving of uncontrollable electric shocks to 150 dogs. These dogs had been restrained and exposed to shocks whose onset, offset, duration and intensity were determined only by the experimenter and not by any voluntary response the dog could make. Thereafter, they were placed in a two-sided chamber in which jumping over the barrier could turn off the shock, or avoid it altogether. Compared with a sample of dogs who had not been subjected to uncontrollable shock, the experimental group behaved in a bizarre fashion, refusing to learn how to avoid the shock and instead lying down to accept it passively time after time. For two-thirds of the group this response persisted. Seligman contends that

> laboratory evidence shows that when an organism has experienced trauma it cannot control, its motivation to respond in the face of later trauma wanes. Moreover, even if it does respond, and the response succeeds in producing relief, it has trouble learning, perceiving and believing that the response worked. Finally, its emotional balance is disturbed: depression and anxiety, measured in various ways, predominate. [1975, pp. 22–3]

Problematic as is the application of these theories to human beings, some observations of babies appear to support the greater helplessness of girls in test situations. Goldberg and Lewis (1969) separated thirteen-month-old babies from their mothers by a wire mesh barrier and found that girls cried more than boys, while boys more often manipulated the catches at the ends of the barrier, apparently trying to escape. Maccoby and Jacklin (1973), repeating the study, found the greater tendency of girls to cry helplessly only happened when the test was preceded by a 'fear stimulus'.

The hypothetical application of the 'learned helplessness' hypothesis to the trauma of first-time motherhood is as follows:

(1) women experience response–outcome independence (failure to control events by their own actions) throughout their lives as members of a subordinate group;
(2) they are therefore more likely to approach childbirth with a weak sense of their own efficacy to control its progress and resolution;
(3) the element of uncontrollability in childbirth itself (e.g. as regards the onset of labour, the number of contractions needed to dilate the cervix, and so forth) acts to confirm the mother's role as helpless victim (or at least calls for a large input of self-confidence and self-esteem if it is not to be experienced as personally depressing);
(4) what doctors do in the name of medical control reinforces the response of learnt feminine helplessness to trauma;
(5) and medical control therefore, through its capacity to reinforce feminine helplessness, intensifies the likelihood of postpartum emotional disturbance.

The essence of uncontrollability is knowing that you have no control; believing that you could have it is therefore another matter altogether. This difference may help to explain the different outcomes of women who become depressed and those who do not: the latter may continue to be impressed with a sense of their own *potential* efficacy even in the face of extreme medical control. Attitudes towards controllability may also act as self-fulfilling prophecies. Thus, women in the Transition to Motherhood study who exhibited deferential attitudes towards medical experts were more likely to meet with a high degree of technology in childbirth. Seligman sums up his theory of depression thus:

> . . . the expectation that an outcome is independent of responding (1) reduces the motivation to control the outcome;

> (2) interferes with learning that responding controls the outcome; and, if the outcome is traumatic, (3) produces fear for as long as the subject is uncertain of the uncontrollability of the outcome, and then produces depression. [1975, pp. 55–6]

Many of the findings of the Transition to Motherhood study fit this interpretation. For example, the relationship between a traditional feminine role orientation and deference towards experts is the modal situation of learned helplessness – a belief in oneself as dependent 'by nature' becomes a belief in the legitimacy of others (representatives of the dominant culture) to determine the contours of one's life experiences. Deference was related to high anxiety about the birth, reflecting fear in relation to outcome uncontrollability. A traditional feminine role orientation was associated with the development of a less than 'good' relationship with the product of medical control, the baby, as also was the imposition of medium or high levels of childbirth technology.

All the dimensions of medicalization shown on the left-hand side of Figure 6.2 are, or reflect, ways in which the control of childbirth is exercised by medical experts. Institutional delivery, epidural analgesia and technology in general interpose medical intervention as a condition for the successful delivery of mother and baby from the perils of childbirth. Low control reported by the mother is a sign of dependence on medical intervention; dissatisfaction with second stage labour and with the management of the birth in general are symptoms of the degree to which medical control was experienced as personally upsetting.

The damage that is done to women by these modes of external control is not, in one sense, any worse or any different from their attributed and induced vulnerability within masculine culture. Both medical control and subordinate group status militate against self-determination and encourage helplessness. But, in another sense, the enforcement of helplessness through the external control and hence (to women) *uncontrollability* of reproduction removes women's modus vivendi in two ways. It disturbs their chief legitimate self-justification as servers of the dominant group's needs, so that they receive a sense of failure in the one activity they are demonstrably able to claim as their own. But more simply than this, they are deprived of one form of achievement human beings are able to experience: the achievement of producing another human being. Lacking this sense of achievement, and exposed to other kinds of vulnerability, women are, as we saw in chapter 7, particularly likely to become depressed. It is because they are so useful as manifestations of human weakness and vulnerability that women are so useless to themselves.

PART III

Conclusion

Seeing how the transition to motherhood is one instance of human life change points to the conclusion that women's responses to this are not primarily shaped by the biology of birth. Social circumstance can protect against the trauma of first birth or create vulnerability; key concepts are those of self-esteem, of loss, of identity. The position of women as a – or the – socially subordinate group encourages the formation of a particular psychology. This is not the psychology of the 'feminine' character but the induced self-negation of an oppressed minority. In the concluding chapter the steps of the argument are summarized. Some problems with motherhood as a cultural theme are discussed: the divergence between image and experience; a conspiracy to present childbirth as a natural and not painful act; the link between these realities and the male idealization of motherhood that is rooted in the gender-divided family. In 'Proposing the Future' the question of future changes in childbearing and childrearing is raised. The suggestions for reform and revolution that are made take account of our whole cultural perspective on maternity. It is not only the statistics of specific medical manipulations that need to be considered, but the social articulation of production and reproduction and, most cogently, the ideological lens through which women's activities as reproducers are viewed.

CHAPTER 11

Mistakes and Mystiques

We tend in our teaching to intellectualize childbirth . . . as if we could not ourselves come face to face with the intensity of the experience . . . we talk hopefully and deceptively about 'discomfort' when we really mean pain: we say 'hard work' when we mean that a woman feels as if she is using her last ounce of strength and is at the limit of endurance; and we talk about maternal feelings as if they involved only a gentle sweetness and not the whole range of human passions.

[Kitzinger, 1977, pp. 51–2]

Veiled by the mystiques of feminine psychology and deterministic biology, mothers' reactions to motherhood have been regarded by medical and social science as in a class of their own: a female secret negotiated by, and on behalf of, hidden personality factors. But because women's biological reproductivity has a social function – the reproduction of a society – any difficulties women have with motherhood constitute a 'social problem'. Science, responding to an agenda of basically social concerns, has provided the label 'postnatal depression' as a pseudo-scientific tag for the description and ideological transformation of maternal discontent. Thus labelled, maternal difficulties remain impervious to male scientific understanding, as we have seen in this book; it is only the alternative approach of considering responses to childbirth as a species of a larger genus, human reactions to life events, that their intrinsic character can be mapped out.

SUMMARY

Previous chapters have argued that any analysis of women's 'adjustment' or 'non-adjustment' to motherhood must proceed on a number of levels if it is to avoid the feminine paradigm mistakes of male science. In the first place, how women feel about their childbirths is not the same as how they feel about their babies, and neither of these is coterminous with their attitudes to the social role of mother – the 'institution' as opposed to the 'experience' of motherhood. Of course there may be connections between these areas of feelings, but it is an error to assume their interchangeability. Second, the kind of 'depression' women may undergo after childbirth has a number of different components: a short-term relief/reaction syndrome (the 'blues'); a state of heightened anxiety on first being alone with and responsible for the baby; a condition of fluctuating depressed mood in early motherhood; and, lastly, a more disabling and clinically definable 'depression' whose characteristic feature is a tendency to interfere with physical well-being and to block feelings about being able to 'cope' with motherhood. Taking these different ways of measuring reactions to childbirth, it is clear that it is normal to experience difficulties. A quarter of the women in the Transition to Motherhood sample had depression, four out of five reported the 'blues', three-quarters anxiety and a third depressed mood. A third had less than 'high' satisfaction with the social role of mother, and two-thirds less than 'good' feelings for the baby five months after the birth. Only two of the fifty-five women experienced no negative mental health outcome, had 'good' feelings for their babies and 'high' satisfaction with motherhood; the reactions of the other fifty-three did not follow this pattern. The labels of outcome selected reflect the idea (which is contrary to the findings) that unproblematic adaptation to motherhood is normal and difficulties are not. The language of 'scientific' assessment is rarely value-free and the terminology of outcome used in the Transition to Motherhood study intentionally follows precedent here – the argument being that of ensuring comparability. Much of our cultural thinking about women is oriented around the standard of conformity to the status quo, and only data that relate to this standard can provide a bridge between old and new interpretations.

In chapters 6 and 7 a model of influences on these six measures of maternal reactions to first birth was presented. The model stressed the interconnections between depression and postnatal blues and a technological experience of birth; between depressed mood and current social environment (not going out to work, having housing difficulties and not sharing interests with the baby's father); between feelings for the baby and the baby's behaviour, the mother's isolation, overwork, restriction and capacity to view herself as a mother; between women's satisfaction and their ideas about themselves as mothers and as women – the extent to which they could make the feminine paradigm and the experience of social motherhood coincide. Extending this analysis, chapter 7 distinguished between 'victims' and 'victors' of childbirth by showing how particular kinds of 'vulnerability' increase the risk of depression after childbirth: not being employed, having a segregated marital role relationship, housing problems and little or no previous contact with babies. All of the women with all four of these factors became depressed, compared with 70 per cent of those with three, 53 per cent of those with two, and 20 per cent of those with one. Given a birth marked by high or medium levels of technology, vulnerability factors are able to discriminate between victims and victors more clearly: all thirteen women who had depression were in the high/medium technology, two or more vulnerability factor group. Finally, if women's own feelings about labour are added to the analysis, it is clear that not enjoying and not experiencing achievement in labour constitute a further deprivation that, cumulatively with high technology and social vulnerability, provides a hazardous start to motherhood.

Moving on from the particularity of childbirth, chapter 8 contended that reproduction is one instance of stress and change occasioned by life events, and that it is in this framework that maternal difficulties are best understood. The social transitions of achieving adult femininity, acquiring the status of mother, retiring from work, changing one's career, undergoing physical (body-shape) transformation, becoming a medical and surgical patient, experiencing a 'disaster' and being institutionalized were discussed and their importance as aspects of the transition to motherhood emphasized. Chapter 9 looked at the psychological losses and gains life events bring in their train, disputing the assumption that childbirth must represent gain whereas other life events (losing a spouse or a limb, gaining a new home or job) are thought necessarily to occasion loss. Removing the obstruction of the feminine paradigm, it is obvious that, on the contrary, what is characteristic of childbirth and becoming a mother today is the tendency for women to feel they have lost something, rather than simply gained a child. What is lost may be one's job, one's life-style, an intact 'couple' relationship, control over one's body or a sense of self, but the feeling of bereavement cannot be cured or immediately balanced by the rewards of motherhood – just as the bereaved person will not cease to feel anguished if offered alternative relationships and occupations. A person's attention to the fact and consequences of loss is deflected not by substitution, only, and if then, by time and a re-ordering of the assumptive world.

Chapter 9 ended by arguing that the primary loss of women in becoming mothers is a loss of identity. Chapter 10 asked what the identity of women is – not within Freudian psychology but in terms of the psychology of women as a subordinate group. The fragility of self-esteem, the tangentiality of the idea and feeling that women can 'master' their own fate – these are contours of female personality as it develops in a male world; they are characteristics of women and their induced subordination to men, and they constitute the special vulnerability of women to the stress of life events. Childbirth is no exception to this general rule, and though it is as an exception that it has been seen, it is in terms of the general rule that its social and psychological trauma to women as human beings ought, more validly, to be investigated.

This interpretation of maternal outcome to childbirth has focused on two sets of factors: childbirth as it is today – its medical definition and manipulation; and women as they are today – in the personal biographic sense and in the larger context of the way female identity is culturally organized under partriarchy. It is on the second 'where we are at' issue that I want to offer some speculations in these last chapters.

MOTHERHOOD AS A CULTURAL THEME

One main finding of the Transition to Motherhood project was the considerable gap that exists between expectations and reality: pregnancy, childbirth and motherhood are not the way most women expect them to be. On the whole they are more uncomfortable and less pleasant than anticipated. Four-fifths of the women said the whole process had contradicted their too-romantic expectations: pregnancy was construed as different from expected for 82 per cent of the sample, birth for 93 per cent, and social motherhood, for 91 per cent of the women, was just not the picture they had gleaned from various sources of the way mothers and babies are supposed to be.

In chapters 8 and 9 we saw how the holding and unlearning of unrealistic expectations is especially inimical to self-esteem, and is potentially an influence on the chances of maladaptation and depression following birth. This is well-recognized outside the childbirth field. In Janis's study of surgical patients (see pp. 221–2), the discrepancy between expectations and reality is a necessary (though not a sufficient) condition for the onset of depression:

> The available evidence suggests that a major consequence of low anticipatory fear is a general lack of psychological preparation for coping with subsequent episodes of stress . . . The unworried person is inclined to develop spontaneously a sense of *blanket immunity* which is readily shattered by the impact of actual stress stimuli; whereas, if motivated by anticipatory fear, he [*sic*] is more likely to develop *partial immunity* reassurances which take account of the actual dangers to which he expects to be exposed. The latter type of reassurances continues to be effective in preventing helplessness at moments of acute crisis, thereby reducing the probability of emotional shock and aggrievement reactions when personal suffering subsequently occurs. A low degree of anticipatory fear can, therefore, be regarded as *pathogenic* in that subsequently, if exposed to severe stress stimuli, the unworried person tends to lose emotional control and becomes adversely sensitized because of his lack of effective inner defenses. [1958, p. 401]

In other words, being prepared is beneficial; not being prepared is not.

Much the same argument is put by Martha Wolfenstein in her account of the psychological impact of disasters. She points out that

> There is likely to be more emotional disturbance following the event on the part of those who beforehand warded off all anxiety, and denied the reality of the threat, than on the part of those who were able to tolerate some anticipatory alarm and to acknowledge that the disaster could happen. Anticipation constitutes a small-scale preliminary exposure on the level of imagination and can have an innoculating effect. By rehearsing and familiarising oneself with the coming event one may reduce the risk of being overwhelmed by the experience. [1957, pp. 25–6]

In a study of air force personnel cited by Wolfenstein, those who were more 'unrealistically enthusiastic' about combat beforehand were more likely than others to 'lose their sense of invulnerability in actual danger situations and to show subsequent neurotic disturbances' (1957, p. 26).

There are two particular ways in which women experiencing childbirth for the first time feel they have been misled by unreal expectations. First, having a baby *hurts* much more than they thought it would: 49 per cent of the Transition to Motherhood sample said the birth was more painful than they had imagined; many more 'gave in' and had epidural analgesia, despite previous intentions not to, because the early contractions proved more unpleasant than anticipated. Where accounts of pain are rendered (see Oakley, 1979b, ch. 5 'The agony and the ecstasy'), they stress its intensity as far greater than any other kind of pain. Second, pregnant women do not envisage the level of medical technology/intervention that currently characterizes the management of birth. Few women expected episiotomies, forceps deliveries, the induction or acceleration of labour with artificially ruptured membranes and hormone drips; many (98 per cent, 52 per cent, 59 per cent and 41 per cent respectively) received them.

These considerations, together with the role of unrealistic expectations as described in other life event literature, suggest that a revision is needed of the goals and content of antenatal education as it is offered to pregnant women today. The aims of antenatal education, as stated in Williams and Booth's *Antenatal Education: Guidelines for Teachers* (1974, pp. 3–4) are:

(1) to build up a woman's confidence in herself 'and in those who are looking after her';

(2) to ensure a healthy and happy pregnancy; 'happy in looking forward with joyful anticipation . . . to the birth';
(3) to be prepared for labour so as to achieve satisfaction 'within the context of safe maternity care';
(4) to promote the airing of problems;
(5) to prepare women for the physical and emotional care of the baby.

The emphasis is on the positive and normative side of producing a baby – the emotional excitement and pleasure of getting and being pregnant and of having and caring for a baby; the contribution of reproduction to the marriage relationship; the achievement of true femininity.[1]

Most guides gloss over the connotations of the word 'pain' as applied to labour – or even do not use it. In the Brants' dictionary of *Pregnancy, Childbirth and Contraception* (1975), there is no heading for pain. Neither in the section devoted to 'Contraction, uterine' nor in the one discussing 'Psychoprophylaxis' is the word 'pain' used, although the 'undoubted difficulties' of labour are referred to (p. 194), and the Brants say 'The accepted and moderate approach is for the woman to be given every help to cope with her labour and to hope for a normal delivery, but to be fully aware that most women need additional help from drugs (see labour, pain relief)' (p. 195). Bourne adopts an even more programmatic line:

> The medical definition of the onset of labour is 'the onset of regular, painful, uterine contractions'. This is really an appalling definition and guaranteed to frighten any pregnant woman. Furthermore, it is not true. The modern teaching and theory is to refer to uterine contractions as 'contractions' and not to call them 'pains'. . . . [1975, p. 332]

The 'pain' of childbirth is due to women's inadequate control over themselves and can be corrected by the strategy of attending classes in 'natural' childbirth. How medicine has thus colonized the natural childbirth movement to associate its regime with *medical* control was a theme of chapter 1. The cultural treatment of reproductive pain is, clearly, one further example of the way in which the difficulties women have are construed as women's difficulties: of all victims, women are the most blamed.

As we saw in chapter 1, medical definitions of women as maternity cases are coloured by the theme of hostility to female culture. This engenders an antagonism between doctors' 'knowledge' and that of women who have already had babies: the doctors are able to say that contractions are not synonymous with 'pains'; women are not able to say this and would not feel a need to dispute accepted views about the physical experience of childbirth were these views not the ideology of male medicine in the first place. The identification of women with other women promotes a wish to share the insights of reproduction since these have a protective value in immunizing against shock. The fact that they also provide a cue to the entire deceit of masculine culture in shaping female lives is not coincidental. Male society idealizes motherhood: that is, it gives rise to, and persistently reinforces, a view of motherhood that is ideal and not actual, the ideality deriving from a male, rather than a female, concept of women and their mothering role.

It is this idealization of motherhood and its ramifications that constitute the greatest problem for women in becoming and being mothers today. The idealization is linked with the fostering of romantic expectations about childbirth: it is part and parcel of the feminine image of women that has been shown empirically to militate against satisfying childbirth and motherhood. Breen's study (1975) concluded that the least culturally feminine women are those who enjoy and participate in their childbirths most – and find the relation of mother and child, the *practice* of motherhood most rewarding. A similar reappraisal of the conventional view can be extracted from the present study. It was those women who were able (enabled) to conduct their labours with least intervention who were least 'depressed': it was those whose view of femininity was most self-aware who could confidently and unreservedly say they loved their babies, but simultaneously cite the *social* conditions of the mother role as antithetical to women's happiness. As one female doctor has summed up the reality of counter-productive femininity:

> Passivity, dependence, ineptness, emotional lability, and sexual inhibition are so exactly opposite to the requirements of good birth experience and good motherhood that one suspects that they are desired because of a poorly worked-through fear of mature women. Excessive dependence on the

> obstetrician or surrogate (including the obstetrician-trained husband as birth coach) could be a temporary substitute for active mastery in childbirth . . . Tough, effective, confidently warm human parenting is not encouraged by beginning with twelve months – or many years – of treating the mother like a puzzled, fragile, dependent creature. [Seiden, 1978, pp. 98, 92]

Two facets of masculine culture make a special contribution to women's difficulties as mothers. There is the widespread belief that a maternal instinct qualifies women for childbearing and childrearing alike. This places women on the same level as animals and exposes them to the devastating discovery that, as is the case with male humans, 'instinct' plays an insignificant part, or even no part at all, in human social life. There is also the peculiar pervasive ambivalence about motherhood that is expressed in the combination of ideological glorification and actual social–economic discrimination.

> This is an anti-child society and anyone who thinks otherwise either hasn't had children or has been duped by the pretty baked bean fed children on television. Children can only be regarded as a nuisance, as a threat to marriages, as a drain on resources and as a restriction on parents' freedom in a society which, physically and psychologically, excludes children . . . We might ask that if bringing up children is really considered as important as the propaganda says, and if it is creative and fulfilling, why is it that men are so reluctant to do it? [Comer, 1974, pp. 178–9]

Bringing up children is held out to be women's greatest achievement; but mothers are a socially and economically impoverished group. Arguments about the 'financial endowment' of motherhood, to borrow Eleanor Rathbone's phrase (1924), are countered by the male ethic of 'devotion is not a monetary concept' – the same formula being applied to other feminine occupations such as nanny and nurse (see, for example, Etkowitz, 1971). The beatific value of loss of self in others' welfare is supposedly reward enough for whatever accompanying deprivations there may be – and these, of course, are not spelt out, in part because they are not recognized.

Having a baby hurts; doctors take over the female body in

childbirth; mothers remain people sensitive to their social situations; the emotional and social relation of mother and child is actually such that hate is engendered as well as love, and selflessness, subordination of self to the child's needs, is only imperfectly and with difficulty achieved. These perceptions are prevented in women whose fulfilment as mothers is yet to come, by, or at least within, a society governed by people who neither have babies nor see their main occupation as rearing them. But we can be more specific than this about the sources of women's idealization as mothers. It is rooted in the development of masculine personality itself.

The male idealization of motherhood proceeds by representing mothers as higher in the scale of core human values than men. Mothers' lives are seen as geared to the production of love and the facilitation of growth in a way that is contrary to the values of the rest of (male) society, which occupies itself in the aggressive pursuit of self-aggrandisement. Mothers are also, and partly for these reasons, the social group that is most different from men: most quintessentially feminine and 'other'. In their femininity mothers thus stand for the purest kind of selflessness; they are symbols of, and carriers for, the motive of altruism in human social organization (Miller, 1977).

Nancy Chodorow (1978) has recently provided an interpretation of how this portrayal of motherhood comes about. She shows how a masculine bias against motherhood is incorporated into masculine personality through the gender asymmetry of the family. The argument runs thus. Women, in contemporary society, rear both female and male children. Children's gender, as it is not biologically given, must be socially differentiated. Competing with this agenda of feminine and masculine personality differentiation is the paradox of the mother's relation to female and male babies: the same, as well as different. An infant's sense of self develops in sustained interaction with consistent others. In 'normal' families, the mother provides the platform of relatedness on which the infant builds an image of itself and then conveys to it the contingency and reality of maternal love by frustrating its expectations of exclusive maternal attention. Such frustration produces anxiety, and anxiety calls forth the need for ego capacities that are able to defend the self against anxiety and more clearly establish the boundaries between the self and others. In this 'normal' family situation, identification with the father is important as a more sophisticated means of differentiating between people and objects, but the important difference is that 'love for the mother is originally a love without a sense of reality' (Chodorow, 1978, p. 80) because it is the first 'love' a baby experiences, whereas love for the father is governed by a more 'real' appreciation of the father's function vis-à-vis children, mothers and family life. The basic unreality of the infant's love for its mother carries the rider that perception of the separateness of infant and mother may remain confused. The mother–infant relationship is pre-social and thus, in some ways, anti-social; fathers intrude on this relationship as representatives of society, which is thus experienced as inherently patriarchal in character.[2] Most people, whether female or male, feminine or masculine, retain a rather naïve and egotistical attitude towards their mothers, even though they have also developed the capacity for a love that recognizes the competition or dual interlocking of two people's equally valid needs and interests.

Chodorow contends that even in early childhood when gender does not 'count' the fact that primary love is felt in the *mother*–infant relationship influences attitudes to women *after* the stage at which gender is established. An idealized sacrificial love is attributed to women whereas no such supposition is made about men. The outcome of this is different in the two genders. Daughters' unrealistic expectations of maternity constitute a problem for them in achieving motherhood themselves, and sons' attributions of maternal love to women sustain the idealization of motherhood as a structural theme in the prolongation of patriarchy.

The other side of the coin is the way mothers feel about sons and daughters. Because of their shared femaleness, mothers are likely to feel 'at one with' their daughters, to regard them as an extension of themselves. Sons, conversely, are felt as 'opposite' and are steered by mothers into a process of differentiation from their female origins. To this maternal disposition are added, so far as the male child is concerned, paternal pressure towards a repeat version of masculinity and the messages of other children, other families and other institutions about the importance of developing a masculine personality configuration and behavioural repertoire. Following the biological model, in which the basic foetal form is female and maleness comes about as a result of the extra influence of the male chromosome, the pattern of infants' psychological individuation requires an additional input of masculinity, and is thus, in a way, more hazardous for the male child:

> For boys, gender identifications are more the issue; for girls, psychosexual development. Because both are originally involved with their mother, the attainment of heterosexuality – achieved with the feminine change of object – is the major traditional oedipal goal for girls. For boys the major goal is the achievement of personal masculine identification with their father and sense of secure masculine self, achieved through superego formation and disparagement of women. [Chodorow, 1978, p. 165]

Frustrated not only by the necessary maternal rejection of infant demands but by maternal non-compliance with masculine dependency needs, boys, rejected by their mothers, in turn reject them. But the sentimentalization of maternal love, derived from early infancy, is preserved alongside this devaluation of femininity, so that the hallmark of masculine attitudes to women is contradiction and ambivalence. Men 'need' women not principally in the sense in which human beings need other human beings, but because their dependency needs continue to be defined in relation to women's mothering and because (a further source of ambivalence) male heterosexuality creates a role for women as sexual servers of men. Coexisting with these needs is the opposed need to do without women altogether – that is, to reject the feminine and further the masculine element in the self and society.

Coming down from the level of theory to the more mundane but challenging level of practice, we can see how this ambivalence is expressed in the words of boys learning to be men. Studying working-class boys and their culture, Paul Willis has documented emergent masculine adolescent attitudes to women:

> Their most nuanced and complex attitudes are reserved for the opposite sex. There is a traditional conflict in their view of women: they are both sexual objects and domestic comfor-

ters . . . The 'girlfriend' is a very different category from an 'easy lay'. . . . She is the loyal domestic partner . . . The common prolepsis of calling girlfriends 'the missus' is no accident amongst 'the lads'. A whole new range of meanings and connotations come into play during serious courting. Their referent is the home: dependability and domesticity – the opposite of the sexy bird on the scene. If the initial attraction is based on sex, the final settlement is based on a strange denial of sex . . . The model for the girlfriend is, of course, the mother, and she is fundamentally a model of limitation. Though there is a great deal of affection for 'mum', she is definitely accorded an inferior role: 'She's a bit thick, like, never knows what I'm on about' . . . And within the home there is a clear sense that men have a right to be waited on by the mother . . . [1978, pp. 43–6]

One mode of dealing with this ambivalence is to establish women's inferiority and status of being controlled by men. Male control effects a rationale of incorporation – the feminine becomes an aspect of the masculine – and an appropriate ideology of women's inferiority and psychological/social/economic dependence on men can be contended as its justification. This is an important issue underlying the move towards the male medical management of childbirth charted in chapter 1. A desire on the part of men to participate in female reproductivity is not hard to discern in nineteenth- and early twentieth-century literature arguing the case for male medicalization, and, as Lomas (1978) and others have said, it is possible to interpret the current treatment of women as reproducers in this light. Freudian psychology, which has become 'our cultural psychology' (Chodorow, 1978, p. 142) in so many important ways, has always concealed the legitimacy of men's envy of women's reproductivity, because such an elementary point against the necessity of patriarchy cannot be conceded. If men want to be women, the world is turned upside down, and psychoanalytic constructions of gender belie a limited imagination of the world the 'right' way up.[3]

All the findings of the Transition to Motherhood study relate to these themes of the idealization and male medical control of motherhood. For example, the associations between depression and little or no previous contact with babies and between feminine role orientation and maternal self-image, on the one hand, and satisfaction with motherhood and feelings for the baby on the other, illustrate the contingency of maternal satisfaction on the closing of options to women through an induced feminization – of personality and occupation. The coexistence of depressed mood with depressing social circumstances maps out the vulnerability of mothering in the nuclear family context – and in a world where being a person and being a mother remain, to some extent, mutually exclusive possibilities. Undoubtedly most impressive of all these connections are those between the medicalization of birth and depression, for here is summed up an account of the manifold injuries imposed on women through the chauvinism of men's ambivalence to motherhood.

These characteristics of the definition of motherhood today point to the influence of a culture where (from women's point of view) the mistake has been to link women's biological reproduction with the social 'mothering' of children. The mistake gives rise to the mystique of childbearing and childrearing as (feminine) self-fulfilling occupations. As the hands that rock the cradle are not those of the people who rule the world, the axiom that it is mothers who oppress women is perhaps not fair – but it is, nevertheless, true. By mothering their daughters, women induce in other women the desire to be mothers and the relational capacities and psychic structures that match this goal. By mothering their sons, women participate in their own subjugation; turning their male children towards masculinity, they turn them away from women and towards a lifelong campaign on behalf of patriarchy. This paradox has a different formulation however: it could also be said that the capacity for loving children is what ensures women's continuing oppression, because the cycle of mothering is constantly reproduced and with it the gender-divisive consequences of maternal love, from men's desire to control the 'giving' of birth to their reluctance to cede to women full citizenship in the male world.

One final paradox: all that has been said derives, in a sense, from a male perspective. I have been describing how women are not the same as men and how not being so and being confined by male images of women has imposed certain limitations on their development. I have not given equal (or any) attention to the pleasures women have, despite or because of this, managed to obtain from motherhood, nor have I included a critique of the male paradigm of identity development and promotion in non-reproductive interaction and activities. I have ended on the most apparently paradoxical and confused point of all – by saying that women are oppressed because they love children; or (alternatively put) that if they didn't have children women would no longer be oppressed.

This is, in fact, the logic of the male perspective on motherhood carried to its most extreme formulation. It strikes me, as a woman who has enjoyed having children, as a reductio ad absurdum in much the same way, I imagine, as Karen Horney found herself unable to come to terms with the role accorded the penis in the Freudian account of feminine personality development (1974, p. 10). And what these contradictions point to, I think, is the considerable task women confront in designing a psychology (not to mention a society) that authenticates a female point of view. Reproduction is not just a handicap and a cause of second-class status; it is an achievement, *the* authentic achievement of women. The particular brand of feminism that flourishes in the second half of the twentieth century does not see this, though earlier versions have done. The problem is to reconcile the feminist political programme of women's advancement with the subjective logic of reproduction stripped of its masculine ideological transformation: childbirth as seen through women's eyes without the obfuscation of masculine ambivalence.

Proposing the Future

Pain, pain that will bring me my son, step through the curtains of the officious housewife nature, and give me the truth first, or give me nothing. Nature for her embryo fights like her tigresses with all her weapons, but my mind is sharp with pain, and gimlets a hole through natural salvation.

[Smart, 1966, p. 114]

Reproduction is one of the structures that make up the 'position' of women. Along with production, sexuality and child-socialization, it expresses and determines a cultural ideology and role for women. It is in, and through, these areas, their concrete historical–social definition, that a theoretical analysis of women's situation must proceed. By examining each of the four key structures we are able to see what makes up the totality and complexity of the oppression of women (Mitchell, 1971).

This book has provided an elaboration of the way in which reproduction and women as reproducers are socially defined in one particular historical period – the advanced industrial society of Britain in the latter half of the twentieth century. It has not systematically linked this analysis with women's treatment in the spheres of production, sexuality and childrearing, though some comment on the interlocking of reproductive attitudes with these other areas has been mandatory at points in the analysis. *Women Confined* is not an account of women's situation – only of one important and often ignored component of it. It is as much a charting of an ideology as it is the dissection of social statistics, and this obligation is imposed by the character of human reproduction itself: a natural act shaped by cultural rhetoric. The encoding of childbirth into the formulae of 'science' is more complete than is the case with work, sexuality or social motherhood (because, I have suggested, the threat female reproduction poses to masculine society is that much greater). Code-breaking is thus the fulcrum of the analysis, and is the prior necessity to which I have directed the content of this book.

Another obvious function *Women Confined* has not claimed is a campaigning one. I have not said, except in a very general way, how the current treatment of reproduction and reproducers might be altered. This is paradoxical, since I have also tried to point out what is wrong with contemporary concepts of childbirth and women's function as childbearers, and how the social categorization of women as subordinate beings underlies their propensity to react as victims rather than victors to the experience of birth.

To reveal the workings of a social process does not *necessarily* imply a responsibility to outline, initiate or effect change. That is, it does not do so in sociology in general: investigations of coalmining (Dennis *et al.*, 1969), fishing (Tunstall, 1962) or managerial work-communities (Clements, 1958) do not propose political agendas for change; volumes on social stratification or class structure (e.g. Parkin, 1974) do not necessarily include graphs of revolution; most ethnographies of the family are reactionary rather than revisionist in character (e.g. Young and Willmott, 1973). The tendency to focus on amelioration of social conditions is not directly derived from the description of the social context offered; some of the most overtly problematic may in fact be the least criticized. What accounts for this feature of sociological work is the infiltration of prevailing social orientations towards conservation and change into sociologists' views of their data. For example, the harsh concomitants of extreme division of labour in the family may be apparent in community studies, but the desirability of mitigating these and their basic causes will only be cited if the sociologist himself or herself sees the family as a problematic institution.[1]

Political agendas are more likely to be a product of sociological analysis where the topic is normatively labelled (by sociologists and other people) a 'social problem'. Thus, surveys of ethnic minorities or attitudes to them (e.g. Banton, 1972), literature on 'working mothers' (e.g. Yudkin and Holme, 1969) or on male adolescent delinquency (e.g. Downes, 1966) are prone to offer not only diagnoses but social treatment programmes. All research and writing on women is subsumed under the same category heading as this 'social problem' literature. Its authors are called upon to voice an opinion as to what can be 'done' about women because the 'problem' of women is not only theoretical but actual: an unsolved and perplexing contradiction. Within this category of literature, feminist social analysts are especially asked to deliver an account of social solutions. They are victims of a prevailing trend. The trend, moreover, adopts a simplistic and over-determined attitude towards the 'problem' of women by taking the view that whatever is wrong with women and their current social situation can easily be put right. A list of particular social manoeuvres can both encapsulate and remove the problem – as the provision of new, more hygienic containers may hold and dispose of an especially intransigent and offensive form of rubbish.

Yet the perversity of women's character under patriarchy is to be perverse: the 'problem' of women is not simple and so cannot be simply eradicated. If any single message has come out of the new scholarship on women of the last decade it is surely this. And that women cannot be isolated from men or from children or from society as a whole, or from the economic productive system of capitalism, or from the web of cultural ideologies that define everyone's place in a materialistic and male-centred world. A 'sociology of women' is a strategic trick. A 'sociology of gender' is not really any better. The 'problem of women' is everyone's problem in a social milieu where they are counted as a second sex.

Having made the point that feminist social analysts are not obliged to provide alternative agendas, I shall end this book by suggesting some guides to one. I do this because feminism implies the social responsibility of sisterhood (a term that need not be vacuous) for conditions that affect women.

PROPOSALS

Birth

1. An end to unnecessary medical intervention in childbirth.

2. The re-domestication of birth.
3. A return to female-controlled childbirth.
4. The provision of therapeutic support for women after childbirth.

Bringing up children

5. More state or community help for parents, and more state/community participation in childcare.
6. The abolition of fixed gender roles especially in the family and pertaining to social parenthood.
7. Less segregation of children into homes, nurseries, schools, etc., and more integration of children with mainstream social concerns and activities.
8. Less privatization and isolation of families.

The wider context

9. The formal and informal teaching of realistic parenthood and childbirth to both females and males from infancy onwards.
10. Woman-centred and woman-controlled reproductive care.
11. Less cultural retreat from confrontation with pain and suffering.
12. The reduction of poverty and class-based inequalities.
13. Restructuring of employment work against the norm of masculine full-time occupational commitment and in favour of more varied and fluid combinations of work and non-work life.
14. An end to all forms of social, economic and legal discrimination against women.

These proposals relate directly to Figure 6.2 (p. 142), which shows diagrammatically the main findings of the Transition to Motherhood project. They are the only ways in which, in the long run, the bias against women as reproducers will be corrected. Since this bias is evident not only in the medical treatment of childbirth but in the socialization of women for motherhood, in the general disjunction between women's opportunities and mothers' options, and in the character of the modern family as a socially divisive institution, it is in all these areas that change is needed.

Some of the proposals are more revolutionary than others. The suggestions that unnecessary medical intervention in childbirth should end, that birth should be returned to the home, and that women need more support after birth than they currently get – these are not new ideas. By 'unnecessary' medical intervention I mean all those strategies that were developed to treat the minority of women having babies who experience problems, but that have increasingly been applied to the majority who do not need them. Induction of labour with oxytocics, forceps deliveries and episiotomies are examples. I have described some disadvantages of one other such development, epidural analgesia, earlier (pp. 143–4). This is a prime example of a technique that is of great benefit to a minority of women being unselectively 'offered' to the majority who are not fully informed of its deleterious side-effects. The technique of giving epidurals varies and is most appreciated by women when it numbs pain but preserves the sensation of the baby coming or being pushed out (see p. 223).

Criticism of current birth technology is often combined with an emphasis on home birth (Proposal 2), and both proposals come from a variety of pressure groups. They seem daily less radical as the basic legitimacy of the position is increasingly ceded by medical authorities – though, of course, not yet incorporated into medical practice on anything other than a very minor scale. Postnatal support groups (one form Proposal 4 could take) are operated by social workers and health visitors in various places under the aegis of the NHS. Although their content and ideological charter may not accord with the diagnosis of this book, their existence promotes the idea that lack of 'adjustment' following childbirth is a normal occurrence. It also recognizes the important clinical observation that the repeating and reliving of a 'bad' experience in a therapeutic context can aid the development of 'mastery': the passivity of the self as victim in the original experience may in this way be surmounted.[2]

Female-controlled childbirth is a more radical idea than the other proposals for the future management of birth. It is an old arrangement, and to see a return to it as liberating for women as reproducers is not to envisage it as a 'golden age'. The problem is that male control and medicalization are closely linked and so long as present versions of masculinity continue to obtain so, in all probability, will this connection. Women are not necessarily more sympathetic attendants in childbirth, but they are probably so, and the traditional occupation of female midwifery has always placed a belief in nature – which amounts to a belief in women as their own deliverers – ahead of the contention that it is the pharmacological and mechanical technologies of medical science that are, in the twentieth century, the true deliverers of childbearing women (see Walker, 1976).

Moving on to the proposals concerned with childrearing, the first seems obvious: more state/community help for parents. This is contended by various government reports and agencies to be a way of patching up holes in the family as a – or rather the – individually supportive structure (Select Committee on Violence and the Family, 1977). It is an extension of this argument to view such help, whether in the form of more state nurseries, subsidized food or increased family allowances, as systems of community support for children that will parallel, rather than shore up, the failing capacity of families to cater on a self-help basis for the entire reproduction of the labour force.

The sixth proposal, about ridding the family of its gender-divisiveness, is revolutionary but not new: feminists are over-familiar with its necessity. It is always in this sense that they have called for the abolition of the family. Nobody minds men, women and children continuing to live together if they do so in a way that frees each from the bonds of culturally imposed gender. Gender typifications constrain because they arbitrate a definition of peoples' 'natures' that is truly limiting of 'human nature'.

As the family is a gender hierarchy, it is also a generation hierarchy. Children, like women, are second-class citizens, and, like women, they are confined to the out-of-sight places where they will, it is hoped, be out-of-mind – that is, invisible to the masculine economics and politics of the production–consumption world. One of women's difficulties is that their lives have to contain the invisibility of children in this way; because such an ethic of segregation obtains, contact with children is reserved as the prerogative of biological mothers. Proposal 7 says that, were social attitudes to children less prejudiced and dismissive, more adults would come to parenthood (or choose not to) knowing what life with children is like. Disputing the current privatization of family life (Proposal 8) follows from what women say about the isolation and unilateral responsibility of motherhood. If such barriers could be broken down, a basis for cooperation between 'families' might be laid.

The having and rearing of children cannot be discussed in isolation from their cultural setting. The last six proposals are addressed to this. Proposal 9, which sets forth a more realistic educational programme for parenthood as a necessary instrument for the fostering of parental satisfaction, is a suggestion that has been made by many people with contrasting political orientations. It is evident to anyone who has worked in this field that not knowing what to expect or expecting something that does not happen is a cause of great personal difficulty. In particular, the Transition to Motherhood study suggests that deliberate misrepresentation of the pain of childbirth adds to the risk of postpartum depression, since it makes realistic anticipation impossible.

The tenth proposal relates the female control of childbirth to its broader 'medical' context, which is that of reproductive care in general – including contraception, abortion and gynaecological disease management. There must be an overall move towards female-centredness here so that the 'nature' of women becomes a premise and not the result (the end ideological construction) of the reproductive care system. Proposal 11, which contends the desirability of confronting pain and suffering as human capacities, is a suggestion that goes beyond childbirth itself and links attitudes to women's reproductive suffering with the nexus of cultural attitudes to human unease. The capacity of people to suffer and survive suffering is as central to childbirth, denuded of its contemporary ideological representation, as it is to illness and death, activities that have been subject to much the same kind of medical manipulation and disposal as has childbirth.

The last three proposals are the most fundamental. To liberate society from gender- and class-inequality would be a transformation that is almost beyond the bounds of imagination and probably, therefore, of possibility. But the more neither women nor working-class people are treated to the derisory privileges of a dependent status, the more their capacities for self-determination are enhanced. It is also essential that the whole balance between work and non-work life should be re-thought (Proposal 13); like the overthrow of class, this probably means the disappearance of capitalism. There is no doubt that the central dilemma of women in becoming mothers, which is their loss of identity, is occasioned by our present opposition between work and family as alternative structures of satisfaction. The masculine ethic is one of the family as a haven from the strain of work, and it is this ethic that women have to stand on its head when they say they go out to work to recover a sense of connectedness to others. But women going out to work is only a way out in a limited sense: the problem of the opposition between work and family and (for women) the competitiveness of the demands of the two structures will remain.

The motive behind these proposals is to enable women to look upon childbirth as a genuine human achievement; one, moreover, that is able to endow a lasting legacy of self-respect and belief in self-determination. I do not mean that every woman should look upon birth as an apotheosis of womanhood; I mean that the way and the context in which childbirth happens should make it possible for women to feel they have achieved something of value to themselves in having a child.

Notes

Chapter 1

1. Some studies of the midwife's role are: Donnison (1977); Walker (1972, 1976).
2. A point that is illustrated by medical responses to the publication of a well-informed letter on induction from the chairperson of the Patients' Association (a woman): it was assumed to come from a male doctor in disguise (*The Lancet* 1975, No. 1, p. 1088).
3. On the history of medicine and women's role see Verbrugge (1976).
4. Hence the feminist politics of self-examination. See Frankfort (1972) and Boston Women's Health Book Collective (1976).
5. He has 'swept the membranes', a procedure that involves interior manual manipulation of the cervix and is used as a covert way of inducing labour.
6. This is a reference to two critical articles on induction and other aspects of modern maternity care published by two medical journalists in the *Sunday Times*, 13 and 20 October 1974.
7. Some work is now being done in this field. Maternal accounts of foetal well-being (based on the number and frequency of movements) have recently been the subject of several studies, two of which are Pearson and Weaver (1976) and Sadovsky *et al.* (1973).
8. On laboratory investigations of the chromosomal effects see Fishman (1973); Galperin-Lemaitre and Kirsch-Volders (1975); Macintosh and Davey (1970).
9. The names of individuals in the Transition to Motherhood study have been changed.
10. As exemplified in intra-professional discussions such as 'A Place to be Born' (1976) pp. 55–6.
11. This figure is cited by the Dutch obstetrician G. J. Kloosterman.
12. It was 162 per 1000 in 1850 and 161 in 1895, though it fell in between: Ryder and Silver (1970).
13. One portrait of this tendency is Poynter and Keele (1961).
14. A recent analysis of mortality differences in eighteen developed countries in relation to health service factors has found a *positive* association between the prevalence of doctors and mortality: Cochrane, St Leger and Moore (1978).
15. This is, of course, a characteristic of 'patienthood' generally.
16. G. Stimson (1976a) discusses the use of marital status in medical advertising for contraceptives and other drugs.
17. For example, the contributions by G. V. Stimson, M. R. Haug, and A. Cartwright and M. O'Brien in Stacey (1976).
18. The medical concept of 'uterine dysfunction' expresses this idea. It is interesting also in this respect to note that the first apparatus used in Britain for the automated induction of labour was known as 'William' not 'Mary'.

19. A point made by Graham (1977a). Antenatal advice literature in the United States has had the same character as in Britain but seems to have moved more quickly towards a legitimation of the idea that women are people too. See Bean (1972); Guttmacher (1973).
20. From the hospital observations carried out in 1974–5 as part of the Transition to Motherhood project.
21. The hazards of epidural analgesia include a higher incidence of forceps deliveries, hypotension, toxic reactions to the local anaesthetic agents used, neurological sequelae 'up to and including paraplegia' (Moir, 1974).
22. In the antenatal education classes observed for the Transition to Motherhood study both doctors and midwives advocated epidurals for this reason.
23. It has been pointed out to me by a doctor that an alternative interpretation is that this position is chosen by the doctor as a less embarrassing one for the woman.

Chapter 2

1. Ideologies of childbearing and childrearing are connected via the notion of 'instinct', which, like 'hormones', is a methodologically empty term: see Oakley (1974a) ch. 8 'Myths of woman's place. Two: Motherhood'.
2. On methodological (and other) problems in the 'sex differences' literature see Maccoby and Jacklin (1974) especially ch. 1.
3. These figures do not, of course, include psychiatrists and psychotherapists in private practice.
4. See also Sherman (1971); Parlee (1975; n.d.). I have drawn extensively on Parlee's valuable critique in this chapter.
5. See also Dalton (1971). Dalton's latest popular book on this subject, *Once a Month* (1978), perhaps significantly omits the topic of postnatal depression altogether.
6. Kaij and Nilsson say: 'systematic investigations of incidence, etiology, prognosis and symptoms of neurotic reactions in pregnancy and puerperium are virtually non-existent' (1972, p. 368). The situation is much the same in 1979 as it was then.
7. For a counter-argument see the reproducers' accounts of reproduction contained in Oakley (1979b).
8. Larsen (1966) asked a sample of women for their descriptions of pregnancy and postpartum stresses and found that many cited stressful experiences associated with hospitalization. Cone (1972), in a study of Cardiff women, found that 64 per cent of hospital-delivered women classed themselves as depressed after delivery compared with 19 per cent of those delivered at home.
9. Some of the best known are Deutsch (1944); Bibring (1959); Bibring *et al.* (1961).
10. Chertok is here summarizing some unpublished work by Pavenstedt.
11. The notion of the 'curse', often interpreted ideologically, can thus alternatively be seen as an expression of concrete, technical liability.
12. See Oakley (1974b) for data on housework hours.
13. A recent British calculation cited in Kenny (1978) p. 150.
14. A concept referred to by Breen (1975) p. 26.
15. Chodorow (1978) discusses the implications of this within the psychoanalytic framework.
16. This label is used by Lomas (1967).

Chapter 3

1. With apologies to C. Wright Mills (1959).
2. A point made by Hochschild (1975); see also Oakley (1974b) ch. 1 'The invisible woman: sexism in sociology'.
3. *Thinking About Children* is an unusual self-critique as well as being an orthodox research report; Busfield and Paddon point out many of the pitfalls of the conventional approach to family intentions.
4. See Gill (1977) on changing explanations of illegitimacy.
5. One of the participants in the Transition to Motherhood study described in Part II. Unidentified names attached to quotations throughout the text come from this source. A list of participants and their social backgrounds is to be found in Oakley (1979b), Appendix, 'List of characters'.
6. This literature is summarized in Reiss (1971) pp. 217–22.
7. These consequences of the marital bias are spelt out by Rapoport and Oakley (1975).
8. Graham (1977b) tested the hypothesis that women's attitudes to subsequent births differ from those to first births and found significant similarities. Sherman (1971) lists some other studies.
9. See Rapoport *et al.* (1977) for a critique of the sociological literature on parenting and childrearing that elaborates these points.
10. Some feminist critiques of functionalism are Millett (1971); Beechey (1978); Oakley (1974a).
11. The major functionalist theorist of the family is of course T. Parsons: Parsons (1964); Parsons and Bales (1956). See Morgan (1975) for an account of the weaknesses of functionalist explanations of the family.
12. See Rapoport *et al.* (1977) and Oakley (1974a) chapter 8 for references to this other side of the picture.
13. These include Mead and Newton (1967); Ford (1945). Oakley (1977) draws on these and other studies.
14. See Bradley (1964) for one contemporary demonstration of the 'animal' ideology of natural childbirth.
15. See Fish (1966) for an illustration of this tendency.
16. See Goldthorpe (1973) for a discussion of the ethnomethodological enterprise.
17. This interpretation is made explicit in a DHSS document (1977) which stresses failure in the mother (to attend early for antenatal care, to cut out smoking, lcohol and other 'drugs' from the diet) rather than inadequacies in, and dissatisfaction with, the maternity services.
18. For example, Cartwright's survey of attitudes to induction (1979).

Chapter 4

1. The US figure (which includes illegitimate births) is 22.1 years: United States Department of Health, Education and Welfare (1977).
2. I use this term to mean the man with whom a woman is living, whether or not she is married to him. However, a terminological problem arises in that there is no equivalent substitute for the terms 'marriage' or 'marital role'. For this reason, these terms are used later in the book to include couples who are not legally married.
3. A term used by Gouldner and discussed in Bell and Newby (1971) p. 17.

4. My motives for publishing two books based on the housework project were similar. The *Sociology of Housework* (1974b) was analytical and *Housewife* (1974a) descriptive.
5. See Dennis Marsden's review of my books on housework in *The Times Higher Education Supplement* 31 January 1975.
6. Platt says the evidence of sex discrimination in research careers is 'scanty', but highly relevant to the question how and to what extent women participate in social research.

Chapter 5

1. For the 'blues': 'Did you feel at all depressed at any time during your stay in hospital?'
   For anxiety on homecoming:
   'What did you feel like when you came home with the baby?'
   'Did you feel at all anxious about looking after the baby on your own?'
   Descriptions of depressed mood could be given at various points in the interviews. Each interview also carried the following questions:
   'How do you feel in yourself apart from the physical side of things?'
   'Are you suffering with your nerves at all?'
   'Are you depressed at all at the moment?'
2. The questions used covered frank feelings of anxiety and/or depression, feelings of tension/inability to relax, undue sensitivity to noise, panic attacks, fear/avoidance of social contacts, self-confidence, concentration, appetite and sleep disturbance, feelings of lethargy and irritability.
3. Tod (1972) talks about 'puerperal depression' as one entity. Bardon (1972) assumes that both psychoses and puerperal depressions are likely to have the same cause (without delineating the meaning of puerperal depression). Pitt (1972) distinguishes between psychoses and the 'blues' but not between anxiety states and depressed mood/clinical depression.
4. I derive this figure in part from a comparison between the women in my sample and those studied by Brown and Harris (1978). In their terms, the discrepancy between 15 per cent and 24 per cent (the 'depression' figure I use in my analysis) would be accounted for under the heading 'borderline' cases. This category would include some of the instances of marked depressed mood in my sample.
5. This is only one of the complex issues raised by, and about, such a difference in perspective between those who experience mental illness and those who diagnose and treat their symptoms. See D. Ingleby (ed.) (forthcoming). It has been pointed out to me that psychiatric definitions of mental illness are likely to reflect psychiatrists' prevailing professional requirements, in the same way that obstetricians' definitions of reproduction have altered historically to fit changes in their professional position.
6. The overall index was based on answers to the questions:
   'How does it feel being a mother?'
   'Do you like looking after the baby?'
   'How do you feel you are coping with the baby generally?'
   These questions were asked at both postnatal interviews. All three components of 'adjustment' were separately rated 1–5 (1 = very satisfied or coping very well). On this basis the women were divided into three groups:
   (a) 'high satisfaction' – a rating of 1 or 2 for satisfaction with being a mother and looking after the baby at both postnatal interviews and a rating of 1 or 2 for coping at five months or of 1–3 at five weeks;

(b) 'medium satisfaction' – more than one rating of 3 but no rating of 4 or 5;
(c) 'low satisfaction' – one or more rating of 4 or 5.

7. 'What do you particularly enjoy about looking after the baby?'
'Is there anything you dislike about it?'
(asked at both postnatal interviews).
'Do you feel you have a relationship with your baby?'
'Do you ever get cross with your baby?'
(asked at the first postnatal interview).
'What sort of relationship do you feel you have with the baby now?'
'Do you feel that the relationship you have with the baby is special?'
'When you compare her/him with other babies, how do you feel?'
'Do you feel relaxed or tense when you're looking after the baby?'
'Do you worry about the baby?'
'Do you ever feel angry with the baby?'
(all asked at the second postnatal interview).

Three groups of women were distinguished, positive feelings, negative feelings and anxiety being rated separately 1 – 5 (1 = high positive feelings, no negative feelings, and no/very little anxiety):
(a) 'good' feelings – a rating of 1 or 2 for positive or negative affect at both postnatal interviews and of 1 or 2 for anxiety at the second postnatal interview;
(b) 'medium' feelings – ratings of 1 – 3 at the second postnatal interview plus one or more rating of 3 – 5 at the first postnatal interview; if positive and negative affect were rated 1 at the second postnatal interview, then a 4 for anxiety was allowed;
(c) 'poor' feelings – one or more ratings of 4 or 5 at the second postnatal interview (excluding the last case above).

8. For example, drawing clear boundary lines between questions/answers of relevance to one rating and those of relevance to another; rating the whole sample for 'adjustment', then for baby relationship, then for depression, and so on, using numbers to identify interviewees and not names.
9. See for instance the newsletters of the Association for Improvements in the Maternity Services.
10. See Huntingford (1978) on the development of official 'place of delivery' policies.
11. The *British Medical Journal* started in 1978 a regular feature called 'Medicine and the Media', which reflects the influence of this 'consumer' movement.
12. The 'technology' score was arrived at thus:

artificial rupture of membranes	1
episiotomy	1
pethidine	1
catheter	1
pudendal block	2
dextrose drip	2
manual removal of the placenta	2
accelerated with syntocinon	3
mechanical monitoring of foetal heart and/or uterine contractions	4
epidural analgesia	4
simple forceps/ventouse delivery	4
difficult forceps delivery	6
induction of labour (including ARM and syntocinon)	6
general anaesthetic	6
caesarean section (including general anaesthetic)	10

A score of 0 – 11 was counted as 'low', 12 – 19 as 'medium' and 20 – 28 as 'high'.

13. On control, the key question was 'Would you say you felt in control of yourself and what was going on throughout the labour or not?'; on the management of the birth, the summary questions were 'What did you feel overall about the way you were treated by the midwives during labour? And what about the doctor(s)?'; on the second stage, 'What was pushing the baby out like?'
14. This distinction was suggested by the sample women themselves. It also relates to some of the earlier sociological literature on women's attitudes to the feminine role: see Seward (1945) and Steinemann (1963).
15. 'Do you think of yourself as a mother?' (interview 1)
'Are you aware of being a mother?' (interview 3)
'Do you feel that you're doing what you always wanted to do in having a baby to look after?' (interview 4)
The extent to which a woman saw herself as a mother was rated 1–5 (1 = a highly maternal self-image) at the first, third and fourth interviews. A composite rating was then used to categorize the women into 3 groups:
    (a) high self-image as a mother – ratings of 1 or 2 from interview 1 through to interview 4;
    (b) medium self-image as a mother – ratings of 1–3 including at least one 3;
    (c) low self-image as a mother – ratings with one or more 4 or 5.
16. On this theme, see Lewis and Rosenblum (1974).
17. This difficulty haunts the 'sex differences' literature: see Maccoby and Jacklin (1974).
18. The argument is that male foetuses are more likely than female foetuses to provoke toxaemic pregnancies: Ounsted (1972).
19. Males weigh on average 150 g more than females at birth: Ounsted (1972) p. 184.
20. Green (1975) discusses these studies.
21. Richards and Bernal found this a problem in their research: see Bernal (1974).
22. It is usually the midwife or the doctor who first identifies the baby's sex. This was so in the delivery observations carried out for the Transition to Motherhood study; see also Macfarlane (1977) ch. 5 'The first minutes'. Many mothers say their first concern is not the baby's sex but its normality. Of course, from the point of view of the medical staff it is safer to make statements about sex than about normality.
23. In the Transition to Motherhood study, partner's occupation and type of marital role relationship are associated ($p < .01$); the association between the mother's own occupation and type of marital role relationship reached a lower level of statistical significance than this.

Chapter 6

1. The relationships between (a) anxiety and social isolation, (b) depressed mood and social isolation, and (c) anxiety and presence of social supports are all in the expected direction, but they do not reach statistical significance.
2. Neither induction nor acceleration of labour were influenced by maternal request in this sample.
3. Shereshefsky and Yarrow's study (1973), which employs the conventional approach of analysing adjustment in terms of 'femininity', finds that adaptation is linked with previous interest in babies, vision of self as a mother and 'nurturance' as a personality factor.
4. See the discussion of social class and domesticity in Oakley (1974b).
5. Breen's findings suggest this interpretation (1975, p. 192).

6. The association is not statistically significant.
7. By mother's occupation, $p < .05$, by partner's, $p < .01$.
8. I develop this point in chapter 11.
9. Thoman, Leiderman and Olson (1972) found more prolonged breastfeeding of female babies in a group of Californian mothers, but they report that the sex difference holds only for primiparous mothers.

Chapter 7

1. This is the interpretation put by Brown and Harris (1978).
2. The segregated/joint marital role relationship measure roughly parallels Brown and Harris's 'intimacy' factor, though it does not, of course, measure an exactly equivalent dimension of couples' relationships.
3. I am not using 'threat' in the technical sense employed by Brown and Harris in their analysis. Nor is my model of vulnerability factors as variables contributing to the likelihood of depression after a technological birth strictly parallel to theirs. For example, housing problems are counted as a provoking agent in their model, a vulnerability factor in mine.
4. i.e. by asking for accounts of birth and following these up with various 'probing' questions.
5. See the accounts in Oakley (1979b).

Chapter 8

1. Rapoport *et al.* (1977) discuss social–scientific and popular ideologies of parenthood.
2. See the data on masculine domesticity in Oakley (1974b) ch. 8 'Marriage and the division of labour' and in Oakley (1979b) ch. 9 'Domestic politics'.
3. See the discussion on retirement in Adams *et al.* (1976) pp. 110–17.
4. Research on women's careers is virtually non-existent.
5. Oakley (1974b) discusses housewives' definitions of their work: ch. 6 'Standards and routines'.
6. This typology draws on Merton's (1949) distinctions between conformity, innovation, ritualism, retreatism and rebellion.
7. Release from the handicaps of social and biological maternity has been central to the women's liberation agenda from its beginnings: the third, fourth and fifth 'aims' of the current British women's liberation movement concern free contraception and abortion on demand, free community-controlled childcare, and legal and financial independence for women.
8. See also Breen (1975) ch. 6 'On the psychology of women and femininity'.
9. In the case of pregnancy nausea, for instance, an excess of oestrogen is held responsible: Lennane and Lennane (1977) pp. 30–8. The Lennanes are concerned to identify the biological basis of pregnancy, delivery and postpartum symptoms throughout their text.
10. This concern is part of the psychoanalytical perspective in which motherhood represents (and therefore replaces other expressions of) female sexual maturity.
11. Hart (1977) makes this point.
12. On the notion of 'consumer' as applied to the health services, see Stacey (1976).
13. The fact that the occupations of the women's partners are here, and elsewhere in the analysis (p. 131), more closely linked with important social and medical factors than those of the women themselves relates to the points made earlier

(pp. 101–2) about the 'meaning' of occupationally based social class in the case of women. The only valid conclusion that can be drawn is that the male-based model taps some socio-economic dimension that is not tapped in the same way by a female-based occupational model. The question remains as to what index of women's social class could be substituted for an occupational one to provide a means of differentiating between groups of women with respect to life chances and life-styles.

14. Deferential/non-deferential attitudes to experts were also not related statistically to the following factors: pregnancy orientation, pregnancy symptoms, feelings of achievement in birth, feelings of being in control over labour, and overall attitude to labour.
15. In the hospital where the Transition to Motherhood study was carried out for example, 45.9 per cent of women having their first babies had forceps deliveries in 1976, compared with 17.3 per cent of those having second or subsequent deliveries.
16. None of the women in the Transition to Motherhood study were offered a 'choice' as to whether the baby should be born in hospital or at home, and most were not able to choose the hospital they would attend. One problem with the notion of 'choice' in this context is that it implies that the patient is well informed about the different options; often, and especially for women having first babies, this is not the case.

Chapter 9

1. Hunt (1968) found that a desire for company and the wish to escape boredom were almost as important as financial motives for going out to work: Volume I, Report, pp. 19–20.
2. It is not, of course, possible to say how far these changes might have occurred over time in the absence of childbirth as a provoking factor. But studies referred to in chapter 3 (pp. 75–8) indicate that the advent of children is responsible for a certain amount of disenchantment in marriage.
3. The idea of women as victims and the philosophy of their need to be 'protected' are closely allied. Women's 'weaknesses' (their socially rooted oppression and depression) are traced to their biological and domestic identities. 'Protective' philosophies produce practices (codified as legislation) that treat women as handicapped and therefore as restricted people. See the contributions in Smart and Smart (1978), esp. A. Sachs 'The myth of male protectiveness and the legal subordination of women: an historical analysis'.
4. Whether by virtue of biological reproduction or social adoption.

Chapter 10

1. Hacker is here citing Louis Wirth.
2. This parallels the autonomy of the housewife role that women value: Oakley (1974b) pp. 22–4.
3. See the notion of 'sensitivity' as used in Ainsworth *et al.* (1974).
4. Although he does mention (pp. 84–5) the greater induced helplessness of black minorities.

Chapter 11

1. In this respect much antenatal literature copies and inflates the feminine paradigm of more 'scientific' studies.
2. Juliet Mitchell argues this in *Psychoanalysis and Feminism* (1974).
3. Hence the dominance of 'penis envy', rather than 'womb envy', as a central psychoanalytic concept.

'Proposing the Future'

1. Dennis *et al.* (1969) and Young and Willmott (1957) are examples. On awareness of these gender implications, see Frankenburg (1976).
2. Freud, in *Beyond the Pleasure Principle*, commented on this (cited in Wolfenstein, 1957, p. 135). On one American experience of postnatal support groups, see Turner and Izzi (1978).

Bibliography

ADAMS, J., HAYES, J. and HOPSON, B. (1976) *Transition: Understanding and Managing Personal Change* London, Martin Robertson

AINSWORTH, M. D. S., BELL, S. M. and STAYTON, D. J. (1974) 'Infant–mother attachment and social development: socialization as a product of reciprocal responsiveness to signals' in Richards (ed.)

AITKEN-SWAN, J. (1977) *Fertility Control and the Medical Profession* London, Croom Helm

ANDREWSKI, I. (1966) 'The baby as dictator' *New Society* 15 December

ARMS, S. (1977) *Immaculate Deception* New York, Bantam Books

ASCH, S. S. (1965) 'Psychiatric considerations: mental and emotional problems' in Rovinsky and Guttmacher (eds)

ASHFORD, J. R. (1978) 'Policies for maternity care in England and Wales: too fast and too far?' in Kitzinger and Davis (eds)

BAKKE, E. WIGHT (1933) *The Unemployed Man* London, Nisbet and Co.

BANTON, M. (1972) *Racial Minorities* London, Fontana

BARDON, D. (1972) 'Puerperal depression' in Morris (ed.)

BARKER, D. (1978) 'Introduction' to N. C. Mathieu *Ignored by Some, Denied by Others: The Social Sex Category in Sociology* London, Women's Research and Resources Centre Publications

BARKER, D. L. and ALLEN, S. (eds) (1976) *Sexual Divisions and Society: Process and Change* London, Tavistock

BARKER-BENFIELD, G. J. (1976) *The Horrors of the Half-Known Life* New York, Harper and Row

BARRETT, M. and ROBERTS, H. (1978) 'Doctors and their patients: the social control of women in general practice' in Smart and Smart (eds)

BEAN, C. A. (1972) *Methods of Childbirth* New York, Doubleday

BECKER, H. S., GEER, B., HUGHES, E. C. and STRAUSS, A. L. (1961) *Boys in White: Student Culture in Medical School* Chicago, Chicago University Press

BEECHEY, V. (1978) 'Women and production: a critical analysis of some sociological theories of women's work' in A. Kuhn and A. Wolpe (eds) *Feminism and Materialism: Women and Modes of Production* London, Routledge and Kegan Paul

BELL, C. and NEWBY, H. (eds) (1971) *Doing Sociological Research* London, Allen and Unwin

BERNAL, J. (1974) 'Attachment: some problems and possibilities' in Richards (ed.)

BERNARD, J. (1973) *The Future of Marriage* London, Souvenir Press
BERNARD, J. (1975) *The Future of Motherhood* New York, Penguin Books
BETTELHEIM, B. (1961) *The Informed Heart* London, Thames and Hudson
BEWLEY, B. R. and BEWLEY, T. H. (1975) 'Hospital doctors' career structure and misuse of medical womanpower' *The Lancet* 9 August, pp. 270–2
BIBRING, G. L. (1959) 'Some considerations of the psychological processes of pregnancy' *The Psychoanalytic Study of the Child* Vol. XIV, New York, International Universities Press
BIBRING, G. L. *et al.* (1961) 'A study of the psychological processes in pregnancy and of the earliest mother–child relationship' *The Psychoanalytic Study of the Child* Vol. XVI, New York, International Universities Press
BLAU, A. *et al.* (1963) 'The psychogenic etiology of premature birth, a preliminary report' *Psychosomatic Medicine* 25
BLOOD, R. O. and WOLFE, O. M. (1960) *Husbands and Wives* Chicago, Free Press
BLOOM, W. L. and CLARK, M. B. (1964) 'Diagnosis and treatment of the obese carboholic' *Journal of Obesity* 1, pp. 10–12
BONDY, C. (1943) 'Problems of internment camps' *Journal of Abnormal and Social Psychology* 38, pp. 453–75
BOSTON WOMEN'S HEALTH BOOK COLLECTIVE (1976) *Our Bodies Our Selves* New York, Simon and Schuster
BOTT, E. (1971) *Family and Social Network* London, Tavistock (revised edn)
BOTTOMORE, T. B. (1962) *Sociology: A Guide to Problems and Literature* London, Allen and Unwin
BOULDING, E. (1977) *Women in the Twentieth Century World* New York, Sage Publications
BOURNE, G. (1975) *Pregnancy* London, Pan Books
BRADLEY, R. A. (1964) *Husband-Coached Childbirth* New York, Harper and Row
BRANT, H. and BRANT, M. (1975) *Pregnancy, Childbirth and Contraception: All You Need to Know* Corgi Books
BREEN, D. (1975) *The Birth of a First Child* London, Tavistock
BROWN, G. W. (1973) 'Some thoughts on grounded theory' *Sociology* 7, 1, pp. 1–16
BROWN, G. W. and HARRIS, T. (1978) *Social Origins of Depression* London, Tavistock
BROWN, W. A. (1972) 'A prospective study of postpartum psychiatric disorders' in Morris (ed.)
BRUCH, H. (1974) *Eating Disorders: Obesity, Anorexia Nervosa and the Person Within* London, Routledge and Kegan Paul
BULLOUGH, V. and BULLOUGH, B. (1977) *Sin, Sickness and Sanity: A History of Sexual Attitudes* New York, Meridian Books
BUSFIELD, J. and PADDON, M. (1977) *Thinking About Children* Cambridge, Cambridge University Press

CARTWRIGHT, A. (1964) *Human Relations and Hospital Care* London, Routledge and Kegan Paul

CARTWRIGHT, A. (1970) *Parents and Family Planning Services* London, Routledge and Kegan Paul

CARTWRIGHT, A. (1979) *The Dignity of Labour?* London, Tavistock

CASS. B., DAWSON, M., RADI, R., TEMPLE, D., WILLS, S. and WINKLER, A. (1978) 'Working it out together: reflections on research on women academics' in C. Bell and S. Encel (eds) *Inside the Whale: Ten Personal Accounts of Social Research* Oxford, Pergamon Press

CASSELL, E. J. (1976) *The Healer's Art: A New Approach to the Doctor–Patient Relationship* Philadelphia, J. B. Lippincott

CHALMERS, I. (1978) 'Implications of the current debate on obstetric practice' in Kitzinger and Davis (eds)

CHALMERS, I. and RICHARDS, M. (1977) 'Intervention and causal inference in obstetric practice' in Chard and Richards (eds)

CHALMERS, I., ZLOSNIK, J. E., JOHNS, K. A. and CAMPBELL, H. (1976) 'Obstetric practice and outcome of pregnancy in Cardiff residents 1965–73' *British Medical Journal* 1, pp. 735–8

CHAMBERLAIN, R., CHAMBERLAIN, G., HOWLETT, B. and CLAIREAUX, A. (1975) *British Births 1970* London, Heinemann

CHAPMAN, J. R. and GATES, M. (eds) (1977) *Women into Wives: The Legal and Economic Impact of Marriage* Beverly Hills, Sage Publications

CHARD, T. and RICHARDS, M. (eds) (1977) *Benefits and Hazards of the New Obstetrics* London, Heinemann Medical Books

CHERTOK, L. (1969) *Motherhood and Personality* London, Tavistock

CHODOROW, N. (1974) 'Family structure and feminine personality' in Rosaldo and Lamphere (eds)

CHODOROW, N. (1978) *The Reproduction of Mothering: Psychoanalysis and the Sociology of Gender* Berkeley, University of California Press

CICOUREL, A. V. (1964) *Method and Measurement in Sociology* Glencoe, Illinois, Free Press

CLEMENTS, R. V. (1958) *Managers: A Study of their Careers in Industry* London, Allen and Unwin

COCHRANE, A. L., ST LEGER, A. S. and MOORE, F. (1978) 'Health service "input" and mortality "output" in developed countries' *Journal of Epidemiology and Community Health* 32, pp. 200–5

COLLVER, A., HAVE, R. T. and SPEARE, M. C. (1967) 'Factors influencing the use of maternal health services' *Social Science and Medicine* 1, pp. 293–308

COMAROFF, J. (1977) 'Conflicting paradigms of pregnancy: managing ambiguity in antenatal encounters' in Davis and Horobin (eds)

COMER, L. (1974) *Wedlocked Women* Leeds, Feminist Books

CONE, B. A. (1972) 'Puerperal depression' in Morris (ed.)

COPPEN, A. J. (1958) 'Psychosomatic aspects of pre-eclamptic toxaemia' *Journal of Psychosomatic Research* 2

COPPEN, A. and SHAW, D. M. (1963) 'Mineral metabolism in melancholia' *British Medical Journal* 2, p. 1439

COSER, R. L. (1960) 'A home away from home' in D. Apple (ed.) *Sociological Studies of Health and Sickness* New York, McGraw-Hill

CRAMMOND, W. A. (1954) 'Psychological aspects of uterine dysfunction' *The Lancet* 2, p. 1241

CRAWFORD, M. (1971) 'Retirement and disengagement' *Human Relations* 24, 3, pp. 225–78

CRISP, A. H., PALMER, R. L. and KELUCY, R. S. (1976) 'How common is anorexia nervosa? A prevalence study' *British Journal of Psychiatry* 128, pp. 549–54

DALTON, K. (1969) *The Menstrual Cycle* Harmondsworth, Penguin Books

DALTON, K. (1971) 'Prospective study into puerperal depression' *British Journal of Psychiatry* 118, pp. 689–92

DALTON, K. (1978) *Once a Month* London, Fontana

DANIELS, A. K. (1975) 'Feminist perspectives in sociological research' in Millman and Kanter (eds)

DAVIS, A. and HOROBIN, G. (eds) (1977) *Medical Encounters: The Experience of Illness and Treatment* London, Croom Helm

DAVIS, A. G. and STRONG, P. M. (1976) 'Aren't children wonderful? A study of the allocation of identity in development assessment' in Stacey (ed.)

DELAMONT, S. and DUFFIN, L. (eds) (1978) *The Nineteenth Century Woman: Her Cultural and Physical World* London, Croom Helm

DELANEY, J., LUPTON, M. J. and TOTH, E. (1977) *The Curse: A Cultural History of Menstruation* New York, Mentor Books

DEMBO, T., LADIEU-LEVITON, G. and WRIGHT, B. A. (1952) 'Acceptance of loss – amputations' in J. F. Garrett (ed.) *Psychological Aspects of Physical Disability* Department of Health, Education and Welfare Office of Vocational Rehabilitation, Rehabilitation Service Series no. 210, U.S. Government Printing Office

DENNIS, N., HENRIQUES, F. and SLAUGHTER, C. (1969) *Coal is our Life* London, Tavistock

DENZIN, N. K. (1970) *Sociological Methods: A Source Book* London, Butterworths

DEPARTMENT OF HEALTH AND SOCIAL SECURITY (1977) *Reducing the Risk: Safer Pregnancy and Childbirth* London, HMSO

DEPARTMENT OF HEALTH AND SOCIAL SECURITY (1978) *Hospital Medical Staff in England and Wales National Tables 30 September 1977*

DEUTSCH, H. (1944) *Psychology of Women* New York, Grune and Stratton

DICK-READ, G. (1942) *Childbirth Without Fear* London, Heinemann

DONABEDIAN, A. and ROSENFELD, L. S. (1961) 'Some factors influencing prenatal care' *The New England Journal of Medicine*, 265, July 6, pp. 1–6

DONNISON, J. (1977) *Midwives and Medical Men* London, Heinemann

DOWNES, D. M. (1966) *The Delinquent Solution* London, Routledge and Kegan Paul

DUFFIN, L. (1978) 'The conspicuous consumptive: woman as an invalid' in Delamont and Duffin (eds)

DUNN, P. M. (1976) 'Obstetric delivery today' *The Lancet* 1, pp. 790–3

DWYER, J. T. and MAYER, J. (1970) 'Potential dieters – who are they?' *Journal of the American Dietetic Association* 56, pp. 510–14

EHRENREICH, B. and ENGLISH, D. (1973) *Witches, Midwives and Nurses* Glass Mountain Pamphlets, New York, The Feminist Press

EHRENREICH, J. (1978) 'The crisis in medical care: beyond socialized medicine' Address to British Sociological Association Medical Sociology Conference, York, 22–4 September

EMERSON, J. (1970) 'Behavior in private places: sustaining definitions of reality in gynecological examinations' in H. P. Dreitzel (ed.) *Recent Sociology No. I* New York, Macmillan

ENGELMANN, G. J. (1883) *Labor Among Primitive Peoples* St Louis, J. H. Chambers (2nd edn)

ENGLEMAN, E. G. (1974) 'Attitudes toward women physicians' *The Western Journal of Medicine* 120, February, pp. 95–100

EPSTEIN, C. (1974) 'A different angle of vision: notes on the selective eye of sociology' *Social Science Quarterly* 55, December, pp. 645–56

EZTKOWITZ, H. (1971) 'The male sister: sexual separation of labour in society' *Journal of Marriage and the Family* 33, 3, pp. 431–4

FAMILY DOCTOR PUBLICATIONS (1977) *You and Your Baby Part I: From Pregnancy to Birth* London, British Medical Association

FEIN, R. A. (n.d.) 'Men's experiences before and after the birth of a first child' unpublished summary of PhD thesis, Cambridge, Massachusetts

FISH, D. G. (1966) 'An obstetric unit in a London hospital: a study of relations between patients, doctors and nurses' unpublished PhD thesis, University of London

FISHER, S. H. (1960) 'Psychiatric considerations of hand disability' *Archives of Physical Medicine and Rehabilitation* 41, pp. 62–70

FISHMAN, H. (1973) 'Ultrasound and marrow-cell chromosomes' *The Lancet* 20 October, p. 920

FLETCHER, R. (1962) *The Family and Marriage* Harmondsworth, Penguin Books

FLEURY, P. M. (1967) *Maternity Care: Mothers' Experiences of Childbirth* London, Allen and Unwin

FONDA, N. and MOSS, P. (eds) (1976) *Mothers in Employment* Brunel University Management Programme

FORD, C. S. (1945) *A Comparative Study of Human Reproduction* New York, Yale University Publications in Anthropology No. 32

FORD, E. S. C. *et al.* (1953) 'A psychodynamic approach to the study of infertility' *Fertility and Sterility* 4

FRANKENBURG, R. (1976) 'In the production of their lives, men (?) . . . sex and gender in British community studies' in Barker and Allen (eds)

FRANKFORT, E. (1972) *Vaginal Politics* New York, Quadrangle Books

FREIDSON, E. (1970) *Profession of Medicine* New York, Dodd-Mead

FROMM-REICHMANN, F. and GUNST, V. K. (1974) 'On the denial of women's sexual pleasure' in Miller (ed.)

GALPERIN-LEMAITRE, H. and KIRSCH-VOLDERS, M. (1975) 'Ultrasound and mammalian DNA' *The Lancet* 4 October, p. 662

GALTUNG, J. (1967) *Theory and Methods of Social Research* London, Allen and Unwin

GAVRON, H. (1966) *The Captive Wife* Harmondsworth, Penguin Books

GENNEP, A. VAN (1960) *The Rites of Passage* London, Routledge and Kegan Paul

GIBBONS, J. L. and MCHUGH, P. R. (1962) 'Plasma cortisol in depressive illness' *Journal of Psychiatric Research* 1, p. 162

GILL, D. (1977) *Illegitimacy, Sexuality and the Status of Women* Oxford, Basil Blackwell

GINSBERG, S. (1976) 'Women, work and conflict' in Fonda and Moss (eds)

GLASER, B. G. and STRAUSS, A. L. (1968) *The Discovery of Grounded Theory* London, Weidenfeld and Nicolson

GLASER, B. G. and STRAUSS, A. L. (1971) *Status Passage* London, Routledge and Kegan Paul

GOFFMAN, E. (1961) *Asylum: Essays on the Social Situation of Patients and other Inmates* New York, Anchor Books

GOLDBERG, S. and LEWIS, M. (1969) 'Play behaviour in the year-old infant: early sex differences' *Child Development* 40, pp. 21–31

GOLDTHORPE, J. H. (1973) 'A revolution in sociology?' *British Journal of Sociology* 7, pp. 449–62

GOREY, E. (1974) *The Listing Attic and the Unstrung Harp or, Mr Earbrass Writes a Novel* London, Abelard

GRAHAM, H. (1977a) 'Images of pregnancy in antenatal literature' in R. Dingwall, C. Heath, M. Reid and M. Stacey (eds) *Health Care and Health Knowledge* London, Croom Helm

GRAHAM, H. (1977b) 'Women's attitudes to conception and pregnancy' in R. Chester and J. Peel (eds) *Equalities and Inequalities in Family Life* New York, Academic Press

GRAHAM, H. (1978) *Problems in Antenatal Care* University of York

GRAHAM, H. and OAKLEY, A. (forthcoming) 'Competing ideologies of reproduction: medical and maternal perspectives on pregnancy and childbirth' in H. Roberts (ed.) *Women and Health*

GREEN, R. (1975) *Sexual Identity Conflict in Children and Adults* Baltimore, Penguin Books

GRIMM, E. R. (1967) 'Psychological and social factors in pregnancy, delivery and outcome' in Richardson and Guttmacher (eds)

GRINKER, R. R. and SPIEGEL, J. P. (1945) *Men Under Stress* New York, McGraw-Hill

GUTTMACHER, A. F. (1973) *Pregnancy, Birth and Family Planning* New York, Viking Press

HACKER, H. M. (1951) 'Women as a minority group' *Social Forces*; reprinted in B. Roszak and T. Roszak *Masculine/Feminine: Readings in Sexual Mythology and the Liberation of Women* New York, Harper and Row, 1969

HAIRE, D. (1972) *The cultural warping of childbirth* Seattle, International Childbirth Education Association

HALLER, J. S. and HALLER, R. M. (1974) *The Physician and Sexuality in Victorian America* New York, W. W. Norton

HAMILTON, J. (1962) *Postpartum Psychiatric Problems* St Louis, Mosby.

HANDLEY, S. L., DUNN, T. L., BAKER, J. M., COCHSHOTT, C. and GOULD, S. (1977) 'Mood changes in the puerperium, and plasma tryptophan and cortisol concentrations' *British Medical Journal* 2, p. 18

HART, N. (1977) 'Parenthood and patienthood: a dialectical autobiography' in Davis and Horobin (eds)

HARVEY, W. A. and SHERFEY, M. J. (1954) 'Vomiting in pregnancy: a psychiatric study' *Psychosomatic Medicine* 16

HAUG, M. (1976) 'Issues in G.P. authority in the NHS' in Stacey (ed.)

HAWKINS, D. F. (ed.) (1974) *Obstetric Therapeutics* London, Bailliere Tindall

HEIMAN, M. (1965) 'Psychiatric complications: a psychoanalytic view of pregnancy' in Rovinsky and Guttmacher (eds)

HEMMING, D. G. (1975) 'The net resource distribution of two-parent low-income families: a regional comparison' *Social and Economic Administration* 9, pp. 207–17

HENLEY, N. M. (1977) *Body Politics: Power, Sex and Nonverbal Communication* Englewood Cliffs, New Jersey, Prentice-Hall

HENSLIN, J. M. and BIGGS, M. A. (1971) 'The sociology of the vaginal examination' in J. M. Henslin (ed.) *Studies in the Sociology of Sex* New York, Appleton-Century-Crofts

HOBBS, D. F. (1965) 'Parenthood as crisis: a third study' *Journal of Marriage and the Family* 27, August, pp. 367–72

HOCHSCHILD, A. R. (1975) 'The sociology of feeling and emotion: selected possibilities' in Millman and Kanter (eds)

HOFFMAN, L. W. and NYE, I. (eds) (1974) *Working Mothers: An Evaluative Review of the Consequences for Wife, Husband and Child* San Francisco, Jossey-Bass

HORNEY, K. (1967) *Feminine Psychology* New York, W. W. Norton

HORNEY, K. (1974) 'The flight from womanhood' in Miller (ed.)

HOUGHTON, H. (1968) 'Problems of hospital communication: an experimental study' in G. McLachlan (ed.) *Problems and Progress in Medical Care* London, Oxford University Press

HOWELLS, J. G. (ed.) (1972) *Modern Perspectives in Psycho-Obstetrics* London, Oliver and Boyd

HUBERT, J. (1974) 'Belief and reality: social factors in pregnancy and childbirth' in Richards (ed.)

HUDSON, L. and JACOT, B. (1971) 'Education and eminence in British medicine' *British Medical Journal* 16 October, pp. 162–3

HUNT, A. (1968) *A Survey of Women's Employment* Government Social Survey, London, HMSO

HUNTINGFORD, P. (1978) 'Obstetric practice: past, present and future' in Kitzinger and Davis (eds)

HUTTON, C. (1974) 'Second-hand status: stratification terms and the sociological subordination of women' Paper given at British Sociological Association conference *Sexual Divisions and Society* Aberdeen, Scotland, 7–10 April

ILLICH, I. (1975) *Medical Nemesis: The Expropriation of Health* London, Calder and Boyars

ILLSLEY, R. (1967) 'The sociological study of reproduction and its outcome' in Richardson and Guttmacher (eds)

'Induction of labour' (1976) *British Medical Journal* 27 March, p. 729

INGLEBY, D. (ed.) (forthcoming) *Critical Psychiatry*

INTERNATIONAL FEDERATION OF GYNAECOLOGY AND OBSTETRICS and INTERNATIONAL CONFEDERATION OF MIDWIVES (1976) *Maternity Care in the World*

JANIS, I. L. (1958) *Psychological Stress* New York, John Wiley

JESSUP, F. (1973) *The Fifth Child's Conception in the Runaway Wife* Harmondsworth, Penguin Books

JORDANOVA, L. (1978), 'Medicine, Personal Morality and Public Order: an Historical Case Study', Paper given at British Sociological Association Medical Sociology Conference, York, 22–24 September

KAIJ, L. and NILSSON, A. (1972) 'Emotional and psychotic illness following childbirth' in Howells (ed.)

KARACAN, I. and WILLIAMS, R. L. (1970) 'Current advances in theory and practice relating to postpartum syndromes' *Psychiatry in Medicine* 1, pp. 307–28

KENNY, M. (1978) *Woman × Two* London, Sidgwick and Jackson

KITSUSE, J. I. and CICOUREL, A. V. (1963) 'A note on the uses of official statistics' *Social Problems* 11

KITZINGER, S. (1962) *The Experience of Childbirth* London, Gollancz

KITZINGER, S. (1977) *Education and Counselling for Childbirth* London, Bailliere Tindall

KITZINGER, S. (1978) *Woman as Mothers* Fontana

KITZINGER, S. and DAVIS, J. A. (eds) (1978) *The Place of Birth* Oxford, Oxford University Press

KLAUS, M. H. and KENNELL, J. H. (1976) *Maternal–Infant Bonding* St Louis, Mosby

KROGER, W. S. and DELEE, S. T. (1946) 'The psychosomatic treatment of hyperemesis gravidarum by hypnosis' *American Journal of Obstetrics and Gynecology* 51

KUHN, T. S. (1962) *The Structure of Scientific Revolutions* Chicago, University of Chicago Press

LARSEN, V. (1966) 'Stresses of the childbearing years' *American Journal of Public Health* 56, pp. 32–6

LEMASTERS, E. E. (1957) 'Parenthood as crisis' *Marriage and Family Living* 19, pp. 352–5

LENNANE, J. and LENNANE, J. (1977) *Hard Labour* London, Gollancz

LESSING, D. (1966) *A Proper Marriage* London, Panther

LEVENSON, B. (1961) 'Bureaucratic succession' in A. Etzioni (ed.) *Complex Organisations* New York, Holt, Rinehart and Winston

LEVI-STRAUSS, C. (1969) *The Elementary Structures of Kinship* Boston, Beacon Press

LEWIS, M. and ROSENBLUM, L. A. (eds) (1974) *The Effect of the Infant on its Caregiver* New York, John Wiley

LINDEMANN, E. (1941) 'Observations on psychiatric sequelae to surgical operations in women' *American Journal of Psychiatry* 98, pp. 132–9

LLEWELLYN-JONES, D. (1965) *Fundamentals of Obstetrics and Gynaecology Vol. I Obstetrics* London, Faber and Faber

LOMAS, P. (1966) 'Ritualistic elements in the management of childbirth' *British Journal of Medical Psychology* 39, pp. 207–13

LOMAS, P. (1967) 'The significance of postpartum breakdown' in Lomas (ed.)

LOMAS, P. (ed.) (1967) *The Predicament of the Family* London, Hogarth Press

LOMAS, P. (1978) 'An interpretation of modern obstetric practice' in Kitzinger and Davis (eds)

LUKER, K. (1975) *Taking Chances: Abortion and the Decision not to Contracept* Berkeley, University of California Press

MCCLEARY, G. F. (1933) *The Early History of the Infant Welfare Movement* London, H. K. Lewis and Co.

MACCOBY, E. E. and JACKLIN, C. N. (1973) 'Stress, activity and proximity seeking: sex differences in the year old child' *Child Development* 44, pp. 34–42

MACCOBY, E. E. and JACKLIN, C. N. (1974) *The Psychology of Sex Differences Volume I Text* Stanford, California, Stanford University Press

MACFARLANE, A. (1977) *The Psychology of Childbirth* London, Fontana

MCGOWAN, P. K. and QUASTEL, J. H. (1931) 'Blood sugar studies in abnormal mental states' *Journal of Mental Science* 77, p. 525

MACINTOSH, I. J. C. and DAVEY, D. A. (1970) 'Chromosomal aberrations induced by an ultrasound fetal pulse detector' *British Medical Journal* 4, p. 92

MACINTYRE, S. (1976a) 'Who wants babies? The social construction of instincts' in Barker and Allen (eds)

MACINTYRE, S. (1976b) 'To have or have not: promotion and prevention in gynaecological work' in Stacey (ed.)

MACINTYRE, S. (1977a) *Single and Pregnant* London, Croom Helm

MACINTYRE, S. (1977b) 'The management of childbirth: a review of sociological research issues' *Social Science and Medicine* 11, pp. 477–84

MCKEOWN, T. (1971) 'A historical appraisal of the medical task' in McLachlan and McKeown (eds)

MCKINLAY, J. B. (1970) 'The new late comers for antenatal care' *British Journal of Preventive and Social Medicine* 24, February, pp. 52–7

MCKINLAY, J. B. (1972) 'The sick role – illness and pregnancy' *Social Science and Medicine* 6, pp. 561–72

MCLACHLAN, G. and MCKEOWN, T. (eds) (1971) *Medical History and Medical Care* London, Oxford University Press

MANDY, T. E. and MANDY, A. J. (1959) 'The psychosomatic aspects of infertility' *Sinai Hospital Journal* 28

MANN, E. C. and GRIMM, E. R. (1962) 'Habitual abortion' in W. S. Kroger (ed.) *Psychosomatic Obstetrics, Gynecology and Endocrinology* Springfield, Illinois, C. C. Thomas

MARKHAM, S. (1965) 'A comparison of psychotic and normal postpartum reactions based on psychological tests' in Société Française de Médecine

Psychosomatique *Premier Congrès International de Medecine Psychsosomatique et Maternité* Paris, Gauthier-Villars
MARRIS, P. (1974) *Loss and Change* London, Routledge and Kegan Paul
MATTHEWS, A. E. B. (1961) 'Behaviour patterns during labour' *Journal of Obstetrics and Gynaecology of the British Commonwealth* 6, pp. 862–74
MEAD, M. (1962) *Male and Female* Harmondsworth, Penguin Books
MEAD, M. and NEWTON, N. (1967) 'Cultural patterning of perinatal behavior' in Richardson and Guttmacher (eds)
MERTON, R. K. (1949) *Social Theory and Social Structure* Glencoe, Illinois, Free Press
MEYEROWITZ, J. H. and FELDMAN, H. (1968) 'Transition to parenthood' *Psychiatric Research Reports* 20, pp. 78–94
MILLER, J. B. (ed.) (1974) *Psychoanalysis and Women* Harmondsworth, Penguin Books
MILLER, J. B. (1977) *Towards a New Psychology of Women* Boston, Beacon Press
MILLETT, K. (1971) *Sexual Politics* London, Rupert Hart-Davis
MILLMAN, M. and KANTER, R. M. (eds) (1975) *Another Voice: Feminist Perspectives in Social Life and Social Science* New York, Doubleday
MINTURN, L., LAMBERT, W. W. *et al.* (1964) *Mothers of Six Cultures* New York, John Wiley
MITCHELL, J. (1971) *Woman's Estate* Harmondsworth, Penguin Books
MITCHELL, J. (1974) *Psychoanalysis and Feminism* London, Allen Lane
MOIR, D. D. (1974) 'Drugs used during labour – analgesics, anaesthetics and sedatives' in Hawkins (ed.)
MOLINSKI, A. (1975) 'Different behavior of women in labor as a symptom of different psychic patterns' in H. Hirsch (ed.) *The Family* 4th International Congress of Psychosomatic Obstetrics and Gynaecology, Basel, Karger
MONEY, J. and ERHARDT, A. A. (1972) *Man and Woman, Boy and Girl* Baltimore, Johns Hopkins
MORGAN, D. H. J. (1975) *Social Theory and the Family* London, Routledge and Kegan Paul
MORRIS, N. (ed.) (1972) *Psychosomatic Medicine in Obstetrics and Gynaecology* 3rd International Congress, London, 1971, Basel, Karger
MOSS, H. A. (1970) 'Sex, age and state as determinants of mother–infant interaction' in K. Danziger (ed.) *Readings in Child Socialization* Oxford, Pergamon Press
MOSS, P. (1976) 'The current situation' in Fonda and Moss (eds)
MURPHY, L. B. (1962) *The Widening World of Childhood* New York, Basic Books
MURRAY, R. M. (1974) 'Psychiatric illness in doctors' *The Lancet* 15 June, pp. 1211–13
MYRDAL, G. (1969) *Objectivity in Social Research* New York, Pantheon

NEWILL, R. (1974) *Infertile Marriage* Harmondsworth, Penguin Books
NEWTON, N. (1972) in Morris (ed.)
NEWTON, N. (1973) 'Interrelationships between sexual responsiveness, birth and breastfeeding' in Zubin and Money (eds)

NEWTON, N. and NEWTON, M. (1972) 'Childbirth in cross-cultural perspective' in Howells (ed.)

NILSSON, A. (1972) 'Paranatal emotional adjustment' in Morris (ed.)

NOTMAN, M. T. and NADELSON, C. C. (eds) (1978) *The Woman Patient: Medical and Psychological Interfaces* New York, Plenum Press

NOTT, P. N., FRANKLIN, M., ARMITAGE, C. and GELDER, M. G. (1976) 'Hormonal changes and mood in the puerperium' *British Journal of Psychiatry* 128, p. 379

OAKLEY, A. (1972) *Sex, Gender and Society* London, Maurice Temple Smith

OAKLEY, A. (1974a) *Housewife* London, Allen Lane

OAKLEY, A. (1974b) *The Sociology of Housework* London, Martin Robertson

OAKLEY, A. (1976) 'Wisewoman and medicine man: changes in the management of childbirth' in J. Mitchell and A. Oakley (eds) *The Rights and Wrongs of Women* Harmondsworth, Penguin Books

OAKLEY, A. (1977) 'Cross-cultural practice' in Chard and Richards (eds)

OAKLEY, A. (1979a) 'A case of maternity: Paradigms of women as maternity cases' *Signs: Journal of Women in Culture and Society* 7

OAKLEY, A. (1979b) *Becoming a Mother* Oxford, Martin Robertson

OAKLEY, A. and OAKLEY, R. (1979) 'Sexism in official statistics' in J. Irvine, I. Miles and J. Evans (eds) *Demystifying Statistics* London, Pluto Press

O'BRIEN, M. (1978) 'Home and hospital: a comparison of the experiences of mothers having home and hospital confinements' *Journal of the Royal College of General Practitioners* 28, pp. 460–6

'Obstetric analgesia and the newborn baby' (1974) *The Lancet* 1 June

OFFICE OF POPULATION CENSUSES AND SURVEYS (1975) *Birth Statistics* London, HMSO

OFFICE OF POPULATION CENSUSES AND SURVEYS (1978) *Population Trends* 11, London, HMSO

ORBACH, S. (1978) *Fat is a Feminist Issue* New York, Paddington Press

ORTNER, S. B. (1974) 'Is female to male as nature is to culture?' in Rosaldo and Lamphere (eds)

OUNSTED, M. (1972) 'Gender and intrauterine growth: with a note on the use of the sex proband as a research tool' in C. Ounsted and D. C. Taylor (eds) *Gender Differences: Their Ontogeny and Significance* Edinburgh, Churchill Livingstone

PARKER, R. and MANGER, S. (1974) 'Anorexia nervosa' *Spare Rib* 28, pp. 6–10

PARKES, C. M. (1971) 'Psycho-social transitions: a field for study' *Social Science and Medicine* 5, pp. 101–15

PARKES, C. M. (1972) *Bereavement: Studies of Grief in Adult Life* London, Tavistock

PARKIN, F. (ed.) (1974) *The Social Analysis of Class Structure* London, Tavistock

PARLEE, M. B. (n.d.) 'Psychological aspects of menstruation, childbirth and menopause' unpublished paper

PARLEE, M. B. (1975) 'Psychology' *Signs: Journal of Women in Culture and Society* 1, Autumn, pp. 119–35

PARSONS, T. (1963) *Social Structure and Personality* Glencoe, Illinois, The Free Press

PARSONS, T. (1964) *The Social System* London, Routledge and Kegan Paul

PARSONS, T. and BALES, R. F. (eds) (1956) *Family: Socialization and Interaction Process* London, Routledge and Kegan Paul

PEARSON, J. F. and WEAVER, J. B. (1976) 'Fetal activity and fetal wellbeing: an evaluation' *British Medical Journal* 29 May, pp. 1305–8

PECK, E. (1973) *The Baby Trap* Bishop's Stortford, Heinrich Hanau Publications

PEEL, J. and CARR, G. (1975) *Contraception and Family Design* Edinburgh, Churchill Livingstone

PITT, B. (1972) 'Neurotic (or atypical) depression following childbirth' in Morris (ed.)

'A Place to be Born' (1976) *British Medical Journal* 10 January, pp. 55–6

PLATH, S. (1971) 'Three women: a poem for three voices' *Winter Trees* London, Faber and Faber

PLATT, J. (1976) *Realities of Social Research: An Empirical Study of British Sociologists* London, Sussex University Press

POYNTER, F. N. L. and KEELE, K. D. (1961) *A Short History of Medicine* London, Mills and Boon

PRINGLE, M. KELLMER (1974) *The Needs of Children* London, Hutchinson

RAPOPORT, R. (1967) 'The study of marriage as a critical transition for personality and family development' in Lomas (ed.)

RAPOPORT, R. and OAKLEY, A. (1975) 'Towards a review of parent–child relationships in social science' Paper given at Ford Foundation conference on *Sex Roles in Sociology* Merrill-Palmer Institute, 10–12 November

RAPOPORT, R. and RAPOPORT, R. N. (1964) 'New light on the honeymoon' *Human Relations* 17, pp. 33–56

RAPOPORT, R., RAPOPORT, R. N. and STRELITZ, Z. (1977) *Fathers, Mothers and Others* London, Routledge and Kegan Paul

RATHBONE, E. F. (1924) *The Disinherited Family: A Plea for the Endowment of the Family* London, Edward Arnold

REISS, I. (1971) *The Family System in America* New York, Holt, Rinehart and Winston

RICH, A. (1977) *Of Woman Born* London, Virago

RICHARDS, M. P. M. (ed.) (1974) *The Integration of a Child into a Social World* Cambridge, Cambridge University Press

RICHARDS, M. P. M. (1975) 'Innovation in medical practice: obstetricians and the induction of labour in Britain' *Social Science and Medicine* 9, pp. 595–602

RICHARDS, M. and BERNAL, J. (1974) 'Why some babies don't sleep' *New Society* 28 February

RICHARDSON, S. A. and GUTTMACHER, A. F. (eds) (1967) *Childbearing – Its Social and Psychological Aspects* Baltimore, Williams and Wilkins

ROLLINS, B. C. and FELDMAN, H. (1970) 'Marital satisfaction over the family life cycle' *Journal of Marriage and the Family* 32, pp. 20–8

ROSALDO, M. Z. and LAMPHERE, L. (eds) (1974) *Woman, Culture and Society* Stanford, California, Stanford University Press

ROSEN, M. (1977) 'Pain and its relief' in Chard and Richards (eds)

ROSENGREN, W. R. (1961a) 'Social sources of pregnancy as illness or normality' *Social Forces* 39, pp. 260–7

ROSENGREN, W. R. (1961b) 'Some social-psychological aspects of delivery room difficulties' *Journal of Nervous and Mental Diseases* 132, pp. 515–21

ROSENGREN, W. R. (1962a) 'Social instability and attitudes towards pregnancy as a social role' *Social Problems* 9, pp. 371–8

ROSENGREN, W. R. (1962b) 'Social status, attitudes towards pregnancy and childrearing attitudes' *Social Forces* 41, pp. 127–34

ROSSER, J. (1978) 'Ultrasound and pregnant women' in Association of Radical Midwives *Newsletter* June

ROSSER, J. E. (1978) 'Sexual identity on becoming a mother: some cultural contradictions' Paper given at British Sociological Association Medical Sociology Conference, York, 22–24 September

ROSSI, A. (1968) 'Transition to parenthood' *Journal of Marriage and the Family* 30, February, pp. 26–39

ROSSI, A. (1973) 'Maternalism, sexuality and the new feminism' in Zubin and Money (eds)

ROVINSKY, J. J. and GUTTMACHER, A. F. (eds) (1965) *Medical, Surgical and Gynecological Complications of Pregnancy* Baltimore, Williams and Wilkins

RUBENSTEIN, B. B. (1950) 'An emotional factor in infertility' *Fertility and Sterility* 2

RYDER, J. and SILVER, H. (1970) *Modern English Society: History and Structure 1850–1970* London, Methuen

SADOVSKY, E., MAHLER, Y., POLISHUK, W. Z. and MALKIN, A. (1973) 'Correlation between electromagnetic recording and maternal assessment of fetal movement' *The Lancet* 26 May, pp. 1141–3

SCANLON, J. W. (1976) 'Effects of local anesthetics administered to parturient women on the neurological and behavioral performance of newborn children' *Bulletin of the New York Academy of Medicine* 52, pp. 231–40

SCHAFFER, R. (1977) *Mothering* London, Fontana

SCHEFF, T. J. (1963) 'Decision rules, types of error and their consequences in medical diagnosis' *Behavioural Science* 8, pp. 97–105

SCULLY, D. and BART, P. (1973) 'A funny thing happened on the way to the orifice: women in gynecology textbooks' *American Journal of Sociology* 78, January, pp. 1045–50

SEGAL, H. A. (1954) 'Initial psychiatric findings of recently repatriated prisoners of war' *American Journal of Psychiatry* 111, 1, pp. 358–63

SEIDEN, A. M. (1978) 'The sense of mastery in the childbirth experience' in Notman and Nadelson (eds)

SELECT COMMITTEE ON VIOLENCE AND THE FAMILY (1977) First Report, Session 1976–7 *Violence to Children Volume I Report* London, HMSO

SELIGMAN, M. E. P. (1975) *Helplessness* San Francisco, W. H. Freeman

SEWARD, G. H. (1945) 'Cultural conflict and the feminine role: an experimental study' *Journal of Social Psychology* 22, pp. 177–94

SHARPE, S. (1976) *'Just Like a Girl': How Girls Learn to be Women* Harmondsworth, Penguin Books

SHAW, N. STOLLER (1974) *Forced Labor* New York, Pergamon Press

SHERESHEFSKY, P. and YARROW, L. (1973) *Psychological Aspects of a First Pregnancy and Early Postnatal Adaptation* New York, Raven Press

SHERMAN, J. A. (1971) *On the Psychology of Women: A Survey of Empirical Studies* Springfield, Illinois, C. C. Thomas

SMART, C. and SMART, B. (eds) (1978) *Women, Sexuality and Social Control* London, Routledge and Kegan Paul

SMART, E. (1966) *By Grand Central Station I Sat Down and Wept* London, Panther

SPENCER, H. R. (1927) *The History of British Midwifery from 1650 to 1800* London, John Bale, Sons and Danielsson Ltd.

STACEY, M. (1976) 'The health service consumer: a sociological misconception' in Stacey (ed.)

STACEY, M. (ed.) (1976) *The Sociology of the NHS* Sociological Review Monograph 22, University of Keele

STACEY, M. with HOMANS, H. (1978) 'The sociology of health and illness: its present state, future prospects and potential for health research' *Sociology* 12, 2, pp. 281–307

STALLWORTHY, J. (1972) 'Management of the hospital confinement' in Howells (ed.)

STEINEMANN, A. (1963) 'A study of the concept of the feminine role of 51 middle class American families' *Genetic Psychology Monographs* 67, pp. 272–352

STEWART, D. and STEWART, L. (eds) (1976) *Safe Alternatives in Childbirth* Chapel Hill, North Carolina, Napsac Inc.

STIMSON, G. V. (1974) 'Obeying doctor's orders: a view from the other side' *Social Science and Medicine* 8, pp. 97–104

STIMSON, G. V. (1976a) 'Women in a doctored world' *New Society* 1 May

STIMSON, G. V. (1976b) 'G.P.'s, "trouble" and types of patients' in Stacey (ed.)

STIMSON, G. V. and WEBB, B. (1975) *Going to See the Doctor* London, Routledge and Kegan Paul

STOLLER, R. (1968) *Sex and Gender* New York, Science House

STOLLER, R. (1974) 'The sense of femaleness' in Miller (ed.)

STOTT, D. H. (1957) 'Psychological and mental handicaps in the child following a disturbed pregnancy' *The Lancet* 1, p. 1006

Sunday Times (1974) 13 and 20 October

SUTHERLAND, A. M. and ORBACH, C. E. (1953) 'Psychological impact of cancer surgery' *Cancer* 6, pp. 958–62

SWINSCOW, T. D. V. (1974) 'Personal view' *British Medical Journal* 28 September

TAKUMA, T. (1978) 'Human behavior in the event of earthquakes' in E. L. Quarantelli (ed.) *Disasters: Theory and Research* Sage Studies in International Sociology, vol. 13, London, Sage Publications

THEOBALD, G. W. (1974) 'The induction of labour' in Hawkins (ed.)

THOMAN, E. B., LEIDERMAN, P. H. and OLSON, J. P. (1972) 'Neonate-mother interaction during breastfeeding' *Developmental Psychology* 6, 1, pp. 110-18

THOMPSON, C. (1941) 'The role of women in this culture' *Psychiatry* 4, pp. 1-8

TIZARD, J., MOSS, P. and PERRY, J. (1976) *All Our Children* London, Maurice Temple Smith

TOD, E. D. M. (1972) 'Puerperal depression' in Morris (ed.)

TOWERS, B. (1971) 'The influence of medical technology on medical services' in McLachlan and McKeown (eds)

TUNSTALL, J. (1962) *The Fisherman: The Sociology of an Extreme Occupation* London, MacGibbon and Kee

TUPPER, C. (1956) 'Conditioning for childbirth' *American Journal of Obstetrics and Gynecology* April, pp. 733-40

TUPPER, C. and WEIL, K. J. (1962) 'The problem of spontaneous abortion' *American Journal of Obstetrics and Gynecology* 83

TURNER, C. (1969) *Family and Kinship in Modern Britain: An Introduction* London, Routledge and Kegan Paul

TURNER, M. F. and IZZI, M. H. (1978) 'The COPE story: a service to pregnant and postpartum women' in Notman and Nadelson (eds)

UNITED STATES DEPARTMENT OF HEALTH, EDUCATION AND WELFARE (1977) *Vital Statistics of the U.S. 1973, volume I, Natality*

VERBRUGGE, M. H. (1976) 'Women and medicine in nineteenth century America' *Signs: Journal of Women in Culture and Society* 4, 1, pp. 957-72

VERSLUYSEN, M. (1977) 'Medical professionalism and maternity hospitals in eighteenth century London: a sociological interpretation' The Society for the Social History of Medicine *Bulletin* 21, December, pp. 34-6

VERSLUYSEN, M. (n.d.) 'Men-midwives, professionalizing strategies and the first maternity hospitals – a sociological interpretation' unpublished paper

WALKER, J. (1972) 'The changing role of the midwife' *International Journal of Nursing Studies* 9, pp. 85-94

WALKER, J. (1976) 'Midwife or obstetric nurse? Some perceptions of midwives and obstetricians of the role of the midwife' *Journal of Advanced Nursing* 1, pp. 129-38

WARRIOR, B. and LEGHORN, L. (1975) *Houseworkers' Handbook* Cambridge, Massachusetts, Woman's Center

WEISSTEIN, N. (1970) '"Kinde, Kuche, Kirche" as scientific law: psychology constructs the female' in R. Morgan (ed.) *Sisterhood is Powerful* New York, Vintage Books

WERTZ, R. W. and WERTZ, D. C. (1977) *Lying-In: A History of Childbirth in America* New York, The Free Press

WILLIAMS, M. and BOOTH, D. (1974) *Antenatal Education: Guidelines for Teachers* Edinburgh, Churchill Livingstone

WILLIAMSON, N. E. (1976) 'Sex preferences, sex control and the status of women' *Signs: Journal of Women in Culture and Society* 1, Summer, pp. 847-62

WILLIS, P. E. (1978) *Learning to Labour* Farnborough, Hants, Saxon House
WOLFENSTEIN, M. (1957) *Disaster: A Psychological Essay* London, Routledge and Kegan Paul
'Women in medicine' (1974) *British Medical Journal* 7 September, p. 591
WOOD, A. D. (1974) '"The fashionable diseases": women's complaints and their treatment in nineteenth century America' in M. Hartman and L. W. Banner (eds) *Clio's Consciousness Raised: New Perspectives in the History of Women* New York, Harper and Row
WRIGHT MILLS, C. (1959) *The Sociological Imagination* New York, Oxford University Press

YALOM, I. D. *et al.* (1968) '"Postpartum blues" syndrome: a description and related variables' *Archives of General Psychiatry* 18, January, pp. 16–27
YOUNG, I. (1974) *The Private Life of Islam* London, Allen Lane
YOUNG, M. and WILLMOTT, P. (1957) *Family and Kinship in East London* London, Routledge and Kegan Paul
YOUNG, M. and WILLMOTT, P. (1973) *The Symmetrical Family* London, Routledge and Kegan Paul
YUDKIN, S. and HOLME, A. (1969) *Working Mothers and their Children* London, Sphere Books

ZAJICEK, E. (n.d.) 'Development of women having their first child' unpublished paper
ZELDITCH, M. (1956) 'Role differentiation in the nuclear family: a comparative study' in Parsons and Bales (eds)
ZUBIN, J. and MONEY, J. (eds) (1973) *Contemporary Sexual Behavior: Critical Issues in the 1970s* Baltimore, Johns Hopkins

Index